LIST OF CONTRIBUTORS

W. I. Acton, *Institute of Sound and Vibration Research, University of Southampton, England.*

G. R. C. Atherley, *Department of Pure and Applied Physics, University of Salford, England.*

D. M. Bruton, *Principal Medical Officer (Ground), Air Corporations Joint Medical Service, London Airport, England.*

M. E. Bryan, *Department of Electrical Engineering, University of Salford, England.*

W. Burns, *Professor of Physiology, Charing Cross Hospital Medical School, University of London, England.*

D. L. Chadwick, *Consultant Surgeon, Department of Otolaryngology, University of Manchester, England.*

R. R. A. Coles, *Institute of Sound and Vibration Research, University of Southampton, England.*

H. Davis, *Former Director, Central Institute for the Deaf, St. Louis, Missouri.*

M. E. Delany, *Environmental Unit, National Physical Laboratory, Teddington, England.*

E. D. D. Dickson, *Chairman, Royal National Institute for the Deaf, London, England.*

J. V. Dunworth, *Director, National Physical Laboratory, Teddington, England.*

M. R. Forrest, *Army Personnel Research Establishment, Farnborough, Hampshire, England.*

A. Glorig, *Director, Callier Hearing and Speech Center, Dallas, Texas.*

J. A. B. Gray, *Secretary, Medical Research Council, London, England.*

T. I. Hempstock, *Department of Pure and Applied Physics, University of Salford, England.*

R. Hinchcliffe, *Institute of Laryngology and Otology, University of London, England.*

G. Holmgren, *The Boden Hospital, Boden, Sweden.*

L. Johnsson, *The Swedish Forest Service, Stockholm, Sweden.*

R. L. Kell, *Department of Social and Occupational Medicine, University of Dundee, Scotland.*

B. Kylin. *Health Department, Sandvikens Jernverks AB, Sandviken, Sweden.*

O. Linde, *National Institute of Occupational Health, Stockholm, Sweden.*

D. A. Nelson, *Hearing Research Laboratory, University of Minnesota, Minneapolis, Minnesota.*

W. G. Noble, *Formerly of the Department of Occupational Health, University of Manchester, England.*

W. Passchier-Vermeer, *Research Institute for Public Health Engineering TNO, Delft, Netherlands.*

J. C. G. Pearson, *Department of Social and Occupational Medicine, University of Dundee, Scotland.*

C. G. Rice, *Institute of Sound and Vibration Research, University of Southampton, England.*

D. W. Robinson, *Head of Acoustics Section, National Physical Laboratory, Teddington, England.*

S. D. G. Stephens, *Medical Research Council Applied Psychology Unit, Cambridge and Teddington, England.*

A. Surböck, *Director, Occupational Diseases Division, Allgemeine Unfallversicherungsanstalt, Vienna, Austria.*

W. Taylor, *Department of Social and Occupational Medicine, University of Dundee, Scotland.*

W. Tempest, *Department of Electrical Engineering, University of Salford, England.*

F. A. Van Atta, *Assistant Director Safety, Bureau of Labor Standards, U.S. Department of Labor, Washington, D.C.*

W. Dixon Ward, *Director, Hearing Research Laboratory, University of Minnesota, Minneapolis, Minnesota.*

OCCUPATIONAL HEARING LOSS

BRITISH ACOUSTICAL SOCIETY SPECIAL VOLUME No. 1

OCCUPATIONAL HEARING LOSS

Proceedings of a conference held at the
National Physical Laboratory, Teddington,
from 23 to 25 March 1970

Edited by

D. W. ROBINSON

National Physical Laboratory,
Teddington, Middlesex

Published for the British Acoustical Society by

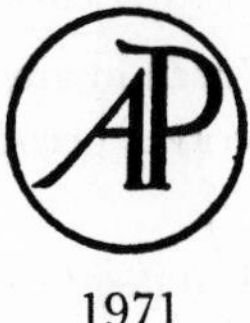

1971

ACADEMIC PRESS

LONDON AND NEW YORK

ACADEMIC PRESS INC. (LONDON) LTD
Berkeley Square House
Berkeley Square
London, W1X 6BA

U.S. Edition published by
ACADEMIC PRESS INC.
111 Fifth Avenue
New York, New York 10003

Library of Congress Catalog Card Number: 71–153523
ISBN: 0–12–590150–X

Printed in Great Britain by William Clowes & Sons, Limited, London, Beccles and Colchester

PARTICIPANTS*

J. A. Adam	Research and Development Department, British Steel Corporation, Moorgate, Rotherham, Yorkshire.
T. W. Aitchison	D.O.R.A. Branch, Board of Trade, Adelphi, John Adam Street, London, W.C.2.
M. D. L. Alton	Imperial Chemical Industries Ltd., Agricultural Division, Billingham, Teesside.
N. Ashworth	Refinery Medical Officer, Shell U.K. Ltd., Shell Haven, Stanford-le-Hope, Essex.
R. H. R. Aston	Chief Medical Officer, Joseph Lucas Ltd., Great King Street, Birmingham, 19.
R. Auerbach	Consultant Surgeon, North Herts Hospital, Hitchin, Hertfordshire.
E. Barker	Medical Officer, British Leyland (Austin-Morris) Ltd., Cowley Division, Oxford.
L. M. Barrett	United Kingdom Atomic Energy Authority, Risley, Warrington, Lancashire.
R. M. Barr-Hamilton	Electrical Engineering Department, The University, Salford, Lancashire, M5 4WT.
H. G. Baxter	Shell U.K. Ltd., Shell Haven, Stanford-le-Hope, Essex.
H. A. Beagley	Consultant Otologist, Institute of Laryngology and Otology, University of London, 330 Gray's Inn Road, London, W.C.1.
L. W. Bean	Department of Mathematics and Physics, Hull College of Technology, Kingston-upon-Hull, Yorkshire.
C. V. G. Behan	Alfred Peters & Sons Ltd., 55 Clarkehouse Road, Sheffield, 10, Yorkshire.
J. Bickerdike	Building and Civil Engineering Department, The Polytechnic, Leeds, 1, Yorkshire.
C. H. B. Binns	Medical Officer, B.P. Chemicals (U.K.) Ltd., Raglan Bay Works, Port Talbot, Glamorgan, South Wales.
K. F. Bishop	Health Physics and Medical Division, Atomic Energy Research Establishment, Harwell, Didcot, Berkshire.

* The names of participants mentioned in the List of Contributors have not been repeated.

A. Blick	Audiology Department, St. James's Hospital, Leeds, Yorkshire, LS9 7TF.
J. M. Bowsher	Department of Physics, University of Surrey, Guildford, Surrey.
A. J. Boyle	National Institute of Industrial Psychology, 14 Welbeck Street, London, W.1.
T. P. C. Bramer	Sound Research Laboratories Ltd., Holbrook Hall, Sudbury, Suffolk.
J. Brebner	Chief Medical Officer (London), Kuwait Oil Company Ltd., 105 Wigmore Street, London, W1H 0AL.
D. E. Broadbent	Director, Applied Psychology Unit, Medical Research Council, 15 Chaucer Road, Cambridge.
W. E. Broughton	Senior Medical Adviser, Shell International Petroleum Company Ltd., Shell Centre, London, S.E.1.
J. Brunt	Imperial Chemical Industries Ltd., Agricultural Division, Billingham, Teesside.
W. D. Buchanan	H.M. Deputy Senior Medical Inspector of Factories, H.M. Factory Inspectorate, Baynards House, Westbourne Grove, London, W.2.
L. F. Christensen	Brüel & Kjær A/S., Nærum, Denmark.
Elizabeth E. Clarke	H. J. Heinz Company Ltd., Waxlow Road, London, N.W.10.
S. W. R. Cox	National Institute of Agricultural Engineering, Wrest Park, Silsoe, Bedfordshire.
D. E. Cuin	B.P.B. Industries (Research and Development) Ltd., East Leake, nr. Loughborough, Leicestershire.
J. Cunningham	Textile Development Unit, Courtaulds Ltd., Queensway, Rochdale, Lancashire.
R. P. G. Dickerson	Divisional Medical Officer, British Rail, Western Region, Exeter, Devon.
P. H. Dinsdale	Textile Development Unit, Courtaulds Ltd., Queensway, Rochdale, Lancashire.
A. R. Dove	H.M. Factory Inspectorate, Engineering Branch, Baynards House, Westbourne Grove, London, W.2.
B. W. Duck	Senior Medical Officer (Occupational Health), B.P. Research Centre, Chertsey Road, Sunbury-on-Thames, Middlesex.
K. P. Duncan	Chief Medical Officer, British Steel Corporation, 33 Grosvenor Place, London, S.W.1.
A. Edmundson	Central Electricity Research Laboratories, Kelvin Avenue, Leatherhead, Surrey.
J. van den Eijk	Research Institute for Public Health Engineering TNO, P.O. Box 214, Delft, Netherlands.

R. W. Ellis	Department of Industrial Health, The Medical School, Newcastle-upon-Tyne.
W. M. Fletcher	Physics Department, The Metal Box Company Ltd., Kendal Avenue, Acton, London, W.3.
D. G. Fowler	Fowler Davies & Company, Consultants, 71 Mayflower Way, Farnham Common, Buckinghamshire.
E. H. Miles Foxen	Senior Surgeon, Ear, Nose and Throat Department, Westminster Hospital, London, S.W.1.
P. R. Gilbert	Senior Medical Officer, Post Office Central Headquarters, Tenter House, 45 Moorfields, London, E.C.2.
J. C. Graham	Principal Medical Officer, H. J. Heinz Company Ltd., Waxlow Road, London, N.W.10.
C. S. Greeves	National Engineering Laboratory, East Kilbride, Lanarkshire, Scotland.
S. A. Hall	Institute of Occupational Health, London School of Hygiene, University of London, Keppel Street, London, W.C.1.
S. Hansen	Brüel & Kjær A/S., Nærum, Denmark.
R. Harrison	Imperial Chemical Industries Ltd., Dyestuffs Division, Hexagon House, Blackley, Manchester, M9 3DA.
G. A. Hedgecock	Medical Centre, Pilkington Brothers Ltd., St. Helens, Lancashire.
J. B. Hibbs	Steel Castings Research and Trade Association, 5 East Bank Road, Sheffield, Yorkshire, S2 3PT.
R. I. Higgins	British Cast Iron Research Association, Alvechurch, Birmingham.
J. D. Hood	Otological Research Unit, Medical Research Council, National Hospital, Queen Square, London, W.C.1.
R. A. Hood	Chelsea College of Science and Technology, Pulton Place Annexe, London, S.W.6.
D. A. Howell	Admiralty Underwater Weapons Establishment (North), Portland, Dorset.
W. J. Hunter	Medical Officer, General Foods Ltd., Banbury, Oxfordshire.
J. E. J. John	Department of Audiology, The University, Manchester, M13 9PL.
R. I. Johnson	The Metal Box Company Ltd., 37 Baker Street, London, W1A 1AN.
H. D. Jones	Medical Officer, Central Medical Department, Courtaulds Ltd., Coventry, CV6 5AE.

H. R. Kemble	Medical Officer, Tractor Plant, Ford Motor Company Ltd., Cranes Farm Road, Basildon, Essex.
P. F. King	Consultant Adviser in Otorhinolaryngology to the Royal Air Force, Central Medical Establishment, Kelvin House, Cleveland Street, London, W.1.
R. Kitchener	GKN Group Technological Centre, Birmingham New Road, Wolverhampton, WV4 6BW.
D. I. Klein	Medical Department, Braidwood Audiology Unit, Inner London Educational Authority, 20 Elmcourt Road, London, S.E.27.
E. König	Ear, Nose and Throat Clinic, The University, 4000-Basel, Switzerland.
J. H. Kuehn	Technical Director, B & K Laboratories Ltd., Cross Lances Road, Hounslow, Middlesex.
G. L. Lee	Hygiene Laboratory, British Leyland (Austin-Morris) Ltd., Longbridge, Birmingham.
W. R. Lee	Department of Occupational Health, The University, Manchester, 13.
R. V. Leedham	Department of Electrical Engineering (Phoenix), The University, Bradford 7, Yorkshire.
R. C. Lemon	Senior Medical Adviser, Shell International Petroleum Company Ltd., Shell Centre, London, S.E.1.
H. G. Leventhall	Department of Physics, Chelsea College of Science and Technology, Pulton Place Annexe, London, S.W.6.
R. M. Lloyd	Hearing Aid Consultant, The Hearing Centre, 40 Lemon Street, Truro, Cornwall.
G. Lorriman	Senior Medical Officer, Medical Advisory Service, Civil Service Department, Tilbury House, Petty France, London, S.W.1.
J. McFarlane	Electrical Engineering Division, GKN Group Technological Centre, Birmingham New Road, Wolverhampton, WV4 6BW.
H. McRobert	Electrical Engineering Department, The University, Salford, Lancashire, M5 4WT.
Jacqueline A. Marsh	Environmental Advisory Service, Pilkington Brothers Ltd., St. Helens, Lancashire.
I. A. Marshall	Extended Service Laboratory, National Coal Board, Wath-upon-Dearne, Rotherham, Yorkshire.
A. M. Martin	Department of Pure and Applied Physics, The University, Salford, Lancashire, M5 4WT.
M. C. Martin	Royal National Institute for the Deaf, 105 Gower Street, London, W.C.1.

C. R. Mayou	Medical Practitioner, "Top Gates", Cherry Hill Avenue, Barnt Green, nr. Birmingham.
Franca Merluzzi	Clinica del Lavoro "Luigi Devoto", University of Milan, Via S. Barnaba 8, 20122 Milan, Italy.
J. T. Morgan, Surgeon Captain, R.N.	Department of the Medical Director-General (Naval), Ministry of Defence, Empress State Building, Lillie Road, London, S.W.6.
J. P. Moore	Shell U.K. Ltd., Stanlow Refinery, Ellesmere Port, Cheshire, L65 4HB.
D. C. Murphy	Medical Department, Esso Petroleum Company Ltd., Victoria Street, London, S.W.1.
C. T. Newnham	Regional Medical Officer, British Rail, Western Region, Paddington Station, London, W.2.
T. P. Oliver, Surgeon Commander, R.N.	H.M. Dockyard, Rosyth, Dunfermline, Fife, Scotland.
R. G. Orr	Medical Officer, Atomic Energy Research Establishment, Harwell, Didcot, Berkshire.
R. A. Owen	Development Coordination Division, The Metal Box Company Ltd., 37 Baker Street, London, W1A 1AN.
G. R. Oxley	The Associated Octel Co. Ltd., Ellesmere Port, Cheshire, L65 4HF.
P. L. Pelmear	Senior Medical Officer, GKN Castings Ltd., P.O. Box 4, Bromsgrove, Worcestershire.
D. F. Percy	Industrial Acoustics Company Ltd., Victor House, Norris Road, Staines, Middlesex.
A. Pérez-López	Centro de Investigaciones Físicas "Leonardo Torres Quevedo", Serrano 144, Madrid 6, Spain.
D. W. Petchey	Research and Development Department, The Metal Box Company Ltd., Kendal Avenue, Acton, London, W.3.
J. E. Peters	Alfred Peters & Sons Ltd., 55 Clarkehouse Road, Sheffield, 10, Yorkshire.
A. M. Petrie	Mechanical Engineering Department, Paisley College of Technology, High Street, Paisley, Renfrewshire, Scotland.
I. Picton-Robinson	Medical Officer, Health Department, British Leyland (Austin-Morris) Ltd., Longbridge, Birmingham.
M. J. Porter	Safety Health and Welfare Department, Department of Employment, Baynards House, Westbourne Grove, London, W.2.

J. A. Powell	Department of Pure and Applied Physics, The University, Salford, Lancashire, M5 4WT.
R. H. Pugsley	Medical Acoustic Division, Amplivox Limited, Beresford Avenue, Wembley, Middlesex.
A. Raber	Allgemeine Unfallversicherungsanstalt, Abteilung Arbeitsmedizin, Webergasse 2, 1200-Wien XX, Austria.
P. Ransome-Wallis	Medical Practitioner, The Corner House, Herne Bay, Kent.
K. Ratcliffe	Perkins Engines Company, Eastfield, Peterborough, Northamptonshire.
W. H. Richardson	Audiology Section, Institute of Naval Medicine, Alverstoke, Hampshire.
Joyce E. Robinson	28 The Drive, Esher, Surrey (Conference Secretariat)
D. F. Rousell	Safety Division, British American Optical Company Ltd., Radlett Road, Watford, Hertfordshire.
Jean Rousell	Audiometric Department, St. Mary Abbots Hospital, London, W.8.
R. Routledge	Senior Medical Officer, Ford Motor Company Ltd., M.S. and B. Division, Chequers Lane, Dagenham, Essex.
J. P. Seller	Tottenham Technical College, High Road, London, N.15.
N. Shah	Consultant Surgeon, Institute of Laryngology and Otology, University of London, 330 Gray's Inn Road, London, W.C.1.
N. L. Spoor	Radiological Protection Division, United Kingdom Atomic Energy Authority, Harwell, Didcot, Berkshire.
J. C. Stead	Technical College, Loughborough, Leicestershire.
R. W. B. Stephens	Physics Department, Imperial College of Science and Technology, Prince Consort Road, London, S.W.7.
Jay Stickings	Wool Textile EDC, National Economic Development Office, Millbank Tower, London, S.W.1.
Jean Stone	Consultant, 47 Loughborough Road, Quorn, Loughborough, Leicestershire.
J. D. Sutcliffe	Noise Reduction Consultants, Del Sasso, Badsworth, Pontefract, Yorkshire.
R. L. Taylor	Scientific Services Department, Central Electricity Generating Board, Portishead, Bristol.
D. Thompson	Medical Centre, Vauxhall Motors Ltd., Luton, Bedfordshire.

A. Trueman	Chief Medical Officer, British Airports Authority, 2 Buckingham Gate, London, S.W.1.
L. E. Tyler	Medical Adviser to GKN Ltd., 2 Lower Prestwood Road, Wolverhampton.
C. Wakstein	Department of Mechanical Engineering, The University, Liverpool.
J. G. Walker	Operational Acoustics and Audiology Group, Institute of Sound and Vibration Research, The University, Southampton, SO9 5NH.
P. R. Waters	Mine Safety Appliances Company Ltd., Taplow, Berkshire.
J. Webber	Admiralty Research Laboratory, Teddington, Middlesex.
L. S. Whittle	Environmental Unit, National Physical Laboratory, Teddington, Middlesex (Assistant Conference Organizer)
J. H. Williams	Navy Department, Ministry of Defence, Whitehall, London, S.W.1.

PREFACE

This volume contains the full text of papers read at the Conference on Occupational Hearing Loss held at the National Physical Laboratory, Teddington, from 23 to 25 March 1970. Thirteen of the papers were presented by invitation, the aim of the organizers being that each contribution should appeal not only to experts and research workers but to all those concerned in one way or another with some facet of the subject. The remaining six papers were accepted at the request of authors, and it is gratifying to record that the diversity of their contents greatly enlarged the scope of the proceedings. Addresses given at the opening and closing of the Conference are also reproduced, as well as the text of the extemporary summing up delivered at the final session by Dr. A. Glorig.

Discussions at the Conference were conducted in three ways: by question and answer on individual papers, in extended periods devoted to groups of papers on cognate topics, and finally in two simultaneous round-table meetings on the specific pre-selected questions of international standardization and on the responsibility of industry for noise reduction. The round-table meetings were presided over by Dr. Hallowell Davis and Mr. M. J. Porter respectively, and the organizers wish to place on record their appreciation of the skilful way in which these sessions were conducted. Apart from the round-table meetings, which were of an informal character, the transactions were recorded and the full discussions in the main sessions, based on verbatim transcripts as edited by the contributors, are reproduced here at the end of the respective sections. Some rearrangement has been made by the Editor in order to juxtapose related contributions on the principal topics of debate, and to place the contributions so far as possible in a logical sequence.

Occupational hearing loss is a rapidly-developing subject in which, until recent times, the difficulties of research have tended to produce information of a somewhat fragmentary kind. As a consequence there has grown a tendency, on the part of those who have to apply the results, towards divergent practices and interpretations, depending on the particular authors that may have influenced their viewpoints. In the last two or three years, however, a great expansion of well-documented research has occurred, from the results of which quantitative relationships between industrial noise exposure and its harmful effects on the normal and pathological ear are beginning to emerge in much more generalized forms. The time, therefore, was an opportune one to bring together the principals engaged in these researches and the representatives of other disciplines concerned with the practical implementation of industrial hearing preservation measures and of hearing loss compensation.

In planning the Conference, the organizers visualized a division of the subject into four parts, three of which correspond to the respective sections of this volume. The first of these was devoted to expositions of the results of field studies and of the conclusions which can be drawn from them regarding the causative relations between noise and hearing loss. The second section was concerned with technical aspects of hearing measurement and protection and with the administration of protective measures. The third section dealt with the implications of occupational hearing loss from the standpoint of social handicap and as seen by the practising otologist. These divisions led on naturally to a fourth, which falls within the medical field, devoted to differential diagnosis and medicolegal problems in the context of compensation. This fourth section became the subject of a related meeting of the joint Sections of Otology and Occupational Medicine of the Royal Society of Medicine, which was held in London in the week following the Conference. The papers given at this meeting have been published separately in the Proceedings of the Royal Society of Medicine.

The organizers of both meetings owe much to the vision of the late Dr. P. O. M. McGirr, who was instrumental in bringing together the members of the British Acoustical Society and of the Royal Society of Medicine responsible for the respective programmes, notably Mr. A. W. Morrison, F.R.C.S., Group Captain P. F. King, Professor W. Burns, Dr. S. Gauvain and the writer. Dr. McGirr was to have given one of the invited papers at the Conference but his tragic death at an early age in 1969 left a gap, and for closing this at short notice the organizers are greatly indebted to Dr. D. M. Bruton from the same organization. The death of Dr. McGirr is a great loss to the world of occupational medicine, notably in the hearing conservation field. The eventual success of the meetings which he inspired is testified by the present volume which is offered as a tribute to his memory.

It is fitting here also to remember another grievous loss to the cause of audiological research and otology which occurred early in 1970 through the death of Sir Terence Cawthorne, F.R.C.S. He was to have presided over the closing session of the Conference. On behalf of all the participants a tribute to his memory has been paid by one of his close associates, Mr. D. L. Chadwick, F.R.C.S., and this appears at the head of Mr. Chadwick's contribution to these proceedings.

On a happier note, the organizers would like to record their appreciation to Dr. J. V. Dunworth, Director of the National Physical Laboratory, for making possible the staging of the Conference and for presiding as host at the dinner held on 24 March; also to Dr. J. A. B. Gray, Secretary of the Medical Research Council, for his personal participation at the

Opening. The Editor would like to express here his very grateful thanks to the chairmen of the sessions; to all those who participated in the organization, particularly his professional colleague Mr. L. S. Whittle and Mr. R. P. Itter, Secretary of the British Acoustical Society; also to the contributors of papers and to speakers in the discussions whose promptitude in submitting their texts was an object lesson; and finally to his wife, Mrs. J. E. Robinson, who served in the varied roles of Conference receptionist, hostess, verbatim transcriptionist and general secretary and without whose ready help the preparation of this book would not have been achieved.

D. W. Robinson

FOREWORD

It gives me great pleasure to introduce this volume as I near the end of my period of office as second President of the British Acoustical Society. The Society is a young one, having grown out of a series of meetings in 1964 convened by the Royal Society under the Chairmanship of Sir Gordon Sutherland, F.R.S., then Director of the National Physical Laboratory and now the Master of Emmanuel College, Cambridge, England.

Acoustics is a very diverse subject with applications in industry, medicine, communications, music, underwater exploration and fishing and in the problems associated with noise. This diversity had previously hindered the creation of a single representative body, and the resulting lack of unity was a contributory factor to the shortage of trained acousticians.

In March 1965 the group of individuals called together by Sir Gordon Sutherland became the Provisional Council of a new Society with Dr. Arthur J. King as its Chairman, and at the first Annual General Meeting later that year Professor R. E. D. Bishop was proclaimed first President of the British Acoustical Society, thus signalling the close link between Acoustics and the subject of Vibrations in which Professor Bishop occupies so eminent a place.

The British Acoustical Society now flourishes, and this is in large measure due to its good fortune to have as its energetic Programme Committee Chairman and President-Elect Professor D. G. Tucker. With each successive year the Council has been able to extend the Society's activities, and its Programme Committee has staged a progressively more ambitious series of science meetings. It is probably no coincidence that the life-time of the Society has also witnessed a remarkable growth of public and official concern with problems of noise and its effects on the community, and a resurgence of interest in Acoustics within British Universities is now to be found more in the engineering and cross-disciplinary faculties than in the departments of pure physics that nurtured the subject in former times.

These movements, together with the culmination of a large piece of research into industrial noise and hearing by the Medical Research Council and the National Physical Laboratory, set the scene in 1970 for a conference the proceedings of which comprise the present volume. This is the first to be so published for the British Acoustical Society by

Academic Press Inc. as a separate book, and so it is a landmark in the Society's history and a major step towards the realization of its larger aims.

E. J. Richards,
Vice-Chancellor,
University of Technology,
Loughborough, England

October, 1970

CONTENTS

SECTION I: FIELD STUDIES

SECTION II: PRACTICAL ASPECTS

SECTION III: ASSESSING HEARING LOSS

Closing Section

EDITOR'S NOTE

In the interests of uniformity, the Editor takes the responsibility for adopting the spelling "presbycusis" throughout this volume. This conforms to the majority usage, though the alternative form "presbyacusis" is preferred by some of the contributors and is perhaps preferable on etymological grounds.

Welcome Speech

By

J. V. Dunworth

Director, National Physical Laboratory

Ladies and Gentleman, this Laboratory does not to any extent produce pieces of equipment but instead provides advice, ideas and information. The only way in which we can justify our existence is by telling people about our work. For this reason we welcome very much receiving visitors to our laboratory.

A characteristic of the National Physical Laboratory, concerned as it is with the whole basis of measurement, is that it must be a place where people are prepared to work on the same problem for many years and to deal with it in depth. The subject of your conference today is of this character.

I hope you will not mind my taking a few minutes of your time to say a few words about the NPL. We have a total staff of about 2000. This includes a Ministry of Works team who provide many of our services. There are some 800 professionally trained staff. There are three sections of the Laboratory. One is concerned with our national remit of being the ultimate arbiter of measurement, and I can in fact describe myself as the ultimate arbiter in this country for any measurement, though fortunately I'm not normally appealed to in person. Another section of the Laboratory is concerned with materials. We have the largest team of people in Britain working in the materials field in Government service. The third section of the Laboratory is concerned more with specific industries. We operated the first computing service in this country, and one of the two founders of modern computing, Turing, was working in this Laboratory at the time. We have also a very fine Mathematics Division. We have the national facilities for the study of both ordinary and high-speed ships in their interaction with water. We have a powerful aerodynamics department which will increasingly be concerned with civil engineering structures rather than aeroplanes. We played an important part, for instance, in the design of the Forth and Severn Bridges, and we influenced the design of the Post Office Tower in London. We played an important part in identifying the cause of the collapse of the cooling tower at Ferrybridge some time ago. Finally there is an acoustics team and Dr. Robinson has played a leading role in it. You will know him and therefore I need say no more about him or his work.

I will now hand over to Dr. Gray, who is the Secretary of the Medical Research Council. It is good of him to spare the time to be here this morning. It has been a very great pleasure for us at NPL to work closely with the Medical Research Council in the study of industrial deafness and I look forward to similar projects on which we can work with the Medical Research Council in the very rapidly growing field of medical engineering.

Opening of the Conference

By

J. A. B. Gray

Secretary, Medical Research Council

Before saying anything else, I would like to thank the organizers of this Conference for inviting me to make these opening remarks, the theme of which follows on—quite by chance—from what Dr. Dunworth has just said and is concerned with coordination and working together in this and other fields of science. There are several reasons why I am particularly happy to do this. There are, first of all, personal reasons; the fact that my own scientific work was in the field of sensory neurophysiology; but much more important, that Dr. Hallowell Davis is here to give the introductory paper. I have known Dr. Davis for a long time and there are many occasions when we have met in scientific discussions, at conferences or in the privacy of our own offices. He is a person for whom I—and I am sure everyone who knows him—have developed a very profound respect, for not only is his research in the highest class but it spans an extraordinarily wide field for a single individual. Because of this he has been able to bring together the diverse threads of this wide field and relate them to the practical problems of preventing and counteracting hearing loss. I would like to give my personal welcome to an old friend and also to add my welcome to the United Kingdom to all our visitors from overseas.

There are also other less personal reasons why I am glad to have the opportunity to speak at this opening. The Medical Research Council has long been concerned with research in this field, and at this present point in time there are a number of reasons why this Conference is of special interest. Occupational hearing loss is one aspect of the social problem of noise and noise is recognized as a physical form of pollution. I mention this because your programme recognizes some of the broad issues involved in this wider context, and for that matter in many others. Amongst the speakers you have both research workers and those responsible for taking effective action on the basis of existing knowledge—and I am not suggesting that these two categories do not overlap. You have also brought together people of many different disciplines: engineers, physicists, psychologists, physiologists, surgeons, to name a few that I recognize on the programme. Knowledge in this field of hearing and in the wider one of pollution cannot grow unless there is active team work between individuals from a wide range of disciplines—something one can describe as a horizontal coordination. But to continue with this terminology, there is also an important element of vertical coordination, that is to say the dependence of studies of occupational hearing loss on studies on sound, on sensation, on behaviour and on the mechanisms of the auditory system. Research is always dependent on knowledge and skills derived from other regions of science, and this interdependence of all parts of science is something which is increasing steadily. Clearly these interrelations demand in the first instance coordination at the bench level on the initiative of individual scientists. It is, however, also necessary that the organization of science should be such as to encourage this collaboration. I would go further—it is necessary for experts in all appropriate areas of science to contribute, at a policy-making level, to each problem.

The subject of this Conference is part of one of the oldest collaborations between Research Councils, that between the old Department of Scientific and Industrial Research, which used to be responsible for the National Physical Laboratory where this Conference is taking place, and the Medical Research Council. I think I am right in saying that this collaboration goes back to the early years of both those bodies—somewhere about 1918. In different ways, this collaboration has gone on ever since. Today the field of research related to pollution is such that it requires the coordinated action of all five Research Councils, the Agricultural, the Natural Environment, the Social Science, the Science and the Medical, in order that a coherent picture of the overall problem can be obtained. Pollution, whether a physical one such as noise, or a chemical one, is a problem on the social scale which, for a physiologist like myself, has similarities to the economy of an individual animal, in which raw materials are converted into the power and products needed and waste products are produced. Elaborate systems have evolved in the biological organism to process and eliminate this waste, and evolution has also produced adaptations by which certain levels of waste can be tolerated. In the physiological situation one thing is certain, that when waste accumulates and rises above certain levels the whole system is likely to become disorganized, and the disorganization can be understood only in terms of the whole system. The same thing is true of social pollution: it cannot be understood within the competence of any one branch of science or within the limit of any one Research Council.

I have mentioned these things briefly because I am convinced that the collaboration between different areas of science, which you have successfully developed on an individual basis, needs to be developed much further on an organizational basis. In this connection it is most important that individual Departments of Government, in their proper desire to organize particular types of work, do not take any major step which would disrupt, to their own ultimate disadvantage, that unity of science which is almost certainly essential for its further development.

Earlier on I referred to the fact that this Conference includes not only research but also problems of action. This is an interface of great importance, but it is an interface and a different type of problem from the intricate interweaving of the pattern of science. Problems can arise here in either direction; for example, administrators may on occasion find it difficult to obtain from the scientists the answers they need; on others, administrators may invoke the need for research when what in fact is needed is action which can be taken on existing knowledge. Much needs to be done to improve communication at this interface, and one thing this Conference is clearly aiming to do is to improve this communication and to do it in a way which, at the same time, is pulling together all those different aspects of science which are relevant. I am sure that designing a conference in this way is something that will make the meeting thoroughly profitable. In contrast, it is sadly not unknown that in attempting to improve communication between science and administration, ways are sometimes proposed which ignore the basic facts of the complex interrelations of the fabric of science.

I wish you a successful meeting and declare the Conference open.

A Historical Introduction

By

Hallowell Davis

Central Institute for the Deaf, St. Louis, Missouri

A survey of the development in the U.S.A. of rules and criteria for hearing impairment will illustrate a series of concepts and basic assumptions pertinent to occupational hearing loss and compensation for it.

The original "Fletcher point-eight rule" (Fletcher, 1929) was intended for otologists, to provide an overall index of a patient's hearing capacity, the percentage hearing loss. In principle the rule divided the normal auditory area (Fig. 1) into cells with the dimensions of decibels and hertz and gave the percentage of cells that had been lost. The concept is atomistic, very much as if we were counting lost anatomical units, such as hair cells. The "point-eight" factor represents the translation of a normal dynamic range of 120 dB to a percentage scale. Fletcher's important simplification, however, was to restrict the frequency range of interest to three major speech frequencies, 500, 1000 and 2000 Hz. Thus some cells of the auditory area became much more important than others, as illustrated in Fig. 1.

Next, the Fowler-Sabine scale, recommended by a sub-committee of the American Medical Association (1942 and 1947), put graded values on the decibel scale. It discounted minor losses within the range of normal hearing and also at very high intensities, and it increased the value of the central frequencies and added 4000 Hz. It introduced also an arbitrary weighting factor of five to one to obtain a binaural evaluation when the two ears were unequally impaired. Its chief weaknesses were the arbitrary assignments of unequal weights, and the complex table of weighting values and calculations (see Fig. 2); and it did not displace the simple Fletcher point-eight rule.

Social legislation related to noise-induced hearing loss began in U.S.A. with the principle of workmen's compensation insurance to repay an injured worker for loss of earning power. New York State and Wisconsin led the way. Through court decisions, which were influenced strongly by the analogy to silicosis, noise-induced hearing loss was recognized as an industrial disease, with a predetermined payment of x weeks' wages for total loss of hearing. Here the analogy is to the loss of *function* of a hand or of vision. Actually, under the Fletcher point-eight rule, with its ceiling of 120 dB hearing loss as 100%, no noise-deafened worker could ever expect to receive more than perhaps 60% of the compensation scheduled for total deafness.

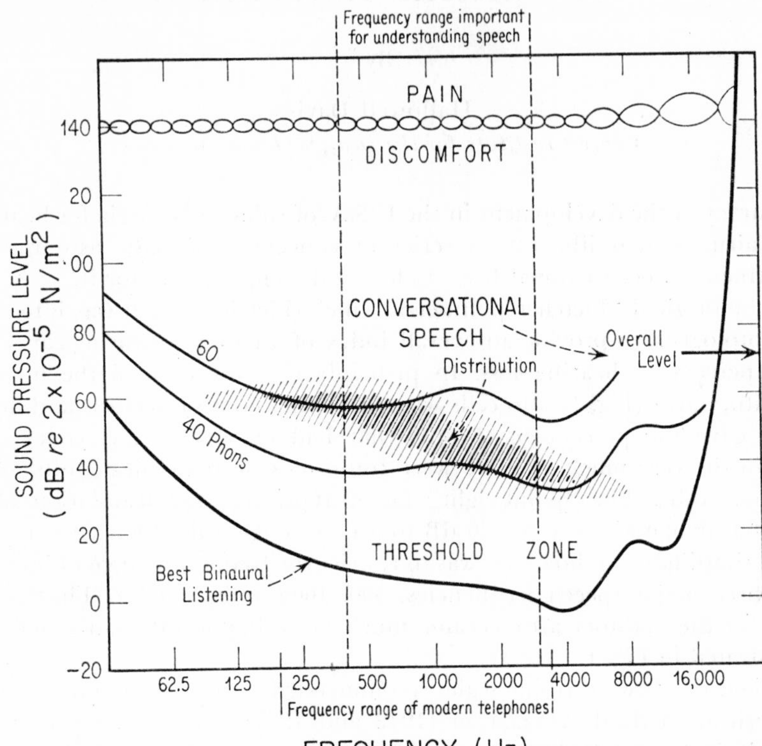

FIG. 1. The speech area. This figure shows the approximate distribution of sound pressure levels with respect to frequency which would occur if brief but characteristic bits of phonemes of conversational speech were sustained like pure tones. The darker shading indicates the greater probability of finding the combinations in that area. The boundaries of the speech area are not sharp. The weaker elements are often masked by background noises. (Reproduced with permission from Davis and Silverman, 1970.)

The Committee on Conservation of Hearing of the American Academy of Ophthalmology and Otolaryngology (1959, 1964 and 1965) developed a rule which is a simplification of the Fowler–Sabine method. It is explicitly related to the sound levels of human speech that are actually encountered in everyday life (not under noisy working conditions). Like the previous rules it disregards any potential benefit from a hearing aid. Only the frequencies 500, 1000 and 2000 Hz are considered. The "high fence" of total impairment or handicap was placed at 93 dB (ISO), average for the

AUDIOGRAM AND HEARING LOSS CHART

(PREPARED BY EDMUND P. FOWLER, M.D. AND P. E. SABINE, PH.D.)

NAME...AGE.........NO.................

ADDRESS...DATE..............................

HEARING LOSS IN DECIBELS	128	256	512	1024	2048	4096	8192
0							
			.2	.3	.4	.1	
10							
			.5	.9	1.3	.3	
			1.1	2.1	2.9	.9	
20							
			1.8	3.6	4.9	1.7	
			2.6	5.4	7.3	2.7	
30							
			3.7	7.7	9.8	3.8	
			4.9	10.2	12.9	5.0	
40							
			6.3	13.0	17.3	6.4	
			7.9	15.7	22.4	8.0	
50							
			9.6	19.0	25.7	9.7	
			11.3	21.5	28.0	11.2	
60							
			12.8	23.5	30.2	12.5	
			13.8	25.5	32.2	13.5	
70							
			14.6	27.2	34.0	14.2	
			14.8	28.8	35.8	14.6	
80							
			14.9	29.8	37.5	14.8	
			15.0	29.9	39.2	14.9	
90							
				30.0	40.0	15.0	
100							

OCTAVE FREQUENCIES

PER CENT HEARING LOSSES

RIGHT EAR		LEFT EAR
	512	
	1024	
	2048	
	4096	
	TOTAL	

COMPUTATION OF PER CENT LOSS OF CAPACITY TO HEAR SPEECH

(A) 7 X TOTAL PER CENT LOSS, BETTER EAR

(B) 1 X TOTAL PER CENT LOSS, WORSE EAR

(C) SUM (A) + (B) =

(D) C ÷ 8, BINAURAL LOSS %

RECORDED BY

INSTRUCTIONS: Plot the hearing losses by air conduction for each ear at the four frequencies shown, and connect contiguous points by straight lines. (solid for right—broken for left) The per cent loss assigned to each interval is the figure immediately above the horizontal line. Set down these figures in the four spaces under right and left ear, in the columns to the right of the chart. Add each column and compute the binaural per cent loss of capacity to hear speech, as indicated.

FIG. 2. Audiogram and Hearing Loss Chart prepared in 1946 for the American Medical Association by Drs. E. P. Fowler and Paul A. Sabine.

three frequencies, because at this level the listener can rarely understand very loud speech at a social distance (see Fig. 3). Beginning handicap was placed at 27 dB hearing level (ISO), where difficulty is encountered with low levels of everyday speech. This "low fence" has become the benchmark for estimating the risk of noise-induced hearing handicap. The AAOO rule now enjoys considerable legal prestige by its incorporation

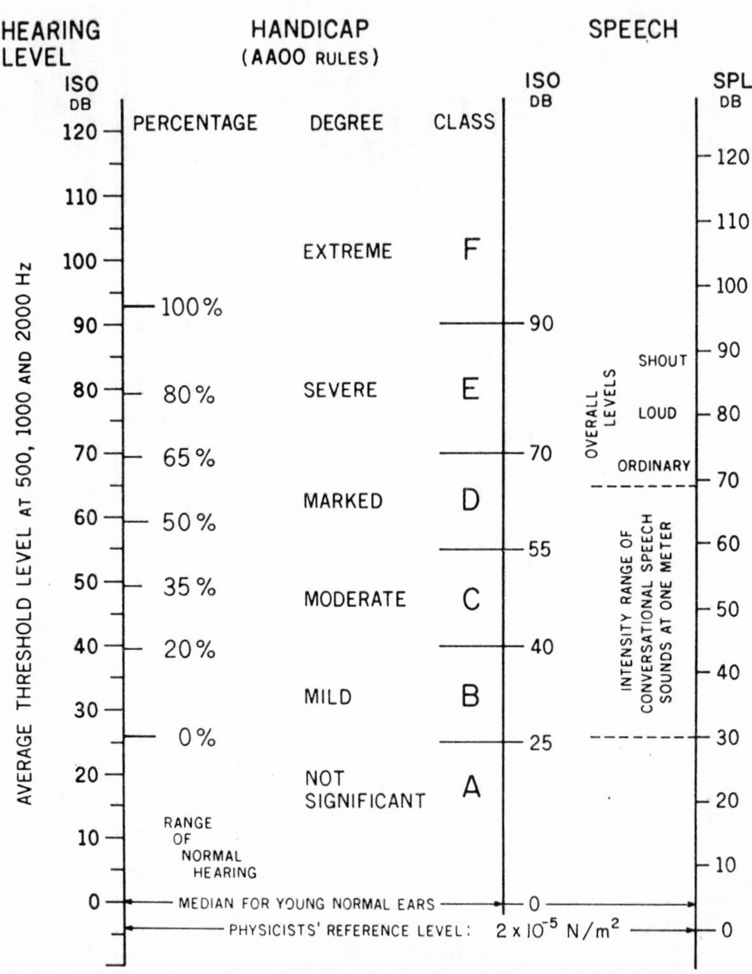

FIG. 3. The scale of percentage handicap in relation to average hearing level (*left*) and the degrees and classes of handicap in relation to the sound pressure levels of speech (*right*), according to the recommendations of the Committee on Conservation of Hearing of the American Academy of Ophthalmology and Otolaryngology.

into many rules or even State laws relating to compensation for hearing handicap, from whatever cause.

The high fence and the low fence were both adjusted deliberately by the Committee to yield a *simple* rule, namely $1\frac{1}{2}\%$ handicap per decibel of hearing threshold level above 26 dB HL. The term "handicap" was substituted for "hearing loss" or "hearing impairment" in order to emphasize the relation of the scale to the physical characteristics of human speech instead of to the extent of anatomical injury to the ear. Handicap relates to social communication. In the interest of simplicity, the AAOO rule introduced unreal abrupt transitions at zero and at 100% handicap. From the point of view of the victim, the rule is harsh at the low fence but lenient at the high fence. Perhaps this should be taken into account if we undertake to set arbitrary limits or criteria for habitual noise exposure in order to reduce the risk of developing a hearing handicap.

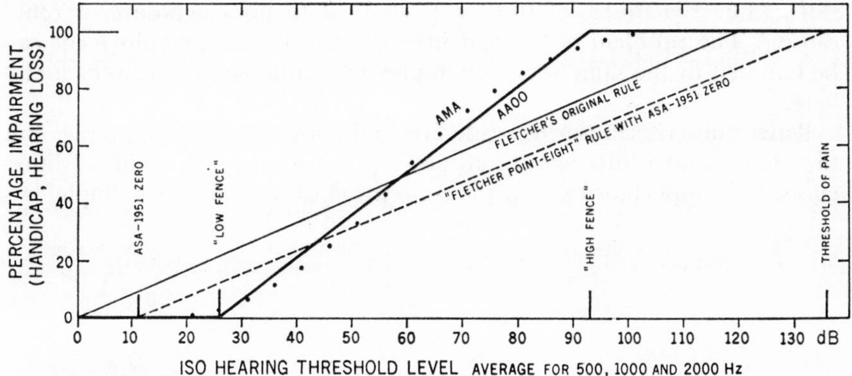

Fig. 4. The relation of percentage impairment (or handicap or hearing loss) to the average of ISO hearing levels at 500, 1000 and 2000 Hz according to four different rules. The faint solid line is Fletcher's original rule, rising with a slope of 0·833 percentage points per decibel. The light broken line is the Fletcher rule, modified by reducing the slope to 0·8 percentage points per decibel and shifting the origin to the right to a zero intercept at the zero of the ASA audiometric scale. The heavy lines show the AAOO rule with its "high fence" and its "low fence" and a slope between them of 1·5 percentage points per decibel. The dots show the results of calculation from the AMA chart (Fig. 2), assuming that the audiogram is always flat. The close correspondence between the AMA and the AAOO rules is not entirely a coincidence.

A comparison of the different percentage scales is made in Fig. 4.

A feature of the AAOO rule that surprises many audiologists is the omission of any allowance for presbycusis. In Wisconsin the rule for presbycusis is to reduce the final monetary award by an arbitrary percentage related to the age of the worker. I personally prefer no reduction at all because advancing presbycusis after retirement will inevitably and predictably increase the handicap. In Missouri a very unjust and illogical rule, intended to allow for "non-occupational causes" of impairment, subtracts a number of decibels *before* the average hearing level is translated into percentage handicap. This procedure ignores the difference in hearing level between "beginning presbycusis" at 0 dB HL and "beginning handicap" at 27 dB HL.

Causes other than noise and presbycusis can contribute to a hearing handicap, including otitis media, trauma, otosclerosis and Ménière's disease. Rules must be devised for dealing with multiple causation, and presbycusis should be handled in this context. The general principle is to estimate first the overall percentage handicap. (See how big the pie is.) Then estimate separately the relative contribution of each of two or more causes to the final impairment. (Cut the pie on this basis.) Fortunately we now have good predictive data for presbycusis in non-noise-exposed populations, as will appear in other papers at this Conference, and we can reasonably estimate its contribution to the total permanent threshold shift. (The remainder of the pie is charged to noise-exposure or other causes.) The problem of "second injury" in a different employment can be handled in the same way. Pre-employment audiograms are very useful here.

Rules and criteria can be made fair and reasonable on the average but they cannot take into account all possible deviations or individual differences. It is important to keep the concepts clear and the rules simple.

Section I

Field Studies

Steady-state and Fluctuating Noise: Its Effects on the Hearing of People

By

Mrs. W. Passchier-Vermeer

Research Institute of Public Health Engineering TNO, Delft, Netherlands

INTRODUCTION

In 1966, the Netherlands working group "Relation between noise and noise-induced hearing loss" of the Research Committee on Occupational Health TNO started an investigation on the effect of noise on the hearing of people exposed to it during working hours. At that time, the International Organization for Standardization was studying draft proposals in which a limit of safe noise was mentioned, the so-called NR 85 limit. As the data of Baughn (1966) were not available then, this limit was based on an assumed relation between PTS and TTS. However, only at 4000 Hz had a clear relation between PTS and TTS been demonstrated. We considered this an unsafe basis for a safe noise limit, and therefore decided to determine the actual permanent threshold shifts caused by exposure to noise for long exposure times. First of all, the work focused on the simplest situation, namely that of continuous exposure for 8 hours a day, 5 days a week to steady-state broad-band noise. Later we extended our research to fluctuating noise.

STEADY-STATE BROAD-BAND NOISE

General Remarks

We collected data from several Dutch industries (van Laar, 1966). Furthermore, literature data were used from Burns *et al.* (1964), Gallo and Glorig (1964), Rosenwinkel and Stewart (1957), Nixon and Glorig (1961), Taylor *et al.* (1964), Kylin (1960) and American Standards Association (1954). We thus had data on 20 groups of people working in noise, comprising about 4500 employees. None of them had been exposed to noise in previous jobs, nor did they display a congenital or sustained hearing damage. In 12 of the groups these people had worked in noise for 10 to 20 years; the exposure times in the other eight groups ranged from several months to 30 or 50 years. The latter groups have been used to examine the way in which hearing levels increase with time. The data of all groups have been analysed to determine a relation between noise and the noise-induced parts of the hearing levels. As we were mainly interested in the effect of noise upon hearing after longer exposure times, we restricted our research to exposure times longer than 10 years.

No details about the method of our investigation will be given here as they have been presented elsewhere (Passchier-Vermeer, 1968). However, before giving the results, we wish to point out the following. When one wants to know the effect of noise upon the hearing of people exposed to it, one first of all needs data on the hearing of people not exposed to noise during working hours. One of the members of our group analysed data from eight publications on the hearing levels of groups of people not exposed to noise and without congenital and sustained hearing damage (Spoor, 1967). He found that the median hearing levels of these groups at frequencies from 250 to 8000 Hz

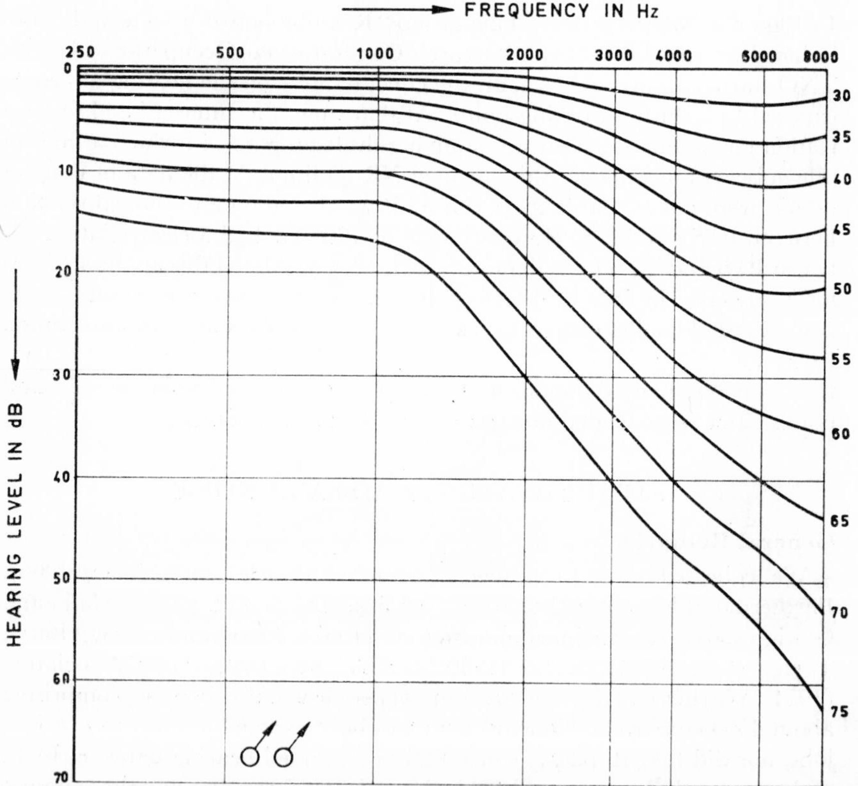

FIG. 5. Median hearing levels of men, not exposed to noise during work-time and without a congenital or sustained hearing damage, as a function of frequency; age in years is parameter.

increase with the logarithm of age. At an age of 25 years, the median hearing levels at all frequencies are taken as zero, according to ISO Recommendation R 389. Figure 5 shows that the median hearing level increases more at the higher frequencies than at the lower ones. At an age of 60 years, for instance,

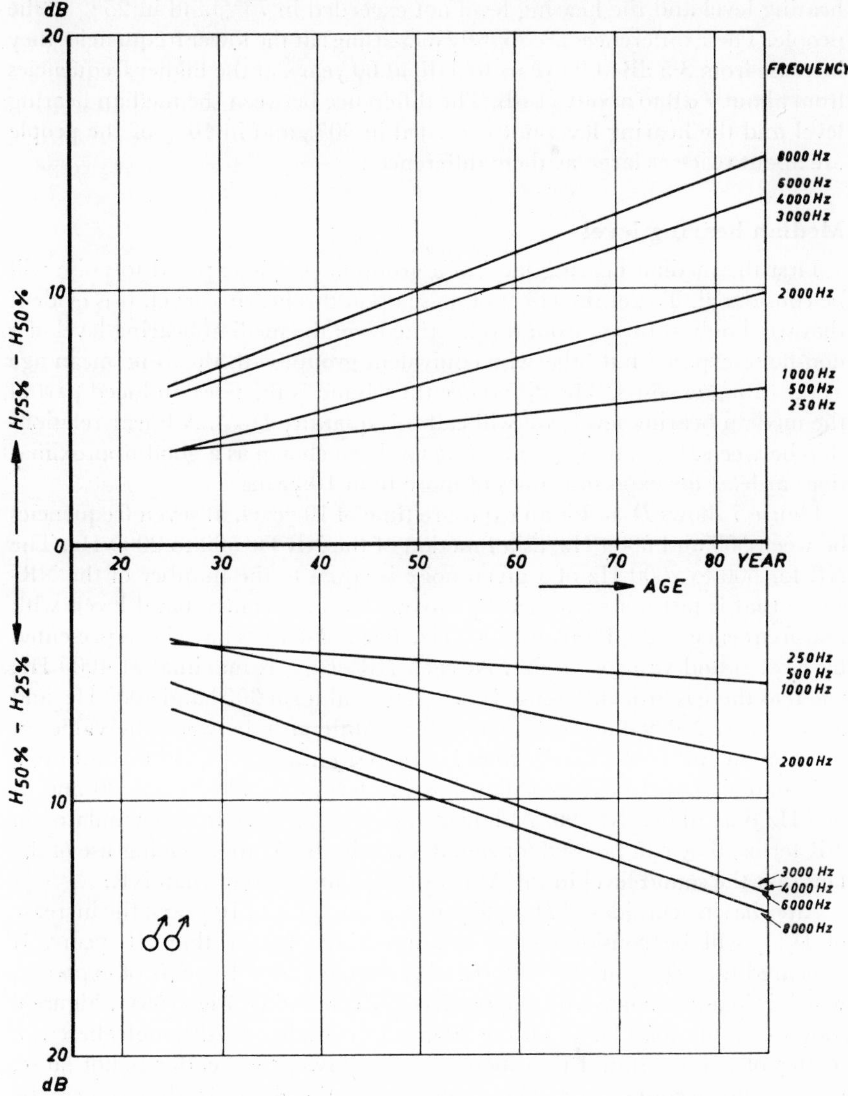

Fig. 6. The difference between the median hearing level of men not exposed to noise ($H_{50\%}$) and the hearing level not exceeded in 75% and in 25% of the people not exposed to noise ($H_{75\%}$ and $H_{25\%}$ respectively), as a function of age; frequency is parameter.

the median hearing levels at 250 to 1000 Hz are about 8 dB and at 6000 and 8000 Hz about 32 dB.

The statistical distribution of the hearing levels of non-noise-exposed people has also been examined (Spoor and Passchier-Vermeer, 1969). Figure 6 shows, as a function of age, the difference between the median hearing level and the hearing level not exceeded in 75% and in 25% of the people. These differences are slightly increasing: at the lower frequencies they increase from 3·5 dB at 25 years to 5 dB at 60 years, at the higher frequencies from about 7 dB to about 11 dB. The difference between the median hearing level and the hearing level not exceeded in 90% and in 10% of the people are about twice as large as these differences.

Median hearing level

First the median hearing level of a group of people exposed to noise will be considered. To get the effect of noise upon this hearing level, it is evident that we should subtract from this hearing level the median hearing level of a non-noise-exposed but otherwise equivalent group, with the same mean age as the group exposed. The difference thus found is the noise-induced part of the median hearing level; we will call this quantity $D_{50\%}$. A linear relationship between $D_{50\%}$ and exposure time has been chosen as a good approximation, at least for exposure times of more than 10 years.

Figure 7 shows $D_{50\%}$ for an exposure time of 10 years, at seven frequencies between 500 and 8000 Hz, as a function of the NR for 500 to 2000 Hz. The NR for 500 to 2000 Hz of a given noise is equal to the number of the NR-curve that is just not surpassed by any of the three octave-band levels with mid-frequencies 500, 1000 and 2000 Hz. The NR-curves have been presented by Kosten and van Os (1962). At each NR, $D_{50\%}$ is maximal at 4000 Hz, whereas there is little difference between the values at 3000 and 4000 Hz, and at the lower NR values there is even little difference between the values at 3000, 4000 and 6000 Hz. At 2000 Hz there is, after 10 years of exposure, a noise-induced part of the median hearing level only above NR 80 and at 500 Hz only above NR 90. Although these results have been formulated in NR terms, they can be used for sound levels in dB(A) too, making use of the fact that the sound level in dB(A) is usually 5 units larger than NR.

After having considered $D_{50\%}$ for an exposure time of 10 years, the increase of $D_{50\%}$ will be considered for exposure times longer than 10 years. It appeared that $D_{50\%}$ at 4000 Hz remains constant after 10 years of exposure, which is in accordance with the results of Nixon and Glorig (1961). Figure 8 shows $D_{50\%}$ at 4000 Hz of all the 20 groups considered. Although there is a scatter of points around the smooth curve drawn, this scatter is not large, taking into account the different origins of the data. It should here be remarked that the data of North-American origin have been transformed to ISO standard.

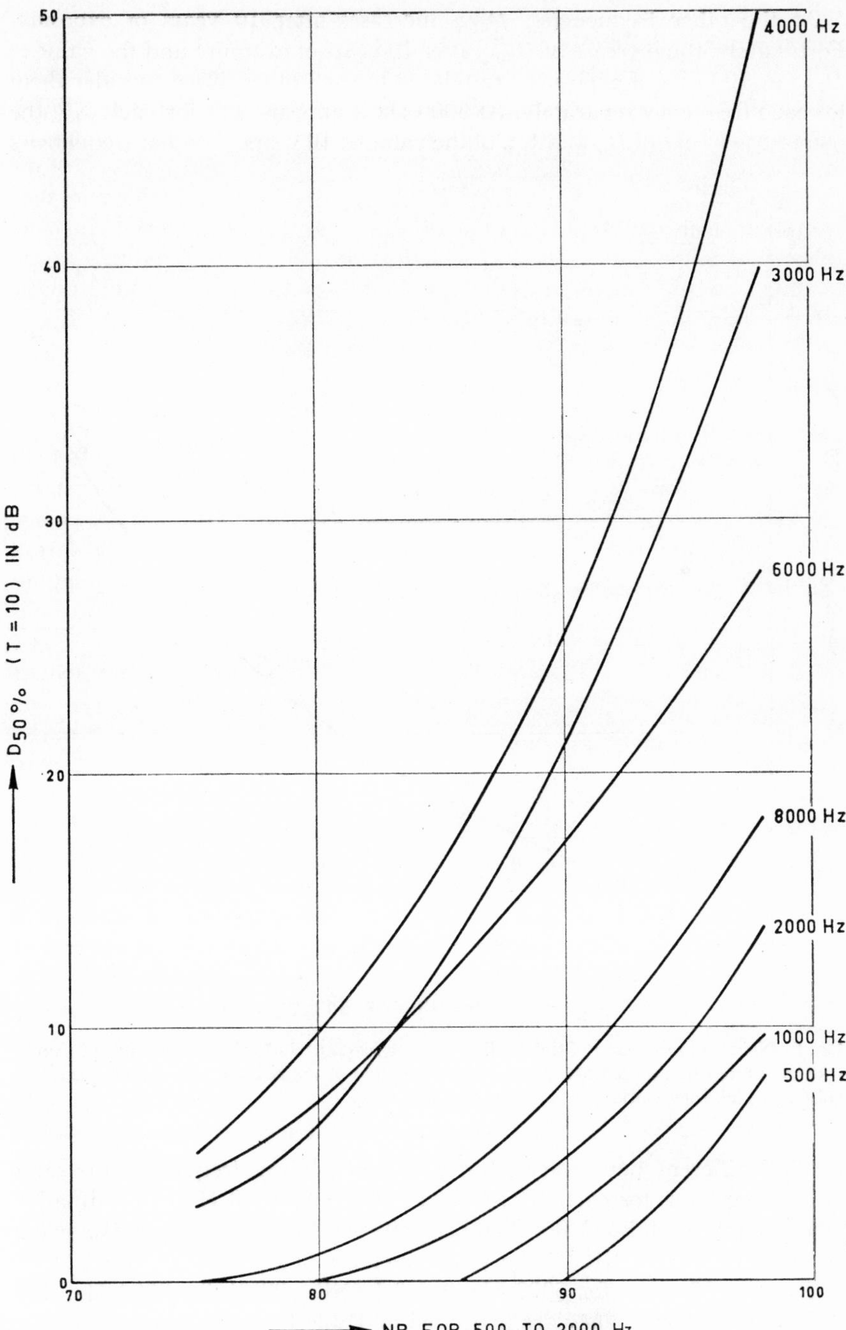

FIG. 7. Noise-induced part of the median hearing level for an exposure time of 10 years, as a function of the NR for 500 to 2000 Hz.

At the other frequencies, $D_{50\%}$ increases after 10 years of exposure. Fortunately, the increase of $D_{50\%}$ after 10 years of exposure and the value of $D_{50\%}$ at 10 years of exposure are related to each other, if we consider them for each frequency separately. At 3000 Hz it appears that for each NR the increase per year of $D_{50\%}$ is 1% of the value at 10 years. At other frequencies

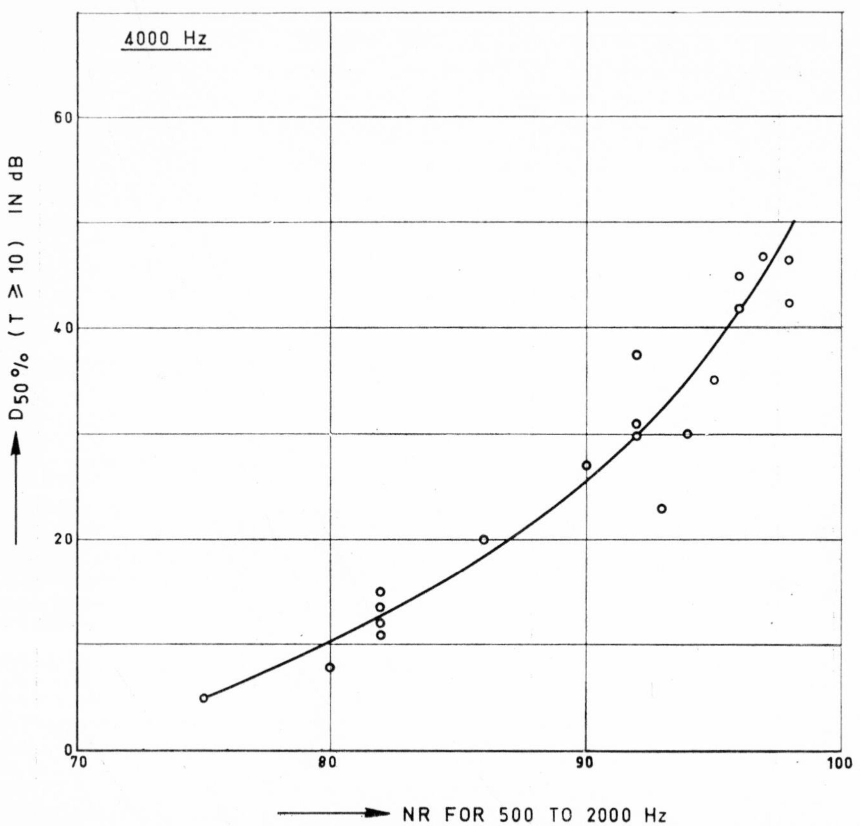

Fig. 8. Noise-induced parts of the median hearing levels at 4000 Hz of 20 groups of people, with exposure times of at least 10 years, as a function of the NR for 500 to 2000 Hz of the noise in which they work.

we find different percentages, but again, at a given frequency, the same percentage holds for each NR. Only at 6000 and 8000 Hz is the situation more complicated. For NR values below 92 we find no increase of $D_{50\%}$ after 10 years and above NR 92 the yearly increase of $D_{50\%}$ is 0·3 (NR − 92)% of $D_{50\%}$ at 10 years for 6000 Hz and 0·4 (NR − 92)% for 8000 Hz. The results for each frequency are presented in Table I.

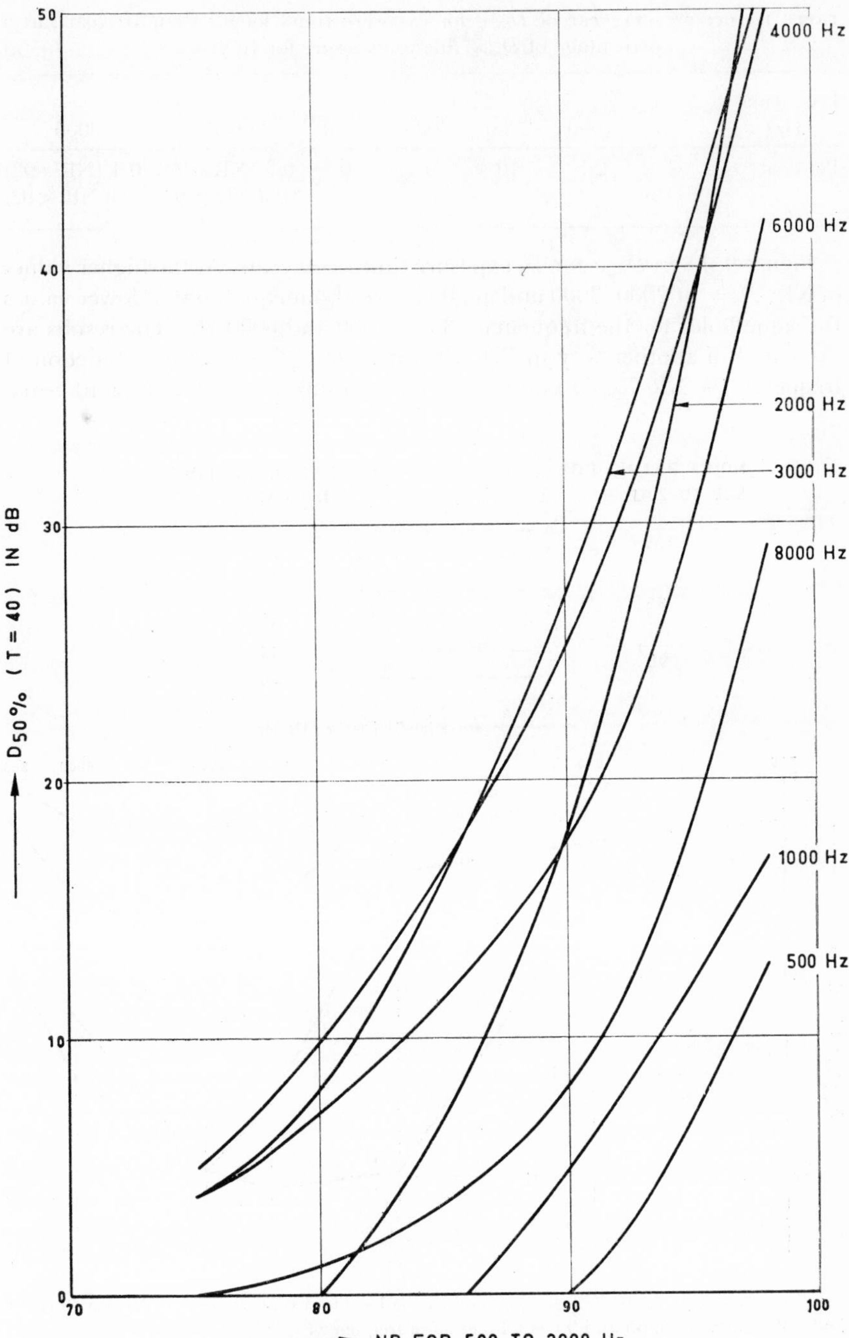

Fig. 9. Noise-induced part of the median hearing level for an exposure time of 40 years, as a function of the NR for 500 to 2000 Hz.

TABLE I. Increase per year of $D_{50\%}$ for exposure times longer than 10 years, as a percentage of $D_{50\%}$ due to exposure for 10 years

Frequency (Hz)	500	1000	2000	3000	4000	6000	8000
Per cent	2	2·5	10	1	0	0·3 (NR − 92) 0 if NR < 92	0·4 (NR − 92) 0 if NR < 92

Figure 9 shows $D_{50\%}$ for an exposure time of 40 years. At the higher values of NR, $D_{50\%}$ at 2000, 3000 and 4000 Hz are about equal, but at lower values the same holds for the frequencies 3000, 4000 and 6000 Hz. The results are presented in another way in Fig. 10, where $D_{50\%}$ is shown as a function of frequency for NR 75, 85 and 95 and for exposure times of 10 and 40 years.

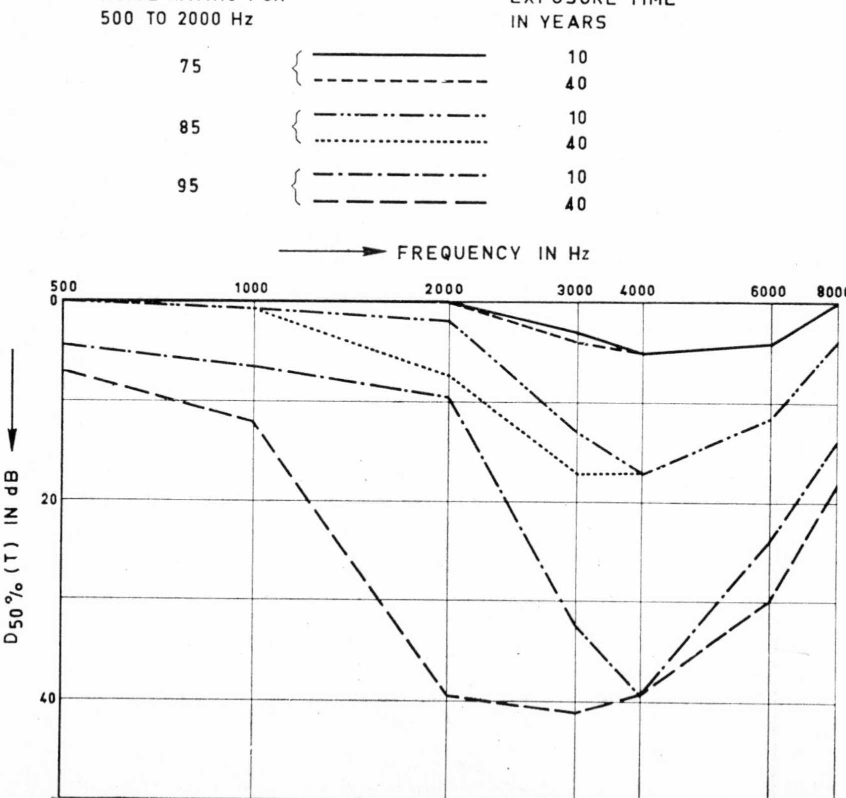

FIG. 10. Noise-induced part of the median hearing level for exposure times of 10 and 40 years and NR values of 75, 85 and 95 as a function of frequency.

At NR 75 there is hardly any difference between $D_{50\%}$ at 10 and 40 years; at NR 85 there is some increase of $D_{50\%}$ at 2000 and 3000 Hz in the course of the years. At NR 95 there is a steep notch at 4000 Hz and 10 years of exposure; this notch has broadened very much after 40 years of exposure.

Above, the results have been presented for the noise-induced part of the median hearing level. From the values of $D_{50\%}$ at 10 years (Fig. 7) and Table I, giving the increase of $D_{50\%}$ after 10 years of exposure, one is able to calculate $D_{50\%}$ at each NR between 75 and 98, or at each sound level between 80 and 103 dB(A), and for exposure times between 10 and 40 years.

Spread in hearing levels

Above, only the effect of noise upon the median hearing level has been considered. Although this gives important information on the effect of noise, it is not sufficient to base on it a limit of safe noise. Therefore, we need data on the effect of noise on the hearing levels that are worse than the median hearing level; for instance the hearing levels that are not exceeded in 75% or 90% of the people. To find the effect of noise upon the median hearing level of people exposed, we subtracted from this hearing level the median hearing level of a non-noise-exposed group with the same mean age. For example, to find the effect of noise on the hearing level just not exceeded in 75% of the people exposed, we have to subtract from this hearing level the one just not exceeded by 75% of the non-noise-exposed people. The difference so found will be indicated by $D_{75\%}$. In an analogous way $D_{90\%}$, $D_{25\%}$ and $D_{10\%}$ have been defined. Our analysis showed that $D_{75\%}-D_{50\%}$ is independent of exposure time at each frequency and for exposure times of at least 10 years. The same holds for $D_{90\%}-D_{50\%}$, $D_{50\%}-D_{25\%}$ and $D_{50\%}-D_{10\%}$. However, these four differences depend upon the NR and frequency. Figure 11 shows that the four differences increase with NR for each frequency, except at 4000 Hz where they are decreasing functions of NR.

If there are no differences between $D_{90\%}$, $D_{75\%}$, $D_{50\%}$, $D_{25\%}$ and $D_{10\%}$ it implies that the whole distribution of the hearing levels of people exposed has increased due to the noise exposure with the same number of decibels. In other words, the spread in the hearing levels of people exposed to noise is just as large as that of non-noise-exposed people. When there are differences between the various $D_{x\%}$ values (with x equal to 90, 75, 50, 25 and 10), the spread in hearing levels of people exposed is larger than that of non-noise-exposed people.

Figure 12 shows $D_{90\%}$, $D_{50\%}$ and $D_{10\%}$ for NR 75, 85 and 95 and an exposure time of 10 years. As has been pointed out already, the differences between $D_{90\%}$, $D_{50\%}$ and $D_{10\%}$ are independent of exposure time. At NR 75, $D_{x\%}$ has different values for different x only at 4000 Hz. This means that, only at this frequency, the spread in the hearing levels has been increased by the noise exposure. At NR 85 the spread in the hearing levels has been

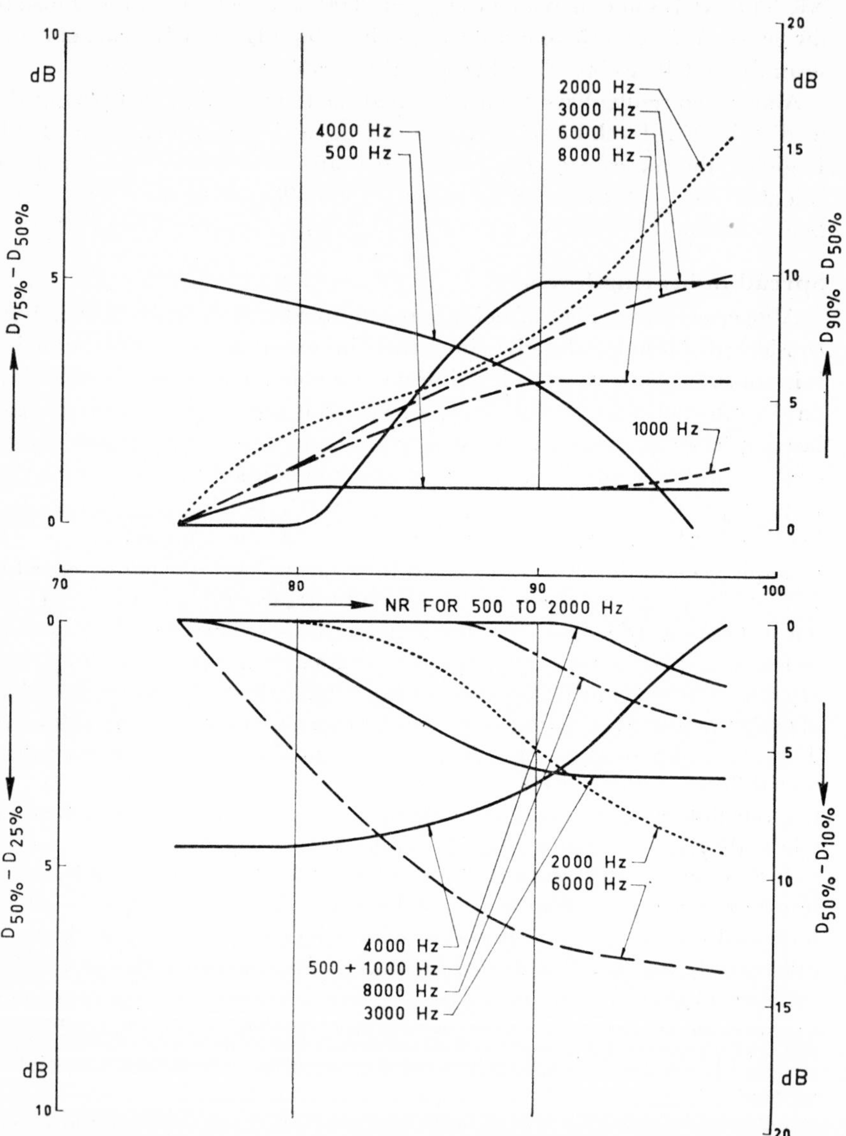

FIG. 11 Differences between $D_{50\%}$ (noise-induced part of the median hearing level) and $D_{90\%}$, $D_{75\%}$, $D_{25\%}$, $D_{10\%}$ (noise-induced part of the hearing level not exceeded in 90%, 75%, 25%, 10% of the people respectively) as a function of the NR for 500 to 2000 Hz. The differences are independent of exposure time for exposure times of at least 10 years.

increased somewhat by the noise exposure at 1000 Hz and above, since the $D_{x\%}$ values differ somewhat in this frequency range. At NR 95 the spread in the hearing levels of noise-exposed people is at any frequency larger than that of non-exposed people, although there is only a slight increase in the spread at 4000 Hz.

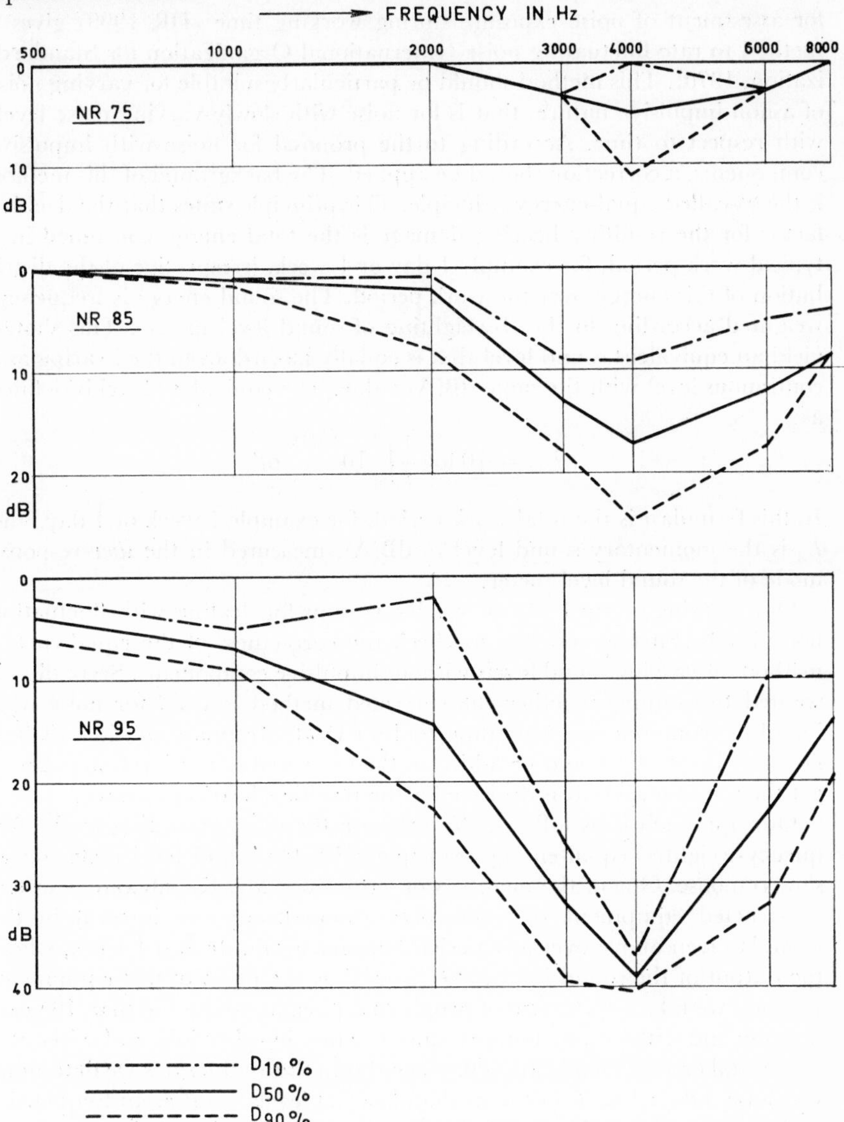

FIG. 12. Noise-induced parts of the hearing levels, not exceeded in 90%, 50% and 10% of the people exposed for 10 years to noise with NR 75, 85 or 95, as a function of frequency.

FLUCTUATING NOISE

General remarks

All the results presented above were for steady-state broad-band noise and for continuous exposure. We will now consider the more complicated situation of fluctuating noise levels. The latest ISO Draft Recommendation for assessment of noise exposure during working time (DR 1999) gives a method to rate fluctuating noise (International Organization for Standardization, 1970). This method should be particularly suitable for varying noise of a non-impulsive nature, that is for noise with slowly-varying noise levels with respect to time. According to the proposal for noise with impulsive components, a correction should be applied. The background of this method is the so-called equal-energy principle. This principle states that the decisive factor for the resulting hearing damage is the total energy consumed in a typical work period, for example 1 day or 1 week, irrespective of the distribution of this energy over the work period. The sound energy is frequency-weighted according to the A-weighting of sound level meters. This should yield an equivalent sound level that is equally hazardous to the hearing as a continuous level with the same dB(A) value. The equivalent level is defined as:

$$L_{eq} = 10 \log \frac{1}{t} \int_0^t 10^{L_A/10} \, dt'$$

In this formula t is the total work-period, for example 1 week or 1 day, and L_A is the momentary sound level in dB(A), measured in the *slow* response mode of the sound level meter.

Our working group had two specific reasons for dealing with fluctuating noise levels. First we wanted to check the correctness of the equal-energy method for varying sound levels without impulsive components. Secondly we wanted to examine whether the corrected method is valid for noise with impulsive components. According to ISO Draft Recommendation 1999, a factor of 10 dB(A) should be added to the measured sound levels in order to get the sound level that is decisive for the resulting hearing damage.

Our approach is as follows. We measure the noise according to the frequency-weighted equal-energy principle, with the sound level meter set at slow response. One of the members of our group, Mr. Kleinhoonte van Os, constructed equipment that measures automatically the integral in the formula given above over any period between 1 minute and 1 week, where the output of the sound level meter is used as the input of this equipment. Further, we take audiograms of people that have worked more than 10 years in noise and without previous exposure to noise in other jobs and without a congenital or sustained hearing damage. From the audiograms we determine the noise-induced parts of the median hearing levels at different frequencies and exposure times. These values are compared with the results for steady-state noise presented above and a theoretical value of the equivalent sound level is calculated. These theoretical values are then compared with the experimental noise measurement results.

Experimental results

So far we have found results for three different groups of people. The first set of results relates to people working in a wood-working factory (Kuiper and Visser, 1969). Although the noise levels vary over the workday, the noise is not of an impulsive nature. The equivalent sound levels measured over the whole workday varied from 98·4 to 100·6 dB(A), depending upon the place of measurement. To get an impression of the fluctuations of the noise during the day, the equivalent sound levels were also measured over periods of $\frac{1}{4}$ hour. At the place where 100·6 dB(A) was measured as the equivalent sound level over the day, the equivalent sound levels in $\frac{1}{4}$-hour periods ranged from 95 to 104 dB(A). If the equivalent sound levels had been measured over even shorter periods, this range would have been still larger. Further, we analysed the audiograms of 144 machine wood-workers, selected according to the criteria already mentioned. The results, presented in Fig. 13, led to an equivalent sound level of 98 to 99 dB(A), which is about the same as the measured equivalent sound levels, which were between 98 and 101

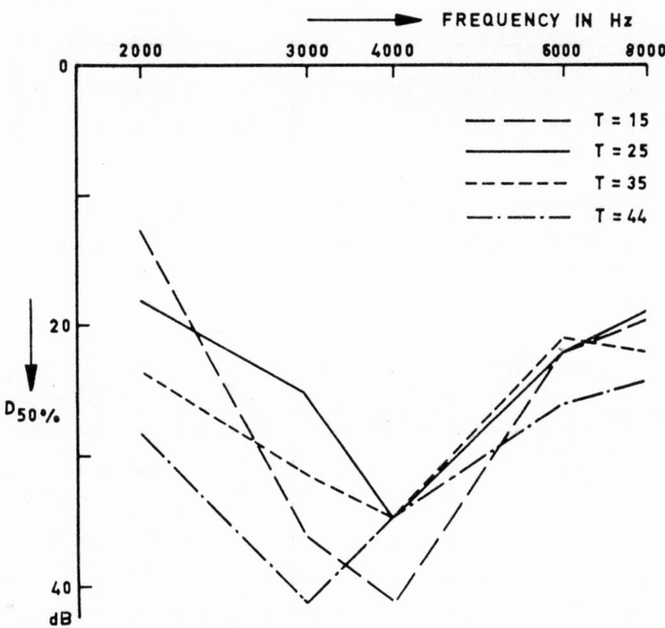

Fig. 13. Noise-induced parts of the median hearing levels of 4 groups of machine wood-workers (in total 144 persons) as a function of frequency. Mean exposure times of the groups are 15, 25, 35 and 44 years.

dB(A). We concluded that, in this case, the equal-energy principle applies and that the sound levels can be measured in the slow-response mode of the sound level meter.

The two other groups worked respectively in the welding shop of a steel construction works and in the shop of the same works where steel plates are pretreated mechanically.

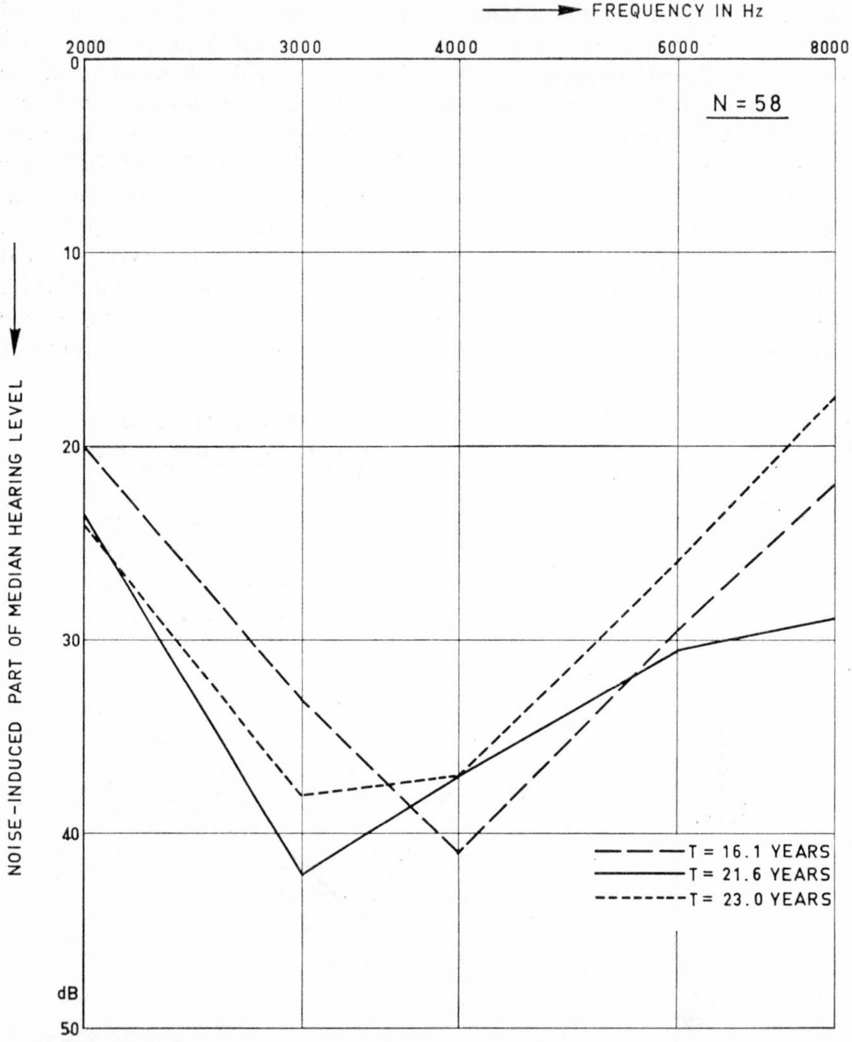

FIG. 14. Noise-induced parts of the median hearing levels of 3 groups of steelworkers (30 persons, 58 ears) as a function of frequency. Mean exposure times of the groups are 16.1, 21.6 and 23.0 years.

In both cases, the noise has impulsive components. The impulses are widely separated in time; these are no more than a few impulses per minute. In the welding shop, two people riveted for about 1 week each year. The group of 30 machine steel workers (58 ears, last case) was split up into three subgroups. Figure 14 shows the noise-induced parts of the median hearing levels of these subgroups. These $D_{50\%}$ values correspond to an equivalent sound level of 100 to 102 dB(A). The equivalent sound levels, measured during 20 workdays for 4 places, ranged from 80·3 to 84·6 dB(A) per day. This gives a difference between measured and theoretical equivalent sound levels of not less than 17 to 20 dB(A). Figure 15 shows the equivalent sound

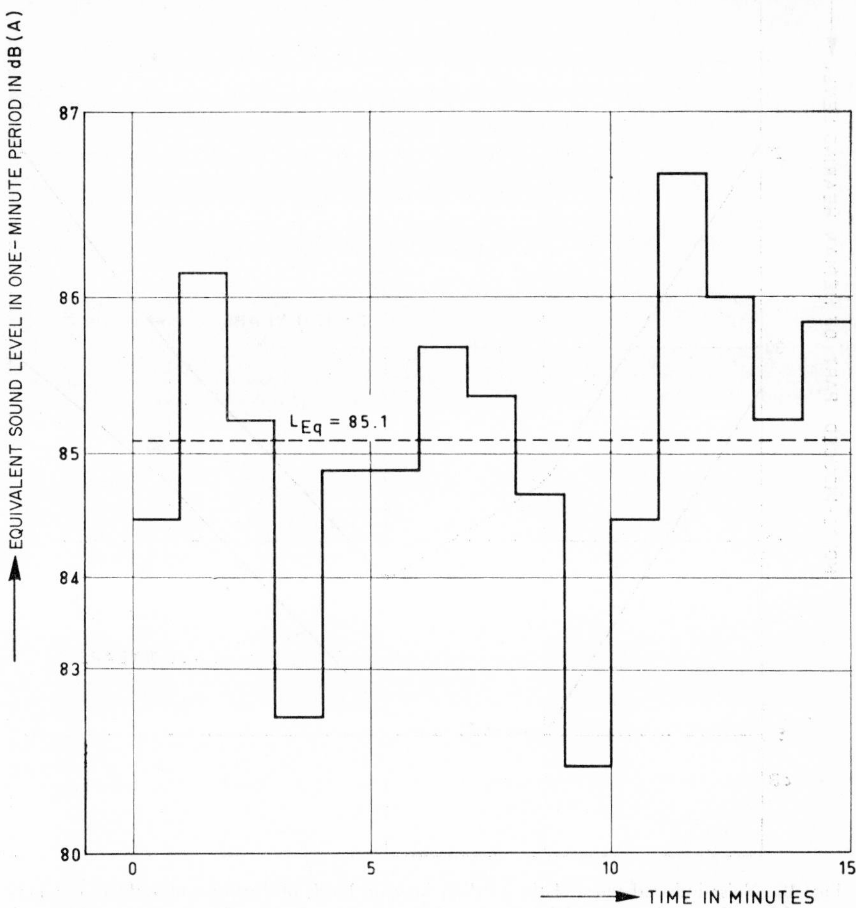

FIG. 15. Equivalent sound levels, measured in 1-minute periods during an arbitrarily chosen quarter of an hour, for machine steel-working. The equivalent sound level for this quarter of an hour is 85·1 dB(A).

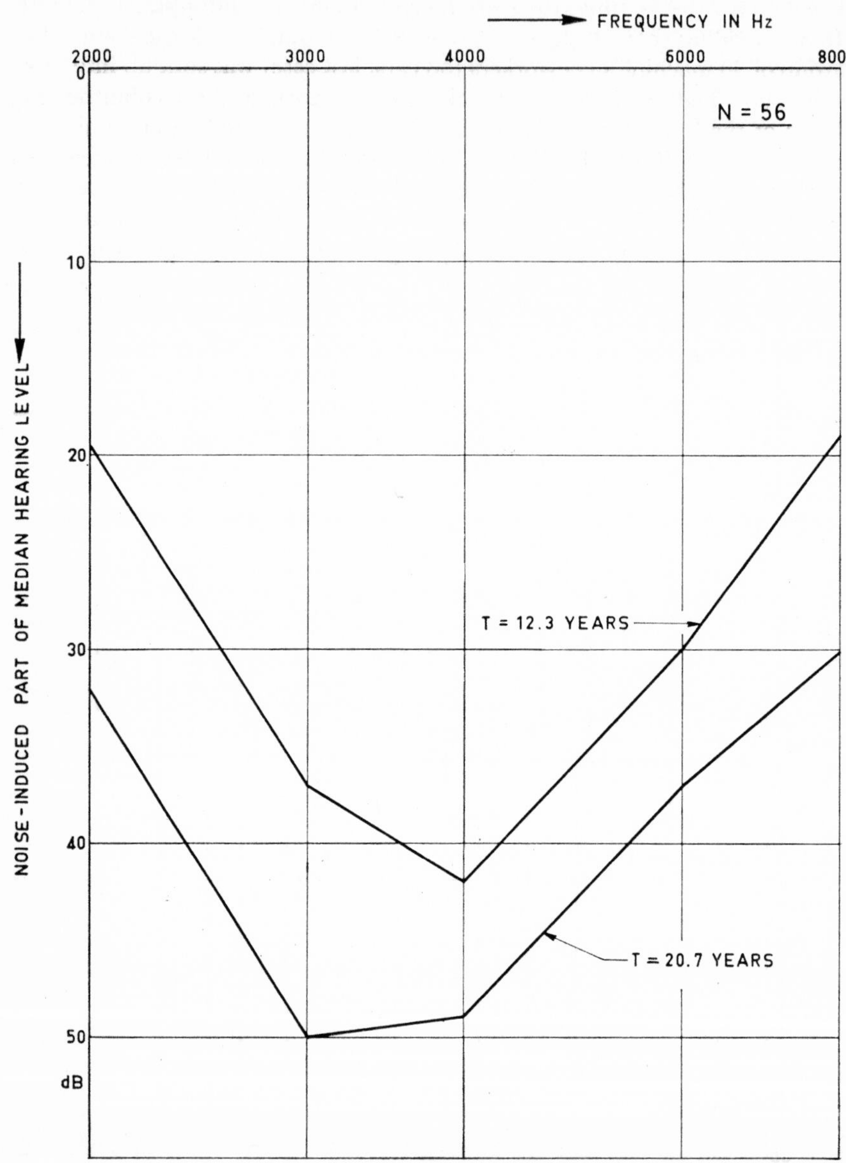

FIG. 16. Noise-induced parts of the median hearing levels of 2 groups of welders (29 persons, 56 ears) as a function of frequency. Mean exposure times of the groups are 12·3 and 20·7 years.

levels measured in 1-minute periods for an arbitrarily chosen period of 15 minutes. The measured equivalent sound levels in 1-minute periods range from about 82 to about 87 dB(A). Even measuring the equivalent sound levels over such a short period does not give a good impression of the impulsive nature of the noise, as the impulses occur in a much shorter period than 1 minute.

Finally, the results for the welding shop. Figure 16 shows the noise-induced parts of the median hearing levels of two subgroups of welders (29 persons, 56 ears). These noise-induced parts agree with an equivalent sound level of 102 to 104 dB(A). The equivalent sound levels, measured

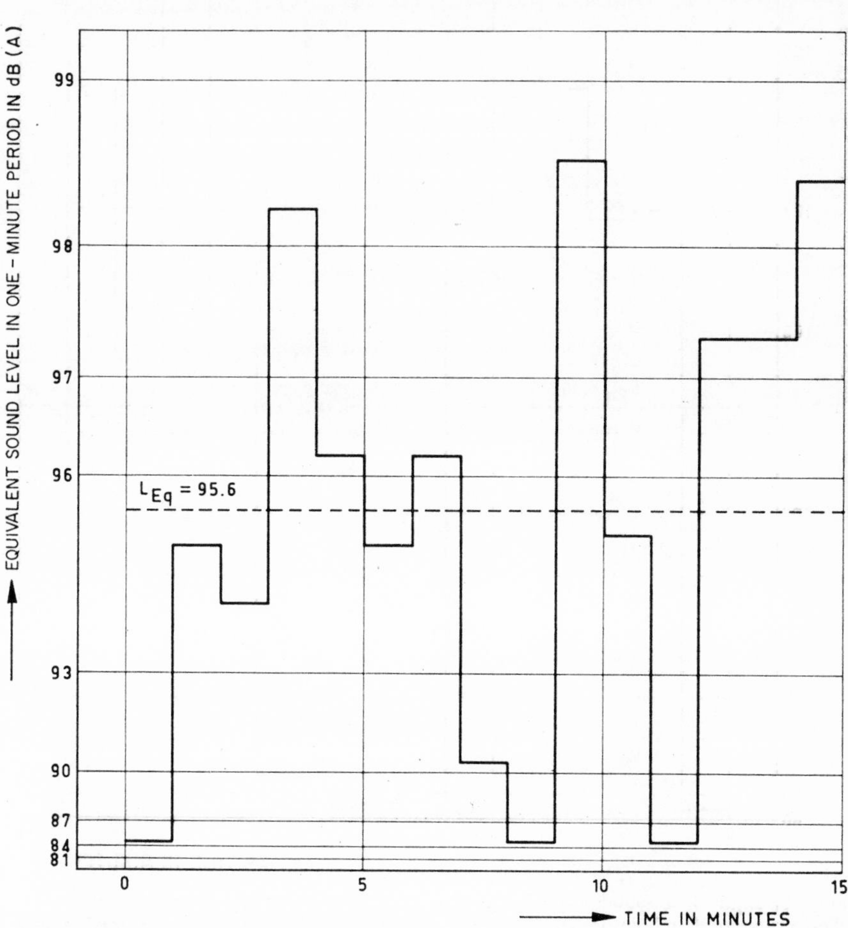

FIG. 17. Equivalent sound levels, measured in 1-minute periods during a rather arbitrarily chosen quarter of an hour, for welding. The equivalent sound level for this quarter of an hour is 95·6 dB(A).

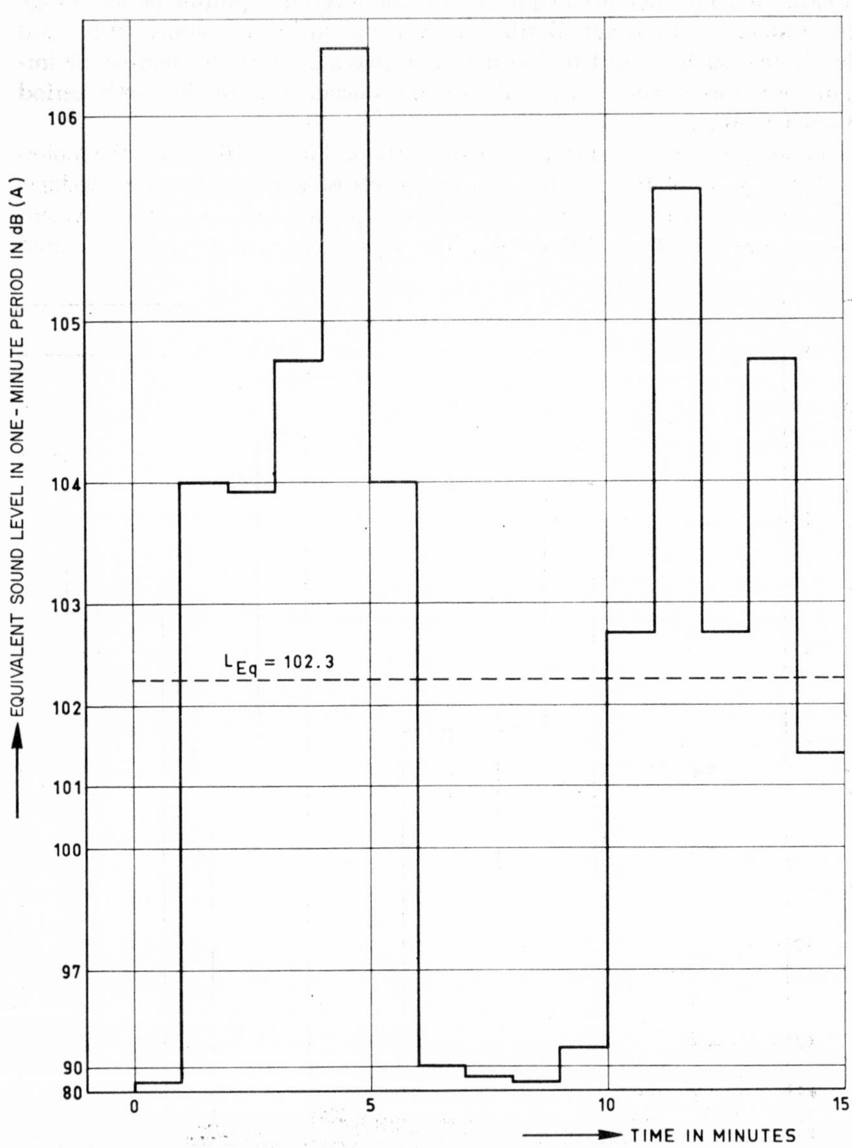

FIG. 18. Equivalent sound levels, measured in 1-minute periods during an arbitrarily chosen quarter of an hour, for riveting. The equivalent sound level for this quarter of an hour is 102·3 dB(A).

during 15 workdays for 3 places ranged from 85.0 to 90·8 dB(A). During these 15 days, the labourers performed their normal duties. Now there is a difference between measured and theoretical equivalent sound levels of 13 to 17 dB(A). Figure 17 shows the equivalent sound levels in 1-minute periods, measured during $\frac{1}{4}$ hour in which a relatively large amount of noise was made. The 1-minute equivalent sound levels range from 84 to about 99 dB(A).

During another 5 days, 2 labourers riveted; this seldom occurs in this shop. The whole-day equivalent sound levels ranged from 92 to 104 dB(A), measured at a distance of 4 to 6 m. from the place of riveting. This gives a difference of up to 10 dB(A) between the measured and theoretical equivalent sound levels. This last figure is quite unrealistic, as riveting takes place only 1 week a year and, furthermore, the place of measurement was in general closer to the place of riveting than the workplace of the people whose audiograms were used. Fig. 18 shows 1-minute equivalent sound levels over an arbitrarily chosen 15 minutes during the riveting period. These 1-minute equivalent sound levels range from 84 to 106 dB(A).

CONCLUSION

The results of audiometric and noise-measurements in a wood-working factory confirm the equal-energy principle. The noise levels varied over the workday, but did not have impulsive components. The sound levels were measured with a sound level meter set at slow response. The results for the two groups of people working in a steel construction works, in noise with impulsive components, show clearly that rating this noise according to the equal-energy principle, and measuring it with a sound level meter set at slow response, yields measured sound levels that are much more hazardous to the hearing than can be expected from the values measured. In these two cases, correction factors of 13 to 20 dB(A) must be applied. Whether the system of noise-measuring—that is to say, measuring impulsive noise with a sound level meter set at *slow* response—or the principle of equal energy, or both, are incorrect is still a point to be settled. In the meantime, our opinion is that a method that needs such high correction factors is unsuitable, the more so as it is not clear yet in which cases these correction factors should be applied.

Noise and Hearing of a Population of Forest Workers

By

G. Holmgren, L. Johnsson, B. Kylin and O. Linde*

Summary

In a hearing study carried out on about 900 forestry workers in northern Sweden about 300 fellers and tractor drivers were submitted to a more thorough examination of the relationship between hearing and exposure to noise. The pattern of exposure for both groups was extremely irregular. As measured by an ISO method for the assessment of an irregular noise with varying level the exposure to the noise from power saws and tractors corresponded to a continuous sound level of about 95 dB and 98 dB, respectively. The results of the hearing tests showed that both groups of forestry workers had a hearing loss typical of noise damage. The loss was largely the same as that recorded in an earlier study of a group exposed to a noise of constant intensity of about 90 dB(A).

INTRODUCTION

A feature of modern occupational health is directed health examinations of groups of employees whose work involves particular exposure to health hazards. In health and environmental studies of forest workers (Hansson *et al.*, 1967; Kylin *et al.*, 1968) it was found that the noise produced by forest tractors and power saws constitutes a risk of hearing damage. An assessment of this risk, however, is complicated by the irregular pattern of exposure in these cases. As there would appear to be no major Swedish study of the hearing of forestry workers in relation to their exposure to noise an account of the results of such a study performed on forestry workers in the Swedish Forest Service might be of interest.

MATERIAL AND METHODS

In 1965 and 1968 hearing examinations were carried out on some 1700 and 1000 forest workers, respectively, in Upper Norrland. About 900 of these were examined on both occasions.

* The Boden Hospital, Boden; The Swedish Forest Service, Stockholm; the Health Department, Sandvikens Jernverks AB, Sandviken; and the National Institute of Occupational Health, Stockholm, Sweden.

The hearing measurements were performed with a Danavox portable audiometer by specially trained staff in a rest cabin at working sites in the forest; the background noise levels were satisfactory for regular audiometry. The audiometers were calibrated in accordance with the ISO standard (International Organization for Standardization, 1964). The study also included the noting of a history including questions relating to previous exposure to noise, subjective symptoms, and prior ear damage. The time elapsing between the most recent exposure to noise from the respective machines and the beginning of the audiometric examination was between 15 and 60 minutes.

From the workers that had been examined on both occasions (about 900) those mentioning no prior ear damage were selected. The final study group comprised 261 fellers and 59 tractor drivers.

For the noise measurements a precision sound level meter (Brüel and Kjær 2203) and a portable tape recorder (Nagra III) were used. The noise was recorded on tape, the meter being used as a calibrated amplifier. Before each set of measurements the equipment was calibrated against a pistonphone signal (124 dB *re* 2×10^{-5} N/m^2). The noise measurements, which were performed under normal working conditions in the winter 6 months, were carried out for 12 fellers, selected at random at different felling sites, and 5 tractor drivers. Five makes of power saw and 5 makes of tractor were used. During the measurement the lumberman usually felled between 3 and 9 trees, which were then trimmed and cut into logs. The feller carried the sound level meter on his back in a special sling and the microphone was fixed at ear level, close to the head.

The measurements on the tractor drivers comprised the whole working cycle, from idling of the engine to loading, hauling and unloading.

The noise recorded on the tape was analysed at the laboratory. A statistical distribution analysis with respect to the different levels occurring during a typical working cycle was carried out. Typical sections from the various lumbering operations were submitted to octave-band analysis.

RESULTS

Exposure analysis

The noise level as measured at the ear of the fellers and tractor drivers for the various working phases is reported in Tables II and III.

As is seen from Fig. 19, the maximum energy of the noise from the power saw lay in the middle frequency range whereas the tractor emitted a predominantly low-frequency noise. Both types considerably exceed the levels that have been recommended by, among others, Swedish researchers (Kylin and Johansson, 1964) as risk values for injurious noise; here, account is taken of the exposure time (Curve A, daily exposure of $\geqslant$ 5 hours; B, 2–5 hours; C, 1–2 hours; D, 20 minutes; and E, 5 minutes).

TABLE II. Sound pressure levels for noise from power saws in various lumbering operations; dB(C)

Power-saw No.	Type	Idling	Felling	Trimming	Cutting
1	Raket 60	85–95	107	97–105	103
2		84–89	104–107	97–103	102
3		81–87	96–101	101–107	96–100
4		89–94	107–109	98–105	105–108
5	Homelite XL-660	93–95	105–110	100–106	100–107
6		83–89	107	94–103	103
7		89–95	101–107	90–105	99–105
8	Partner R 14 S	90–93	110–112	99–108	106–109
9		87–90	97–106	87–99	100–106
10	Husquarna 65	81–88	101–105	92–102	101–104
11		91–95	91–101	93–101	93–102
12	McCulloch 4-10	87–95	107–110	90–105	107

TABLE III. Sound pressure levels for noise from tractors during various operations; dB(C)

Type	Idling	Loading	Hauling	Unloading
SMV Drivax	113–114	112	103–113	106
Hemek	110–112	98–99	108–110	no record
VMV Stalo C	110–113	98–111	99	107–109
Nalle SM 660	106	101	108	100
Timberjack 230	114–115	114	110–111	no record

These risk values, however, apply to continuous noise where the intensity does not vary appreciably with time.

In the present case the noise experienced by both forest fellers and tractor drivers was extremely irregular. The sound level was often low, for instance, when the power saw was idling. The different working operations for the tractor driver also imply a large fluctuation in noise level. The ISO is at present working on a proposal for the assessment of occupational noise exposure according to which it would be possible to estimate an irregular noise with varying sound pressure levels (International Organization for Standardization, 1970). Here a conversion function is used whereby the irregular noise is converted, through a time integration of the sound intensity, to an equivalent noise level in dB(A).

A statistical distribution analysis of the noise level from the power saws and tractors expressed in dB(A) in relation to time for typical working cycles is presented in Figs. 20 and 21.

According to the above procedure the total noise exposure, calculated

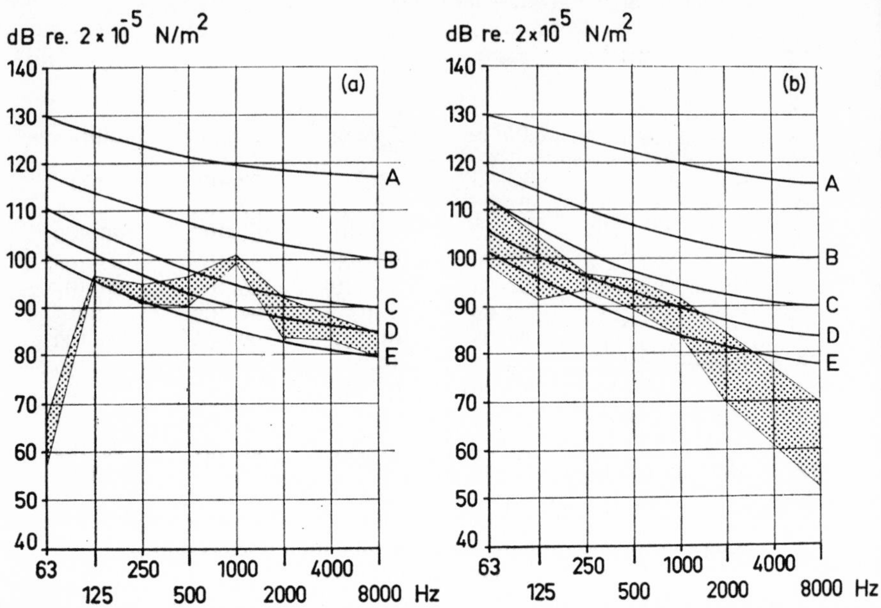

FIG. 19. Octave-band spectra of the noise of (a) a power saw during cutting and (b) tractors.

...... Experimental results
——— Risk curves A–E (see text)

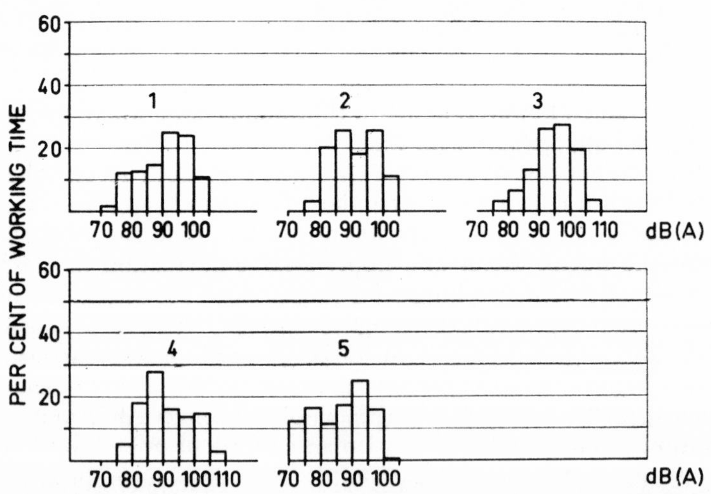

FIG. 20. Distribution analysis of the noise level of power saws during a typical working cycle.

1, Raket 60 (4 saws). 2, McCulloch 4–10 (1 saw). 3, Homelite XL-600 (3 saws). 4, Partner R 14 S (2 saws). 5, Husquarna 65 (2 saws).

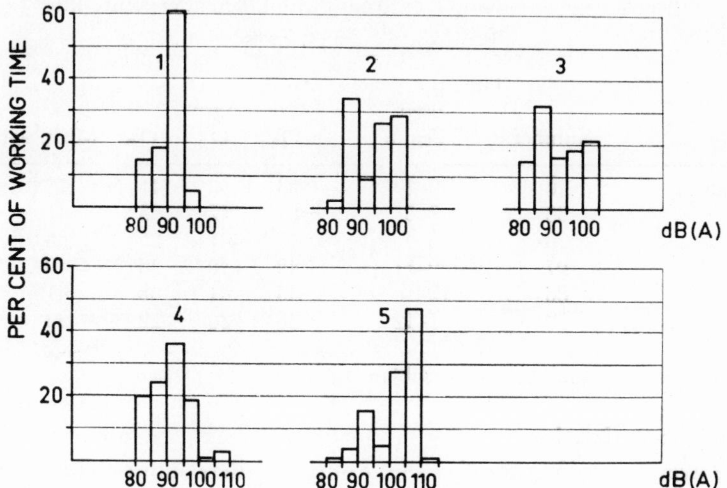

FIG. 21. Distribution analysis of the noise level of tractors during a typical working cycle. 1, SMV Drivax. 2, Hemek. 3, VMV Stalo C. 4, Nalle SM 660. 5, Timberjack 230.

over a 40-hour working week and converted to the equivalent continuous noise level for the respective sources is, on average, as follows:

Power saws	95·3 dB(A)	range 90–99
Tractors	97·8 dB(A)	range 92–106

These values considerably exceed the recommended level of 85 dB(A) above which, according to a Swedish Standard (Svenska Elektriska Kommissionen, 1969) measures should be taken to protect hearing.

At the time of the 1965 study the 261 fellers had used power saws for on average about 10 years and the 59 tractor drivers had driven tractors in forest work for about 8 years. The median age for the fellers was 41 years (lower and upper quartiles 33 and 48 years, respectively) and for the tractor drivers 38 years (29 and 46 years). An analysis of the age distribution for the fellers in groups with different exposure times showed that the mean age for these was roughly the same (Table IV). This may be due to the fact that during the last years there had been a considerable rationalization and mechanization of forestry work in Sweden, with the result that the fellers have been recruited largely from other categories of forestry sectors (drivers of horse-drawn transport) who, moreover, were of higher ages. The group of tractor drivers was too small for such a grouping to be practicable.

Incidentally, this rationalization also resulted in a considerable increase in the daily use of the power saw in forestry work, since it is now also used for trimming.

TABLE IV. Age distribution for groups with different exposure time up to the 1965 examination

	Number	Time power saw used (Years)	Age[a] Q_1	Q_2	Q_3	Mean age
Fellers	20	0–2	53	46	41	46
	30	3–5	51	42	33	41
	28	6–8	47	41	25	38
	97	9–11	48	40	36	40
	86	12–	45	41	38	41
Tractor-drivers	59	1–12	46	38	29	38

[a] Q_1, Q_3; upper and lower quartiles: Q_2; median.

Hearing examination

The average audiograms for the group of fellers showed (Fig. 22) the typical pattern of noise-induced permanent threshold shifts for frequencies between 3000 and 8000 Hz. There was a deterioration in the hearing between the two occasions of examination but it was of negligible degree.

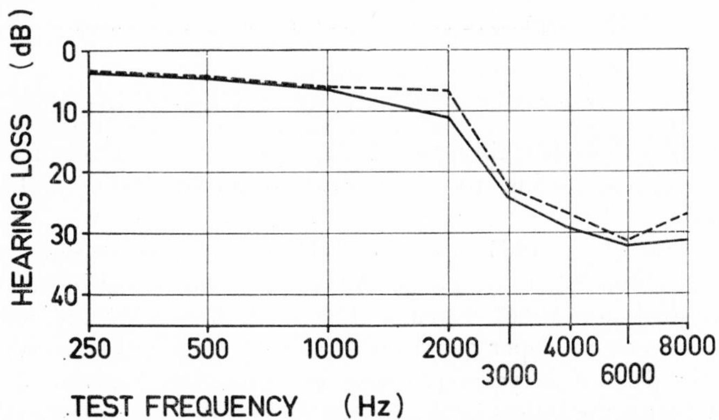

FIG. 22. Average group audiograms of fellers (right ear, $N = 261$).
- - - - - examined in 1965
——— examined in 1968

The tractor driver group also showed a hearing loss between these frequencies (Fig. 23) but there was no worsening between the two examinations—in fact, for certain frequencies (including 6000 Hz) an improvement was noted. This may have been due to more widespread use of ear protectors following the first study in connection with which they were recommended.

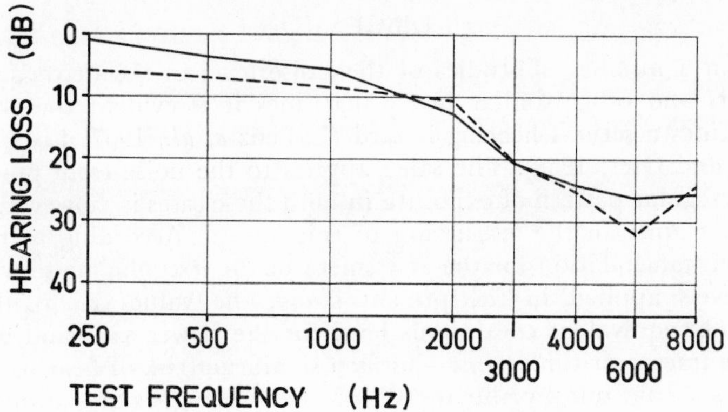

FIG. 23. Average group audiograms of tractor drivers (right ear, $N = 59$).

- - - - - examined in 1965
———— examined in 1968

Finally, in the feller group there was only a weak correlation between the times for which the power saw had been used and the hearing level, the persons that had used the machines longest having the poorest hearing (Fig. 24).

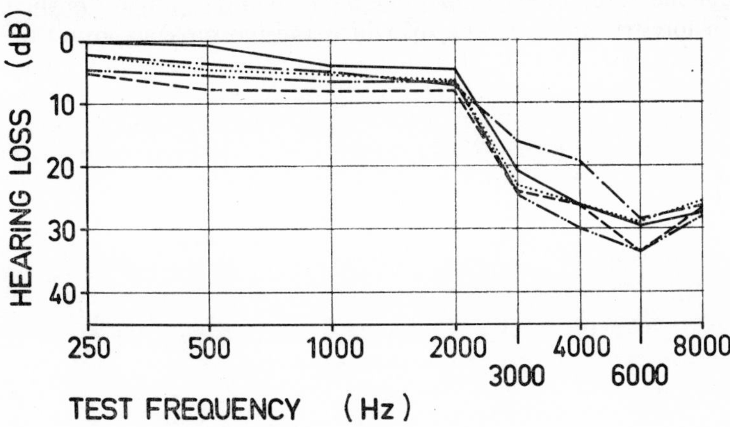

FIG. 24. Average group audigrams of fellers with different durations of working with power saws.

———— 0–2 yr ($N = 20$)
——·—— 3–5 yr ($N = 30$)
- - - - - - 6–8 yr ($N = 28$)
········· 9–11 yr ($N = 97$)
—··— ⩾ 12 yr ($N = 86$)

DISCUSSION

From a number of studies of the noise level in the driver's cabin of tractors and other similar heavy machines it is evident that the noise constitutes a serious hearing hazard (LaBenz *et al.*, 1967; Lisland, 1967; Jones and Oser, 1968). The same applies to the noise from power saws. The irregular pattern of exposure in both these cases is, however, a factor of uncertainty in the evaluation of this hazard. According to the draft ISO recommendation for the assessment of the irregular noise with varying levels applied in the present study, the values recorded—about 95 dB(A) equivalent continuous level for the power saws and 98 dB(A) for the tractor driver's cabin—imply a significant risk of hearing damage. This is borne out by the results of the hearing examinations, which showed that both the power-saw operators and tractor drivers had a moderate hearing loss typical of noise damage. If these results are compared with those obtained in an investigation of the hearing in a population exposed to a steady industrial noise (Kylin, 1960) over a period of about 12 years. it is found that the hearing loss for the power-saw operators and tractor drivers was nearly the same as that for the group exposed to the corresponding steady-state noise of 90 dB(A). The method of evaluating the irregular noise associated with these occupations thus gives a measure of the risk that is slightly on the high side—that is to say, the hearing was better than would correspond to the calculated equivalent continuous noise level of about 95 dB(A). This might be due in some measure to the considerable increase in the daily use of the power saw in forestry work, because of which the measured exposure to noise does not correspond to the true exposure in this retrospective study.

Estimating the Risk of Hearing Loss due to Exposure to Continuous Noise

By

D. W. Robinson

National Physical Laboratory,
Teddington, England

Summary

From the results of the joint MRC–NPL hearing and noise survey it is possible to estimate the magnitude of the permanent threshold shift that will be induced by exposure to a known noise immission level, as a statistical distribution in a population without aural pathology. It is shown that by making a comparatively small allowance for the other auditory deficits that occur in an unselected population, in the form of an additional statistical distribution, the results are in close agreement with those of incidence studies in America. The risk of a specified hearing level being exceeded can be obtained by calculation which also takes into account the effect of age. Numerical examples of the procedure are given, and the implications for damage-risk criteria for steady noises are discussed.

INTRODUCTION

The relationships between noise and the irreversible changes in hearing acuity (NIPTS) that result, in long-term situations of repeated daily exposure, have been the subject of many field studies. However, the number of variables is large, so that, in spite of a degree of uniformity in the basis of measurement of the hearing changes, namely the use of pure-tone audiometry, the various results have remained difficult to compare and appraise.

One fact that always emerges is a wide variation of individual susceptibility, and for this reason the right approach to experiments intended to elucidate the cause–effect relationships must take into account the manner in which the results are to be put to use. Interest may centre on the individual, as in that aspect of hearing preservation which monitors the hearing of workers by periodical audiometry, or in the context of compensation for hearing loss already sustained. On a more general footing, however, much can be done in advance of actual damage occurring by ensuring a safe working environment. Individual audiometry may, in this way, be confined to workers in places of known high risk. It is this more general preventive aspect to which the present paper is devoted.

DAMAGE-RISK CRITERIA

The so-called damage-risk criteria that have appeared in the literature over the past two decades seek to specify a maximum safe noise level for the working environment. The concept being a rather vague one unless more closely defined, it is not surprising that criteria have varied in substance as well as in form, for example in the manner of describing the noise level: sound level *A*, noise rating number, octave band sound pressure levels and so on. Implicit in each criterion is a set of value judgements superimposed on the cause–effect relationships.

The methodical formulation of a damage-risk criterion would explicitly recognize at least five considerations, judgements upon each of which entail certain socio-political implications. They are these:

(a) a species of disability; for example, loss of the capacity to understand conversational speech in quiet surroundings.

(b) a degree of that disability; for example, a just-beginning mild impairment.

(c) a percentage of persons regarded as an acceptable risk even if the specified impairment is attained. In present conditions the ideal of no impairment at even a mild level appears unattainable.

(d) a base-line of reckoning. Shall the population at risk be defined as one suffering no impairments of hearing other than that due to the presumptive cause, noise, and possibly also natural ageing? Or shall it be a representative population with an admixture of auditory pathology and hearing impaired by extraneous but socially accepted acoustic overload from non-occupational pursuits? As will be seen, this distinction greatly affects the occupational noise risk.

(e) the time element. For how long shall the noise exposure be presumed to persist into the future? A natural answer to this would be a working lifetime; periods of 10 or of 20 years have also been discussed in this connection. This aspect is an important one for the following reason. NIPTS grows rapidly at first and thereafter more slowly, whereas ageing exhibits exactly the opposite characteristics. Thus, after a sufficiently long time the expectation of a hearing loss is not much different whether NIPTS has been sustained or not. Yet over the whole of the intervening time the hearing of the noise-exposed person is manifestly impaired relative to the non-exposed. Logically, therefore, the noise risk should be related to the time when its differential effect is at its greatest. This point is developed in the final section of the paper.

Hitherto, global judgements on these considerations have been incorporated in damage-risk criteria, demanding the implicit faith of the user. This is not to say that the varying criteria issued by highly reputable authorities are erroneous, but it is perhaps easier with the above analysis to understand wherein the differences may reside. Furthermore the acquisition of the necessary experimental data to enable a detached view to be taken on each of the five considerations separately, and on some others so far unmentioned such as the role of intermittency in the noise exposure, is difficult and excessively demanding of time and resources. By adding insight to unavoidably incomplete evidence, great impetus has already been given to the preventive aspect of industrial noise damage by authors such as Rosenblith and Stevens (1953), Glorig and his associates (1962), Kryter and other members of CHABA (1963, 1966), Burns and Littler (1960, 1968). At the same time, it cannot be denied that acousticians come under a not altogether unjustified criticism for disagreeing amongst themselves.

Though much remains to be done before a generalized noise-risk criterion can be rigorously established, particularly in regard to such factors as (a) and (b) above, there has recently been a considerable expansion in the volume of experimental data relating noise level and time to the resultant hearing changes in otherwise unimpaired ears, as well as massive surveys of the "incidence" type, in both cases reinforced by information on the statistical distributions of these changes which measure the spread of individual susceptibilities. A better basis now exists for separating matters of fact from those of value judgement.

SCOPE OF NEW BRITISH DATA

The work recently reported by Burns and the writer (Burns and Robinson, 1970) permits a systematic approach to predicting the percentage risk of occurrence of any stated hearing level due to NIPTS in an otherwise unimpaired population of any stated age, for a wide range of acoustic conditions. In itself, this work takes us no nearer to a specification of risk in terms of social or occupational handicap. Accordingly in what follows we shall assume, for the sake of illustration, the AAOO speech impairment basis (Committee on Conservation of Hearing, 1964). Specifically this means that the impairment can be handled in terms of a purely audiometric quantity, namely the mean of the hearing levels at the three frequencies 0·5, 1 and 2 kHz. This is not an essential limitation since our data are given in algebraic form for various frequencies, and it would be a simple matter to recalculate the results given below when and if some other audiometric disability rating becomes established.

The concept of risk can now be given concrete numerical expression: it is defined as that percentage of a population whose hearing level, as a result of a given influence, exceeds the specified value, minus that percentage whose hearing level would have exceeded the specified value in the absence of that influence, other factors remaining the same. Thus we may speak of the risk due to age, to pathology, to noise, to any pair of these influences acting together, or to the combined effect of all three.

The underlying principle is that the components of threshold shift due to the successive influences are arithmetically additive; for this there is some experimental evidence though it may be violated in certain circumstances. It is important to note that the resulting risk values are far from being proportional to the component threshold shifts. They do, however, obey the rules of ordinary arithmetic if due attention is paid to the definition; otherwise paradoxical results can be made to appear. The correct way to interpret risk values is further discussed below. Thus, care is needed in combining component risks at the arithmetical stage, but the concept, as defined, has undoubted utility in so far as its meaning is readily comprehended by the non-specialist. Moreover, by admitting risk (or, more strictly, percentage exceedence) as an independent variable along with the noise level and exposure duration, complete freedom is conferred on administrations who may wish to draw up codes of noise practice suited to their own particular needs and embodying their own value judgements.

The new experimental data permit straightforward calculations of noise risk to be made in the following range of conditions:

(a) noise level reasonably steady and continuous (8 hours per day) in the range up to 120 dB(A); spectrum immaterial within slope limits of ± 5 dB per octave.

(b) exposure 5 days per week, for periods from 1 month to 50 years.

(c) population free from aural pathology and from other non-noise impairments, but subject to normal ageing.

(d) entry into noisy occupation at any specified age. Previous noise exposure, if known in noise level and duration, can be allowed for.

(e) by a conservative extension, exposures of less than 8 hours per day or less than 5 days per week, but otherwise regular, can be accommodated by applying the equal-energy rule. The distribution of hearing levels is then given by the formula:

$$H'(p) = 27{\cdot}5\left\{1 + \tanh \frac{E_A - \lambda(f) + u(p)}{15}\right\} + u(p) + F(N),$$

where N is the age in years

$$F(N) = \begin{cases} 0 & \text{when } N \leqslant 20 \\ C(f)\,.\,(N-20)^2 & \text{when } N > 20 \end{cases}$$

$C(f)$ has the values given in Table V

$$u(p) = 6\sqrt{2}\,.\,\mathrm{erf}^{-1}\left(\frac{p}{50} - 1\right)$$

p is the centile of population for which $H' \geqslant H'(p)$

$E_A = L_A + 10 \log (T/T_0)$ is the A-weighted noise immission level. This quantity is the measure of total noise exposure that uniquely determines the NIPTS.

L_A is the A-weighted sound pressure level of the noise, in dB(A)
T is the duration of exposure, in calendar years
T_0 is the reference duration, 1 year
$\lambda(f)$ is a parameter depending on the audiometric frequency, as given in Table V.

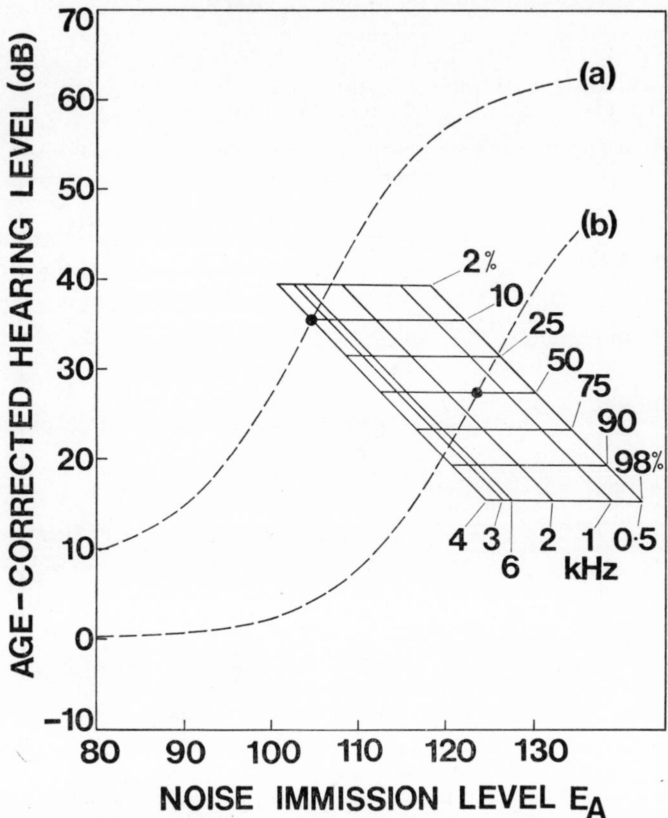

FIG. 25. Diagram for determining the hearing level at various frequencies of given centiles of a non-pathological noise-exposed population, excluding the component due to presbycusis. The procedure is as follows:

(i) Select audiometric frequency and centile of population and locate appropriate datum point on inset grid. Note that the frequency scale folds back above 4 kHz.
(ii) Place curve so that the ● (which is fixed with respect to the curve) coincides with the datum point. Note that the shape of the curve is invariable; shifts to left or right correspond to different frequencies, shifts along the north-west/south-east diagonal correspond to different centiles.
(iii) Read component of hearing level on ordinate scale against noise immission level E_A on abscissa scale.

The examples shown are: (a) 10% of population, frequency 4 kHz; (b) 50% of population (median), frequency 1·5 kHz.

TABLE V. Values of the parameters λ and C

Frequency (kHz)	0·5	1	2	3	4	6
C	0·0040	0·0043	0·0060	0·0080	0·0120	0·0140
λ (dB)	130·0	126·5	120·0	114·5	112·5	115·5

Tables XI, XII and XIII are given later to facilitate calculations by means of the above equation, which is also illustrated graphically in Figs. 25 and 26.

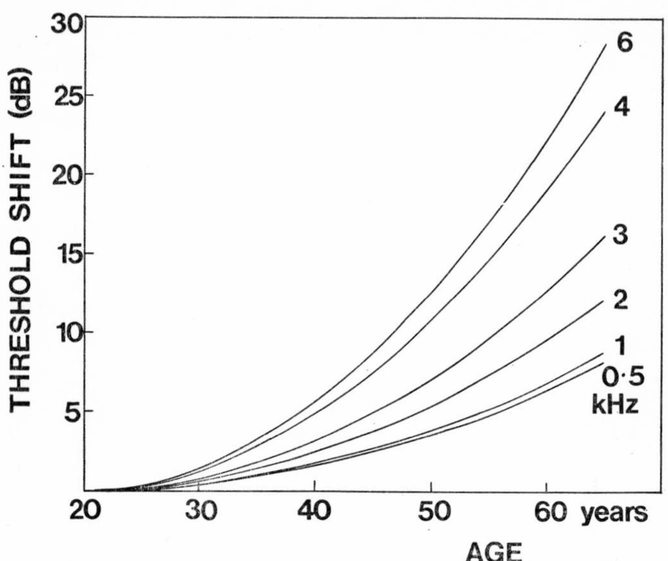

FIG. 26. Median threshold shift due to age (presbycusis correction) relative to age 20 years, based on Hinchcliffe (1959a). The value for the appropriate frequency, added to the ordinate of Fig. 25, gives the expected hearing level of the corresponding centile of a non-pathological noise-exposed population.

NUMERICAL ILLUSTRATIONS OF RISK VALUES

Entry into a uniform noise occupation at age 20, and a 40-hour week, will be assumed, though these limitations are not essential. As already stated, the audiometric quantity concerned is the mean value of H' for 0·5, 1 and 2 kHz. Results will be illustrated for the age span of 40 years from age 20 to 60. For any stated value of $H'_{\overline{0\cdot5\,1\,2}}$, the percentage exceedence p may be found using the formula. Thus, to find exceedence for the unimpaired 20-year-old population, set T equal to zero ($E_A \rightarrow -\infty$) and $F(N)$ equal to zero, so that $H'(p) = u(p)$. This relation being independent of frequency, determine

p directly from the value of $H'_{\overline{0\cdot5\,1\,2}}$, using Table XII. To find the exceedence due to noise, insert the selected value of E_A, set $F(\mathcal{N})$ equal to zero, and calculate H' for each frequency and for a series of values of p. Take the average of H', and determine that value of p for which the average has the desired value. Noise risk is then given by the difference of the two exceedences. The calculation of age risk proceeds on similar lines, this time keeping the noise term zero and inserting the appropriate values of $F(\mathcal{N})$; likewise the combined risk, by inserting both noise immission and age data. It will be evident that the component risks are not independent of each other. For example, a value of noise risk is given by the difference between the combined age-plus-noise exceedence and the age exceedence alone, and this is not the same as the noise risk calculated for the 20-year-old group. This reflects the observation already made, that the effect of noise, as such, declines as other influences, in this case age, mount.

Noise-risk values calculated from the formula, as above, tend to be smaller than other published results, particularly for higher frequencies, and there is little doubt that the exclusion of subjects with "other pathology" is responsible. Clearly an absolute separation of the "pathological" and "noise-induced" components in the hearing levels of experimental subjects is unattainable. In incidence surveys of the type reported by Baughn (1966) no such separation is even attempted, the objective being a different one from ours. Other investigations, including that of Burns and Robinson (1970), upon which this paper is based, have attempted a separation by means of anamnestic data and otological examination. The identification of pathology, using this term in a general sense to include any non-noise-induced impairment other than presbycusis, has doubtless varied from one investigation to another. It is reasonable to assume, however, that a lower bound to noise risk must exist even if it cannot be directly observed, and that the study yielding the lowest noise-risk values is likely to have been the one in which the noise factor was most successfully isolated.

It is true that the condition of "no other pathology" does not occur naturally, and is even difficult to satisfy under controlled experimental conditions. It may be asked why, then, has it been sought after? The reason is the same as that accepted for the establishment of reference standards of the threshold of hearing, namely that an otologically-normal population is the natural base-line for the measurement of impairments. Any unselected population will no doubt exhibit an appreciable admixture of pathology; the problem is to determine how much. A typical non-noise-exposed industrial population may appear a more attractive concept for the prediction of the added noise risk in real-life situations, but it must surely be admitted that it is a far from promising concept from the standpoint of rigorous definition, or as the basis of a standard.

Scattered data exist, for non-noise-exposed groups, which point to the possibility of defining a "typical population", albeit somewhat arbitrarily, through comparison of hearing level surveys with the internationally standardized thresholds of hearing for selected subjects. Differences of audiometric procedure, unfortunately, cloud the issue. There is scope for further study here; however, in order to illustrate the order of magnitude of the influence of pathology on the risk, an arbitrary incidence of "pathology" will be assumed for present purposes. Specifically, the non-noise-exposed pathology-free population is taken to be that implicit in the formula above, having a median hearing level of zero at each frequency at age 20 and a standard deviation of 6 dB. The pathological overlay is represented by a Gaussian distribution with mean value 10 dB and standard deviation 8 dB. The convolution of these distributions then assigns to the 20-year-old "incidence" group a mean hearing level of 10 dB with a standard deviation of 10 dB. The rationale of this particular choice is that it yields results that are in harmony with Baughn's incidence study. An additional touch of realism has been imparted by assuming the pathological overlay to grow with the years, so that at age 60 it has attained a mean value of 12·5 dB with a standard deviation of 9.

The effect of age from 20 to 60 years and for the mean of the three frequencies 0·5, 1 and 2 kHz is, according to the formula, 7·5 dB for the median. The presbycutic overlay has, again somewhat arbitrarily, been assumed to grow with a Gaussian distribution, standard deviation 2·5 dB at age 60. Thus, the non-noise-exposed non-pathology group at age 60 has a median hearing level of 7·5 dB with standard deviation 7 dB.

The effect of noise has been calculated for noise immission levels of 103, 108 and 113 dB, using the formula. In the case of NIPTS, the distribution does not remain Gaussian, but becomes skewed. Figure 27 shows, for the case of NIL 108, the cumulative distributions of hearing levels for the eight groups defined by the permutations: age 20 or 60; normal or pathological, as defined; noise-exposed or otherwise. From the intersections of the curves with verticals drawn at each of a number of hearing levels, which we shall refer to as "fence heights", the exceedences are obtained for each group. By difference, the value of each component risk, each paired risk or all three risks is obtained. There are 12, 6 and 1 of these combinations respectively but those which concern us are the following nine:

noise risk for 20-year-old normals,
noise risk for 20-year-old pathological population,
as above at 60 years of age,
combined risk of noise and age on normals,
combined risk of noise and age on pathological population,
combined risk of noise and pathology on 20-year-olds,
combined risk of noise and pathology on 60-year-olds,
total risk from noise, age and pathology.

Table VI lists the values of the exceedences, together with the median values of hearing level, in the various hypothetical groups. The notation used is: $-$, influence absent; $+$, influence present.

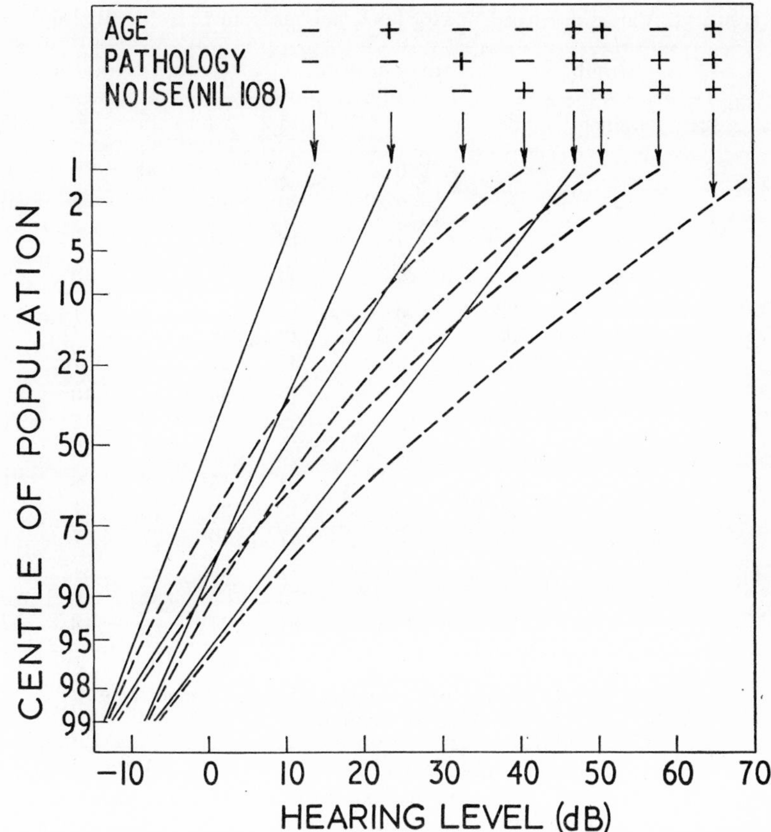

FIG. 27. Cumulative distributions of the hearing levels (average at 0·5, 1 and 2 kHz) of various populations defined by the following eight permutations:

age 20 years	$(-)$; age 60 years	$(+)$
pathology-free	$(-)$; with pathological overlay as defined in text	$(+)$
non-exposed	$(-)$; noise-exposed, NIL 108	$(+)$

From Table VI, values of the noise risk (Table VII), and of the composite risks (Table VIII) are obtained.

INTERPRETATION OF THE CALCULATIONS

It should first be noted that the eight groups have so far been defined without reference to the epochs when the various influences occurred, except that the progress of ageing is inexorably linked to the calendar. The 20-year-old normal group A is self-explanatory, likewise the 20-year-old pathology group B. By a 20-year-old noise-exposed group (E or F) we mean one whose

TABLE VI. Values of exceedence for fence heights from 15 to 35 dB (ISO)

Key	Group: Age	Group: Pathology	Group: Noise	Median hearing level (av. at 0·5, 1, 2 kHz)	Percentage exceedence: 15	20	25	30	35
A	–	–	–	0	1	0	0	0	0
B	–	+	–	10	30	15	6	2	0
C	+	–	–	7·5	13	4	1	0	0
D	+	+	–	20	66	50	33	19	9
			103	3	10	4	2	1	0
E	–	–	108	5·5	22	13	7	4	2
			113	9·5	33	21	13	7	4
			103	13	44	30	18	10	5
F	–	+	108	15·5	53	39	27	18	11
			113	19·5	63	50	37	26	18
			103	10·5	32	17	8	3	1
G	+	–	108	13	45	30	18	11	6
			113	17	57	40	27	17	11
			103	23	71	59	43	31	20
H	+	+	108	25·5	73	63	52	40	30
			113	29·5	81	71	60	48	37

TABLE VII. Values of noise risk for various groups at fence heights from 15 to 35 dB

Key	Base-line: Age	Base-line: Pathology	Noise immission level	Noise risk (%): 15	20	25	30	35
			103	9	4	2	1	0
E–A	–	–	108	21	13	7	4	2
			113	32	21	13	7	4
			103	14	15	12	8	5
F–B	–	+	108	23	24	21	16	11
			113	33	35	31	24	18
			103	19	13	7	3	1
G–C	+	–	108	32	26	17	11	6
			113	44	36	26	17	11
			103	5	9	10	12	11
H–D	+	+	108	7	13	19	21	21
			113	15	21	27	29	28

noise exposure commenced at age 20 and which was complete within a period so short that accretions of pathology and presbycusis can be neglected. For example, this group with NIL 108 might have sustained 6 years' noise exposure at a level of 100 dB(A), 2 years at 105 dB(A), etc., or any such comparatively brief exposure as amounts to a noise immission level of 108. In case of the composite risk (G–A) (Table VIII), it is immaterial whether the

TABLE VIII. Values of composite risk

Key	Joint influences	Base-line	Noise immission level	Composite risk (%)				
				15	20	25	30	35
G–A	Noise plus age	Normals, age 20	103	31	17	8	3	1
			108	44	30	18	11	6
			113	56	40	27	17	11
H–B	Noise plus age	Patho-logicals at age 20	103	41	44	37	29	20
			108	43	48	46	38	30
			113	51	56	54	46	37
F–A	Noise plus pathology	Normals, age 20	103	43	30	18	10	5
			108	52	39	27	18	11
			113	62	50	37	26	18
H–C	Noise plus pathology	Age 60 non-patholog.	103	58	55	42	31	20
			108	60	59	51	40	30
			113	68	67	59	48	37
H–A	Noise plus age plus pathology	Normals at age 20	103	70	59	43	31	20
			108	72	63	52	40	30
			113	80	71	60	48	37

noise exposure occurred early, late or evenly spread out over the 40 years, although, of course, this would affect the corresponding calculations for some intermediate age. In the case of the 60-year-old noise group, case (G–C) of Table VII, the noise exposure must be understood to have occurred in a comparatively brief period just before the age of 60. Similar considerations apply whether the pathological overlay is present or not.

The data in the Tables may be cross-plotted in numerous ways, and the features that are found may be summarized in the following statements.

1. Different risks vary with the fence height in quite different ways; compare, for example, the third and fourth blocks of Table VII. If the values are calculated for a wider range of fence heights, each risk exhibits a maximum somewhere in the range. For (G–C), for instance, it is below 15; for (H–D) it is around 32. Thus, over the range of interest in hearing preservation, some risks continually increase whilst others continually decrease as the fence height is raised.

2. In consequence of 1, the conclusions to be drawn concerning the relative magnitude of risks due to different causes depend on the particular fence height set. For example, at 25 dB the noise risk is greater for the pathology group or the 60-year-old group than it is for 20-year-old normals. At 15 dB, on the other hand, the risk is greater for the 20-year-old normals than for the 60-year-old pathology group. At the conventional "low fence" of 25 dB, a rough rule may be deduced that the risk grows at a rate of about 1% per decibel for normals and 2% per decibel when an additional influence is at work.

3. Care is needed in handling component risk values. An example of correct and incorrect interpretation is illustrated below for fence height 25 and NIL 108.

Source of risk	*False analysis*		*Correct analysis*	
	Risk (%)	*Key*	*Risk (%)*	*Key*
Noise alone	7	(E–A)	7	(E–A)
Age	1	(C–A)	11	(G–E)
Noise plus age	8		18	(G–A)

In the symbolic form given under Key, it is easy to see how to avoid the false result. The noise risk having been entered first, the incremental risk due to age must be taken for the appropriate group, i.e. the noise-exposed and not the normal group. The true total risk of 18% can, of course, be obtained with the order of the items reversed, thus:

Age alone	key (C–A) . .	1
noise	key (G–C) . .	17
combined risk	. . .	18%

4. Whilst it occasions no surprise that the composite risks in Table VIII exceed the risks due to noise alone, it is not so obvious that the simple noise risk itself varies greatly according to the conditions under which it is reckoned, as may be seen in Table VII. Referring to NIL 108 for illustration, the simple noise risk for young otologically-normal persons is seen to be 7% (E–A). The same noise immission applied to persons already aged 60 (or rather, in the neighbourhood of 60 since the noise immission cannot be sustained instantaneously) represents a much greater risk, namely 17% (G–C). Likewise the noise risk to 20-year-old "pathologicals" is also increased, in this case to 21% (F–B). The risks inherent in the age span and the pathological overlay are only 0 and 6% respectively, if these influences are acting alone. It is interesting to note that the noise risk, in the simultaneous presence of advanced age and pathological overlay, may be less than in the presence of

only one of these conditions, thus risk (H–D) is 19%, intermediate between (F–B) and (G–C).

5. The numerical values are sensitive to the assumptions made in respect of age range and "pathology" though the general pattern would be preserved in different examples. When one of the exceedences involved in a risk is in the region 40 to 60%, the value varies rapidly with fence height. The right-hand curve of Fig. 27, for example, has a slope of about 2·5% per decibel. In calculations of risk therefore, a high premium is set on the reliability of the underlying scientific data, and on a close specification of all the conditions pertinent to the group considered.

6. It is instructive to note the risk values that are predicted by the above scheme in relation to a criterion that has acquired currency in recent times, namely a maximum of 90 dB(A) noise level and the "just-beginning mild impairment" level of 25 dB ISO fence height on the AAOO scale (15 dB ASA in the terminology of the AAOO recommendation). Over the 40-year span this criterion permits a noise immission level of 106, and the relevant risks are either (G–C) or (H–D), according to whether or not unimpaired hearing is taken as the base. Table VII shows that the risks are then around 13 and 15% respectively. If the pathological overlay is acquired between the ages of 20 and 60, the much higher figure of 47% applies (H–C), but in this case the risk would be 32% in the absence of noise anyway. For this reason it is perhaps unfair to compare the 47% with the lower values, and yet it does not seem altogether unreasonable to attribute some part of the acquired "pathological" threshold shift to occupational causes other than noise. Mass surveys of hearing tend to show that males, that is broadly the working population, progress to higher threshold shifts than females even when noise is not inculpated. If the same example is worked on the 10- or 20-year-span basis, the risk (E–A) applies in place of (G–C), and (F–B) in place of (H–D), since the effect of age is very much less in these cases. The results are 1 and 8% for 10 years and 2 and 12% for 20 years respectively. Under a wide variety of different assumptions, therefore, the criterion under consideration seems to represent a finite risk according to AAOO usage, but in assessing the significance of this conclusion it should be borne in mind that the 25 dB ISO fence implies only incipient difficulty with the understanding of conversational speech in quiet.

7. An incidence study on 6835 persons by Baughn (1966), mentioned above, forms the basis of the current draft ISO recommendation (International Organization for Standardization, 1970), thus implying a preference on the part of the committee concerned for a base-line of unselected hearing. In an unpublished report, Baughn (1968) has developed his experimental results into a series of curves of percentage exceedence for noise levels from 80 to 115 dB(A) and for fence heights (0·5, 1, 2 kHz average) from 15 to 50 ISO (5 to 40 ASA, as given by Baughn). The curves for fence height 25 ISO have been taken over without alteration into the ISO document.

TABLE IX. Comparison of percentage exceedences after 40 years' exposure

Source	Key (see Table VI)	Median hearing level $H'_{\overline{0\cdot512}}$	NIL	Exceedence at fence height 25	35 (ISO)
This paper	C	7·5	no noise	1	0
This paper	D	20	no noise	33	9
Baughn		22	no noise	33*	9
This paper	G	10·5	103	8	1
This paper	H	23	103	43	20
Baughn		25	103	47*	16
This paper	G	13	108	18	6
This paper	H	25·5	108	52	30
Baughn		27·5	108	57*	24
This paper	G	17	113	27	11
This paper	H	29·5	113	60	37
Baughn		30·5	113	67*	33

Notes. Cases C and G refer to the pathology-free population in the investigation of Burns and Robinson. Cases D and H are for hypothetical groups derived from C and G, see text. Baughn's data are for an unselected population. Entries marked * may be found in draft ISO Recommendation DR 1999 under "40 years" and for noise levels of ≤80, 87, 92 and 97 respectively, by interpolation.

TABLE X. Comparison of noise risks due to 40 years' exposure

Source	Key (See Table VI)	NIL	Noise risk (%) at fence height 25	35 (ISO)
This paper	C–A	no noise	1	0
This paper	D–A	no noise	33	9
Baughn		no noise	33[a]	9
This paper	G–C	103	7	1
This paper	H–D	103	10	11
Baughn		103	14[a]	7
This paper	G–C	108	17	6
This paper	H–D	108	19	21
Baughn		108	24[a]	15
This paper	G–C	113	26	11
This paper	H–D	113	27	28
Baughn		113	34[a]	24

[a] These values also appear in draft ISO Recommendation DR 1999. See Note to Table IX.

Baughn first used a large unselected non-noise-exposed population (2518 persons) studied by Glorig as the base-line of reckoning for various ages, and thus deduced noise risk values from the raw exceedences of his own study. However, those of his own group having less than 80 dB(A) noise level are virtually indistinguishable from Glorig's controls, and may equally well be taken as the non-exposed base-line.

Baughn's data may be compared with those presented in this paper in order to gain an impression of the role played by "selection" (that is, the elimination of other pathology) in the reduction of apparent risk. Table IX compares the percentage exceedences and Table X the noise risks. The upper block of each table refers to non-noise-exposed and the lower three blocks to noise-exposed groups for noise immission levels of 103, 108 and 113 as before. The comparisons are shown for two fence heights, 25 and 35 dB ISO. Baughn's curves, and hence the draft ISO Recommendation, take 18 as the starting age, instead of 20 as here, but this has only a minor effect on the comparison. Comparing the non-noise-exposed groups first, Baughn's median hearing level at age 58 ($H'_{\overline{0 \cdot 5\,1\,2}}$) of 22 dB (12 ASA in the original report) falls close to that of our hypothetical pathology group; the percentage exceedence and noise risk are practically identical. Considering the noise-exposed groups, the comparison between Baughn's results and our "pathology" group is again remarkably close, his median hearing levels being within 1 to 2 dB, and the percentage figures interlacing with ours. Slightly smaller values are predicted for our hypothetical group at the 25 dB fence and slightly greater ones at 35 dB. In contrast to these similarities, however, there are gross discrepancies between our actual experimental results and those of Baughn.

Thus we are driven to the conclusion that, for all practical purposes, there is complete harmony between Baughn's experimental findings and ours if one is prepared to accept that 10 dB is a reasonable estimate of the median difference of hearing levels between a wholly-unselected and a highly-selected population. Due to the differing aims of the two investigations and consequent differences of procedure the opportunities for testing this proposition directly by retrospective re-examination of the data are, unfortunately, limited.

CALCULATION OF NIPTS FOR A NON-PATHOLOGICAL POPULATION

To spare the reader the task of looking up original tables of the hyperbolic tangent and inverse error functions, the terms in the formula involving these functions are tabulated below at convenient values of the arguments.

TABLE XI. Values of the function

$$y = 27{\cdot}5\left(1+\tanh\frac{x}{15}\right)$$

x	y	x	y	x	y	x	y
−45	0·1	−25	1·9	−5	18·7	15	48·5
−44	0·2	−24	2·1	−4	20·3	16	49·2
−43	0·2	−23	2·4	−3	22·1	17	49·8
−42	0·2	−22	2·8	−2	23·9	18	50·5
−41	0·2	−21	3·2	−1	25·7	19	51·0
−40	0·3	−20	3·6	0	27·5	20	51·4
−39	0·3	−19	4·0	1	29·3	21	51·8
−38	0·4	−18	4·6	2	31·1	22	52·2
−37	0·4	−17	5·2	3	32·9	23	52·6
−36	0·4	−16	5·8	4	34·7	24	52·9
−35	0·5	−15	6·5	5	36·3	25	53·1
−34	0·6	−14	7·4	6	38·0	26	53·3
−33	0·7	−13	8·3	7	39·5	27	53·5
−32	0·8	−12	9·2	8	40·9	28	53·7
−31	0·9	−11	10·3	9	42·3	29	53·9
−30	1·0	−10	11·5	10	43·5	30	54·0
−29	1·1	−9	12·7	11	44·7	31	54·1
−28	1·3	−8	14·1	12	45·8	32	54·2
−27	1·5	−7	15·5	13	46·8	33	54·3
−26	1·7	−6	17·1	14	47·6	34	54·4

TABLE XII. Values of the function

$$u = 6\sqrt{2}\,.\,\mathrm{erf}^{-1}\left(\frac{p}{50}-1\right)$$

p	u	p	u	p	u	p	u	p	u
1	13·9	12	7·1			70	−3·1	90	−7·7
2	12·3	14	6·5	35	2·3	72	−3·5	91	−8·0
3	11·3	16	6·0	40	1·5	74	−3·9	92	−8·4
4	10·5	18	5·5	45	0·8	76	−4·2	93	−8·9
5	9·9	20	5·1			78	−4·6	94	−9·3
				50	0				
6	9·3	22	4·6			80	−5·1	95	−9·9
7	8·9	24	4·2	55	−0·8	82	−5·5	96	−10·5
8	8·4	26	3·9	60	−1·5	84	−6·0	97	−11·3
9	8·0	28	3·5	65	−2·3	86	−6·5	98	−12·3
10	7·7	30	3·1			88	−7·1	99	−13·9

TABLE XIII. Average of the median NIPTS at 0·5, 1 and 2 kHz in terms of the parameter $k = E_A + u(p)$

k	$\overline{H'}_{0\cdot512}$	k	$\overline{H'}_{0\cdot512}$	k	$\overline{H'}_{0\cdot512}$	k	$\overline{H'}_{0\cdot512}$
75	0·1	95	1·1	115	11·6	135	42·1
76	0·1	96	1·2	116	12·9	136	43·4
77	0·1	97	1·4	117	14·2	137	44·5
78	0·1	98	1·6	118	15·5	138	45·6
79	0·1	99	1·8	119	16·9	139	46·5
80	0·2	100	2·1	120	18·4	140	47·4
81	0·2	101	2·3	121	20·0	141	48·2
82	0·2	102	2·6	122	21·6	142	49·0
83	0·2	103	3·0	123	23·2	143	49·6
84	0·2	104	3·4	124	24·9	144	50·2
85	0·3	105	3·8	125	26·6	145	50·8
86	0·3	106	4·3	126	28·3	146	51·2
87	0·4	107	4·8	127	30·0	147	51·6
88	0·5	108	5·4	128	31·7	148	52·1
89	0·5	109	6·1	129	33·3	149	52·4
90	0·6	110	6·9	130	34·9		
91	0·6	111	7·6	131	36·5		
92	0·7	112	8·5	132	38·0		
93	0·8	113	9·5	133	39·5		
94	1·0	114	10·5	134	40·8		

Examples in the use of the Tables

1. Calculate the hearing level at 4 kHz that will be exceeded by 10% of a normal population at age 40, after exposure to noise of 95 dB(A) for 20 years.
   (a) $E_A = 95 + 10 \log 20 = 108$
   (b) $\lambda = 112{\cdot}5$ (Table V).
   (c) $p = 10$; hence $u = 7{\cdot}7$ (Table XII)
   (d) $x = 108 - 112{\cdot}5 + 7{\cdot}7 = 3{\cdot}2$; hence $y = 33{\cdot}3$ (Table XI)
   (e) $C = 0{\cdot}0120$ (Table V) and $N = 40$; hence $F(N) = 0{\cdot}0120 \times 20^2 = 4{\cdot}8$
   (f) $H' = y + u + F = 33{\cdot}3 + 7{\cdot}7 + 4{\cdot}8 = 45{\cdot}8$ dB.
2. The same as Example 1, but calculate the mean of the hearing levels at 0·5, 1 and 2 kHz.

   Method 1 Proceed as in Example 1 for the three separate frequencies, using the appropriate values of λ and C; take the mean of the results.

   Method 2 Table XIII has been prepared for calculations with this commonly-used combination of audiometric frequencies.

(a) $E_A = 108$ and $u = 7{\cdot}7$, as before
(b) $k = 108 + 7{\cdot}7 = 115{\cdot}7$; hence $\overline{H'}_{\overline{0{\cdot}5\,1\,2}} = 12{\cdot}5$ (Table XIII)
(c) $C_{\overline{0{\cdot}5\,1\,2}} = 0{\cdot}0048$ (Table V, average for the 3 frequencies)
(d) $F(N) = 0{\cdot}0048 \times 20^2 = 1{\cdot}9$
(e) $H' = \overline{H'} + u + F = 12{\cdot}5 + 7{\cdot}7 + 1{\cdot}9 = 22{\cdot}1$ dB.

3. Calculate the noise risk for Example 2, in relation to the 25 dB (ISO) fence on the AAOO impairment basis.

Method Example 2 predicts that 10% will exceed 22·1 dB hearing level. Calculate similarly for $p_1 = 9, 8, 7, 6\ldots$

p_1	10	9	8	7	6	5	4
H'	22·1	22·5	23·4	24·1	24·6	25·4	26·2

Select the value of p_1 that predicts $H' = 25$, i.e. 5·5%. Repeat this procedure with the noise-induced component of H' suppressed. Thus Example 2 predicts that the age effect alone will cause 10% of the population to exceed the hearing level $(22{\cdot}1 - 12{\cdot}5) = 9{\cdot}6$ dB. Proceed similarly:

p_2	10 ... 3	2	1 ...
H'	9·6...13·2	14·2	15·8...

In this Example, less than 1% attain 25 dB, so that $p_2 = 0$. The risk is given by $p_1 - p_2 = 5{\cdot}5\%$.

THE CONCEPT OF MAXIMUM RISK

It has been pointed out that NIPTS grows rapidly at first and thereafter progressively more slowly, for continued exposure to the same noise; whereas presbycutic threshold shift begins slowly and then accelerates, eventually catching up with or overtaking the NIPTS. The noise risk as defined, depends upon the difference between these two processes. Thus it starts, and in principle ends, with zero values, and is therefore greatest at some intermediate stage. To illustrate this, the time course of the noise risk has been calculated from age 20 to age 70, this span being assumed coterminous with the period of exposure to noise. Levels of 87, 92, 97 and 102 dB(A) have been assumed, these corresponding to NIL values of 103, 108, 113 and 118 respectively after the first 40 years, that is, at age 60. The calculations are made for fence heights from 10 to 45 ISO, on the same basis as before, namely in terms of exceedence of the $H'_{\overline{0{\cdot}5\,1\,2}}$ value. The values, as tabulated, are for a pathology-free population but the influence of a pathological component in the hearing level of 0, 5, 10 dB etc., may be inferred approximately by selecting the appropriate fence. Thus, for a true fence of 25, in the presence of say 10 dB of "pathology", select fence 15. The refinement of an age-linked growth of the pathological overlay, used in constructing Tables V, VI and VII, is omitted, the computations being greatly simplified thereby.

The results are given in Table XIV which shows the pattern of events clearly. For normal ears exposed to noise at any of the levels shown, the noise

TABLE XIV. Noise risk for a non-pathological population at various ages, for exposure at constant noise level commencing at age 20

Noise level dB(A)	Fence height (ISO)	Noise risk (%) at age 21	22	25	30	40	50	60	70
87	10	2	3	5	8	14	17	18	11
92		4	6	10	15	22	28	28	17
97		7	11	18	24	36	42	38	24
102		14	19	30	40	52	56	49	30
87	15	1	2	2	4	7	13	19	20
92		2	3	5	8	15	23	31	32
97		4	7	10	17	26	37	45	43
102		8	13	20	29	44	56	61	54
87	20	0	0	1	2	4	7	13	20
92		0	1	2	4	8	14	24	33
97		1	2	5	9	17	27	38	48
102		3	6	12	17	32	46	57	65
87	25	0	0	0	0	1	3	7	13
92		0	0	1	2	4	8	14	24
97		0	1	2	4	10	17	27	40
102		1	3	6	10	21	33	46	58
87	30	0	0	0	0	0	1	3	7
92		0	0	0	0	2	4	7	15
97		0	0	1	2	5	10	17	28
102		0	1	3	6	14	22	33	48
87	35	0	0	0	0	0	0	1	3
92		0	0	0	0	1	2	4	8
97		0	0	0	1	3	6	10	19
102		0	0	2	4	8	15	23	35
87	40	0	0	0	0	0	0	0	1
92		0	0	0	0	0	1	2	4
97		0	0	0	0	1	3	6	11
102		0	0	0	2	5	9	15	26
87	45	0	0	0	0	0	0	0	0
92		0	0	0	0	0	0	1	2
97		0	0	0	0	0	1	3	7
102		0	0	0	0	2	5	9	17

risk in terms of the AAOO fence (ISO 25) grows progressively with age and is still rising at age 60. The same is true in the presence of a uniform pathological overlay of 5 dB. However, with 10 dB "pathology" (fence height 15) the risk is maximum at about 60 years of age, and at 15 dB (fence height 10) it has already passed through the maximum by about the age of 50.

The conclusion from this analysis is that the "catching-up" process has barely set in before the end of the normal working life of persons with "otherwise unimpaired" hearing, and enters in as an important factor only in the presence of a median value of 15 dB or more of overlaid pathological threshold shift, which is believed to be greater than is met with in ordinary circumstances. Slightly different results would be obtained if the audiometric criterion were changed, by inclusion of higher frequencies, for example. However, both the presbycutic and noise-induced threshold shifts increase with frequency, though not to corresponding extents, so that the broad conclusion would remain the same. Therefore it is clear that the proper basis for constructing a damage-risk criterion, in respect of the time element, is to determine the acceptable risk at the end of the working life.

ACKNOWLEDGEMENT

The work described has been carried out as part of the research programme of the National Physical Laboratory.

The Relation of Temporary to Permanent Threshold Shift in Individuals

By

W. Burns
Charing Cross Hospital Medical School
University of London, England

Summary

Using the data obtained in the joint MRS–NPL survey of hearing and noise exposure, indices of individual susceptibility to permanent and to temporary threshold shifts have been compared. Numerically low but statistically significant values of the correlation coefficient are found. Reasons for the low values and possibilities of their improvement to a degree adequate for a prognostic test of susceptibility to noise-induced hearing loss are discussed.

The existence of considerable variation in individual susceptibility to noise-induced hearing loss was recognized long before quantitative confirmation was obtained. The knowledge of this variability stimulated a quest for a test of susceptibility to noise-induced hearing loss; and, in response, there emerged the hypothesis that susceptibility to temporary threshold shift (TTS) is related directly to susceptibility to permanent noise-induced threshold shift (PTS). Despite the lack of evidence in favour of such an hypothesis, its validity has been persistently, if sometimes tacitly, assumed for many years; and many tests for susceptibility to TTS have been described, in the hope that they could somehow identify those individuals most vulnerable to noise-induced hearing loss. In 1956, however, Jerger and Carhart showed a positive correlation, with fairly low values of the correlation coefficient, but nevertheless of high statistical significance, between a measure of TTS and subsequent noise-induced hearing loss, in individuals. In addition, impetus was given to the use of TTS as a guide to the formulation of acceptable levels of occupational noise exposure by the finding (Glorig, Ward and Nixon, 1962) that the average TTS resulting from an exposure of 8 hours, in young, normal ears was quantitatively about the same as that produced on average by about 10 years of occupational exposure to the same noise as produced the TTS. This group result, of course, does not automatically mean 

that it applies to individuals, and for that reason it is not immediately useful in the present context. In this connection Ward (1965) concluded, after extensive studies of susceptibility to TTS, that the best that could be expected was that susceptibility to noise-induced permanent threshold shift from a particular noise might possibly be predicted "from knowledge of susceptibility to TTS from that same noise".

The studies by D. W. Robinson and the author (Burns and Robinson, 1970), now being reported, were envisaged over 10 years ago to include a systematic examination of TTS in the context of the field study of hearing and noise in industry. Since the aim was to obtain data to assess the situation for the purposes of legislation, the potential use of TTS in predictive tests for susceptibility to noise-induced hearing damage was a natural corollary to the main field study. We do not thereby imply that we regard TTS as the only possible basis for predictive tests; on the contrary, other possibilities exist (Hood, 1969). However, on grounds of existing knowledge, convenience of acquisition of the data, and ease of accommodation in the main field study, TTS tests easily qualified for inclusion. Our approach and findings are described briefly here, and more fully elsewhere (Burns, Stead and Penney, 1970).

PRINCIPLE

Two approaches were used. In both, an index of susceptibility to TTS for each individual was determined. This index was then correlated with a number of indices expressing either rate of hearing deterioration, or its extent. The former approach used serial audiometry data, the latter, data on hearing levels from the retrospective part of the main study.

METHODS

Index of susceptibility to TTS (D_T)

The first step towards this index was a measurement of TTS as a result of exposure for 1 working day, to the particular occupational noise of the individual concerned. The measurements by self-recording audiometry were started $6 \pm \frac{1}{4}$ minute post-exposure, and any of the audiometric frequencies, or combinations thereof, could be used in deriving the index. These data were then subjected, in effect, to two stages of refinement, since direct comparison of TTS values is only meaningful in certain conditions. One restriction is that the subjects should be exposed to the same noise or at least to the same noise level. In the conditions of the field study this does not apply, and so the subjects were assembled into 3 groups according to their occupational noise levels. The classification was by a statistical derivative of sound level A, designated L_{A2}, specifically the level in dB(A) exceeded for 2% of the exposure time. The composition of the groups is shown in Table XV.

TABLE XV. Groups of subjects classified by sound level L_{A2}

Group	Sound level L_{A2} (dB)	Number of subjects
A	99–104	53
B	94–98	82
C	88–93	83

Having grouped the TTS data on this basis, the second stage of refinement was introduced for the following reason.

Ward (1965) demonstrated that in a noise-exposed population TTS is inversely related to hearing level. Thus some correction to the recorded TTS values must be applied if, as in this case, the individuals comprising each group differed considerably in exposure history, doubtless in pre-exposure hearing level, in individual susceptibility and thus in recorded hearing level at the time of the test. Accordingly, each individual's recorded TTS was corrected to apply to 0 dB hearing level relative to the British Standard audiometric zero (BS 2497:1954) by the use of the regression of TTS (at each audiometric frequency) on hearing level (at the same frequency) for the whole group. These corrected TTS values, within each group, were then expressed as deviations in dB, positive or negative, from their mean for the whole group. This operation can be very simply done graphically by plotting TTS against hearing level, and drawing the regression line. The deviations of the individual points, positive or negative, in dB, on the ordinate scale, constitute the values of D_T. In practice a computer programme extracted these values. A relative index of susceptibility to TTS is thus obtained, thereby eliminating the difficulty of absolute values. Figure 28 shows this procedure, for group A, using the average values of TTS at 1 and 2 kHz.

Indices of susceptibility to PTS

For correlation with the index D_T, a number of possibilities exist for the quantitative expression of the susceptibility to PTS. The most direct approach would consist of an initial TTS measurement followed by monitoring of hearing over a prolonged period. This procedure has limitations both ethical and practical. In this investigation, small short-term deterioration, quantified by a number of numerical indices indicating rate of deterioration, was correlated with the index D_T, as one approach to the assessment of PTS.

The main index of PTS used in this investigation (symbol D_P) is defined as the deviation, in decibels, of the individual's age-corrected hearing level from the predicted median value for persons of the same age and noise exposure. The prediction method is that described by Robinson (1968). The index D_P is thus a relative and not an absolute value, and it thereby permits subjects of various hearing levels, ages and exposure histories to be grouped for purposes of correlation with the index D_T.

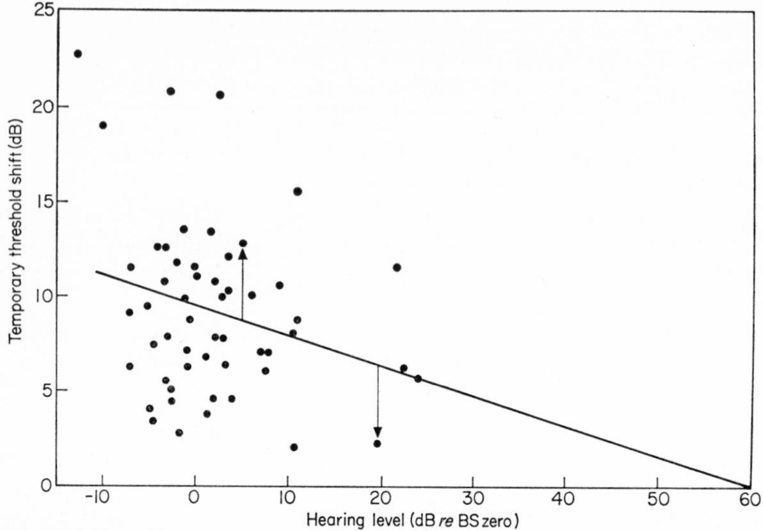

FIG. 28. Derivation of the index of susceptibility to TTS (D_T). The deviations from the regression line of TTS on hearing level, positive or negative (as illustrated by the arrows), constitute the values of D_T. Data from group A; L_{A2}, 99–104 dB. Values of TTS and of hearing level are averages of 1 and 2 kHz audiometric frequencies.

Basis of correlations

Any or all of the audiometric frequencies could be used in a number of combinations for the correlations of the indices of TTS and PTS. Those employed for the correlation of D_T and D_P are shown in Table XVI.

TABLE XVI. Frequency, or mean of frequencies (indicated by bar) used for regression of D_T on D_P, and corresponding correlation coefficients (r), for group A

D_T (kHz)	D_P (kHz)	r	D_T (kHz)	D_P (kHz)	r
1	$\overline{46}$	0·229	$\overline{23}$	$\overline{234}$	0·197
1	$\overline{346}$	0·279	$\overline{23}$	$\overline{346}$	0·290
$\overline{12}$	$\overline{12}$	0·072	$\overline{123}$	$\overline{234}$	0·215
$\overline{12}$	$\overline{234}$	0·288	$\overline{123}$	$\overline{346}$	0·299
$\overline{12}$	$\overline{346}$	0·340	$\overline{346}$	$\overline{12}$	−0·105
$\overline{12}$	$\overline{46}$	0·297	$\overline{346}$	$\overline{346}$	0·064
$\overline{12}$	$\overline{12346}$	0·289	$\overline{12346}$	$\overline{12346}$	0·101

RESULTS

Mean TTS values

The actual mean values of TTS, measured as described under Methods for each of the 3 groups are shown in an audiogram-like presentation in Fig. 29.

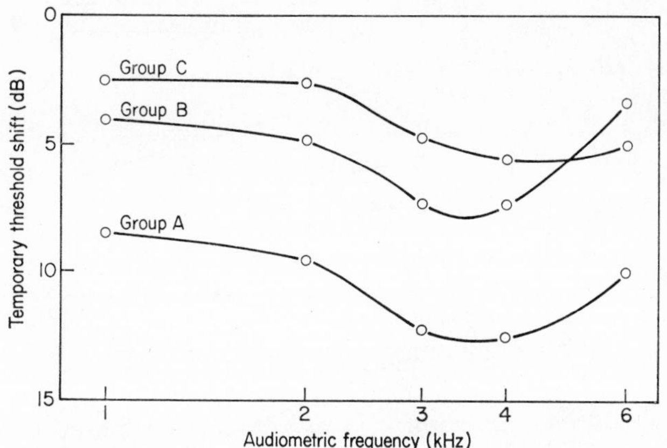

FIG. 29. Values of TTS for a nominal 8-hour (one work day) exposure for groups A, B and C. For details of groups see Table XV. Measurement methods described in text.

Regression of TTS on hearing level: D_T

D_T was derived for seven frequencies or frequency combinations, for groups A, B and C. On average, statistically significant values of the correlation coefficient were obtained for the regression in groups A and B, but did not reach significance in group C. This could be expected from the low slope values of group C and considerable variability of the TTS and hearing level values. Regressions of TTS on hearing level for 3 frequency combinations, in the 3 groups, are shown in Fig. 30.

Correlation of D_T with indices of PTS

(a) DETERIORATION INDICES

Various indices for rate of deterioration were used in correlations with D_T. The correlation was positive in all cases but the results were numerically disappointing, the best correlation coefficient being $+0{\cdot}28$, significance $P = 0{\cdot}10$. This aspect will not be discussed in detail.

(b) INDEX D_P

The regression of D_T on D_P was determined for the frequency combinations shown in Table XVI. The correlations were predominantly positive for group A.

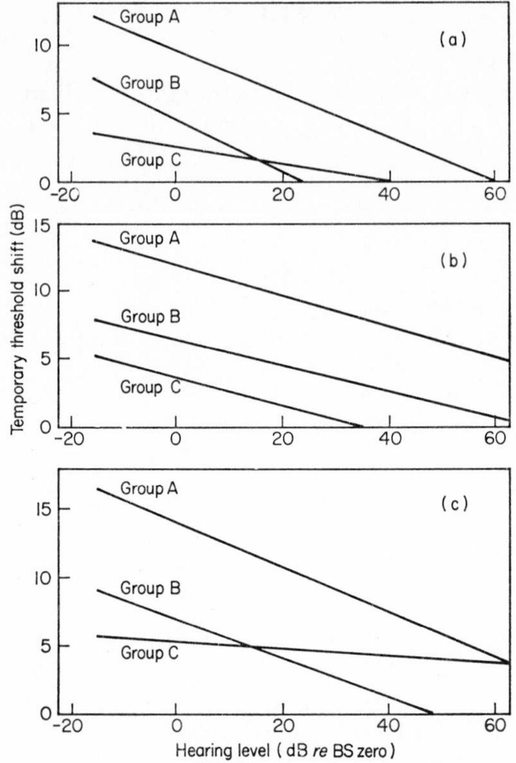

FIG. 30. Regressions of TTS on hearing level in groups A, B and C for 3 frequency combinations: (a) average of 1 and 2 kHz; (b) average of 2 and 3 kHz; (c) average of 3, 4 and 6 kHz. In each case TTS and hearing level are both derived from these combinations of frequencies.

A clear advantage lay with an unexpected combination: low frequencies for D_T, high frequencies for D_P. The best combination was when D_T was derived from the average of the TTS at 1 and 2 kHz ($D_{T\overline{12}}$), and D_P from the average of 3, 4 and 6 kHz ($D_{P\overline{346}}$). For this combination the correlation coefficient was +0·34, statistical significance, $P = 0{\cdot}02$. These results, for groups A, B and C, are seen on a three-dimensional plot in Fig. 31.

DISCUSSION

In all, 42 correlations were made for D_T and D_P (14 frequencies or frequency combinations ×3 groups). Of these 6 were negative, and none of these were in the category of low-frequency D_T and high-frequency D_P. The frequency combinations yielding negative coefficients were in fact in groups A, B and C for the regressions $D_{T\overline{346}}$ on $D_{P\overline{12}}$ and in group B for the regressions $D_{T\overline{12}}$ on $D_{P\overline{12}}$, $D_{T\overline{346}}$ on $D_{P\overline{346}}$, and $D_{T\overline{12346}}$ on $D_{P\overline{12346}}$. All the

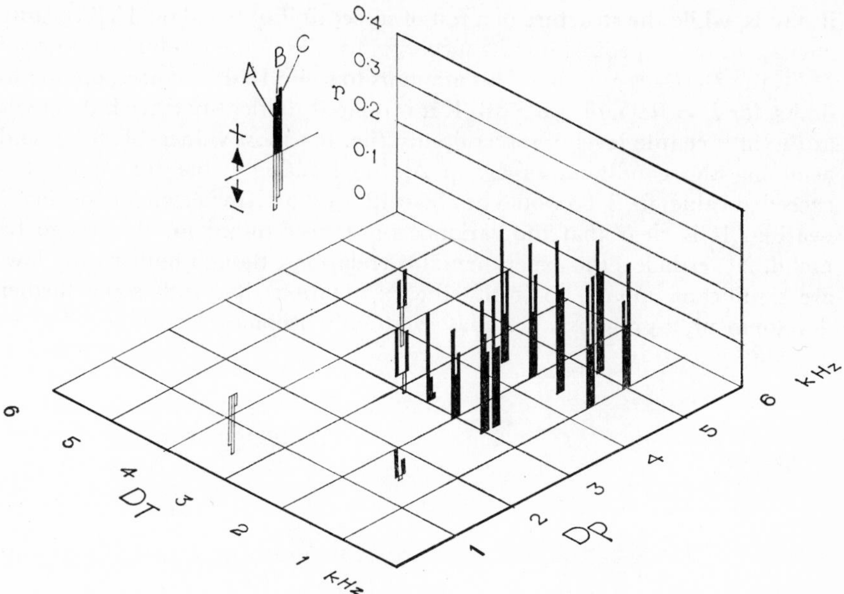

FIG. 31. Values of the correlation coefficient r for regressions of D_T on D_P.

The position of the bars (one each for group A, B and C) on the horizontal surface indicates the frequency or average of the frequency combination used for deriving the indices that are correlated. The height of the solid bars indicates, on the vertical scale, the positive value of r. Negative values of r are shown, on the same scale, as open bars pointing down below the horizontal surface.

remainder of the regressions yielded positive correlations. The reason for the optimum combination occurring with D_T for low frequencies and D_P for high remains obscure. The reason for the low value of r (+0·34) is less so; it must in part be in the considerable variances of both D_T and D_P, and in turn this must be attributed to the intrinsic features of pure-tone audiometry. The effect of reducing the variance can be seen if instead of individual values, the mean of groups of 9 or 10 individuals is used in estimating the regression of group A for $D_{T\overline{12}}$ on $D_{P\overline{346}}$. The result is that the correlation coefficient is raised from +0·34 to no less than +0·74, but of course this is not helpful if it is prediction for individuals which is sought. Reverting to the individual case, if the size of the "4 kHz dip" is used, rather than the absolute hearing level, in calculating D_P (i.e. mean hearing level of 3, 4 and 6 kHz minus mean hearing level of 1 and 2 kHz), the coefficient of +0·34 becomes +0·38. Other possibilities for improvement exist, such as by using repeated estimations of D_T, with various possible refinements. In this study the majority of subjects had only one measurement of TTS, and the use of the mean of several measurements would obviously reduce the variance. As it stands, while the structure of a test of susceptibility based on TTS is easily envisaged, the impediment to its successful use lies in the residual variance of D_T in the D_T/D_P regression. This amounts to some 18 dB^2, corresponding to limits, for $P = 0{\cdot}05$, of $\pm 8{\cdot}5$ dB. If it is desired to identify those individuals at the fifth centile level of susceptibility (i.e. the most vulnerable 5%), and assuming the conditions of group A, the limiting value (i.e. not-to-be-exceeded value) for TTS would be about $12{\cdot}5 \pm 8{\cdot}5$ dB in persons of "normal" hearing. It is clear that the variance must be reduced for the test to be useful. Nevertheless the experimental correlations, though numerically low, are significant enough to justify the expectation that with some further development, a prognostic test may eventually become practicable.

Assessment of Risk of Hearing Loss due to Impulse Noise

By

R. R. A. Coles and C. G. Rice

Institute of Sound and Vibration Research, University of Southampton, England

INTRODUCTION

The measurement and evaluation of impulse noise has long been the largest area of uncertainty in knowledge and insufficiency in guidance in hearing conservation matters, although in recent years the situation is improving considerably. It is appropriate therefore to collate recent data and the methods that are either used in practice or are recommended, and thereby to look at the impulse noise problem as a whole.

There are two principal methods of dealing with impulse noises (i) with an ordinary sound level meter followed by comparison with damage-risk criteria intended for steady-state noises, or (ii) with a pressure/time history display with an oscilloscope and evaluation by criteria such as those recommended by Coles *et al.* (1968). A third method, not to be discussed further because of lack of data connecting physical measurements and auditory hazard, is to use an impact sound analyser of some kind.

In discussing the two principal methods mentioned, it is helpful to classify impulses into three main types, according to the pressure/time histories of the impulse wave envelopes (Fig. 32).

First, *Type* (*a*); these are occasional widely-separated impulses, typified by gunfire and other very intermittent explosive noise sources. In *Type* (*b*), there are repetitive but discrete impulses covering ratios of peak-to-background level in the wave-envelope pattern of not less than about 6 dB and impact rates of about 0·5 to 10 per second; examples would be blanking processes, manual hammering of metal plates, etc. Finally, *Type* (*c*); these are highly repetitive noises, in which the repetition rate is greater than about 10 per second and the ratio of peak to minimum level in the wave-envelope pattern is less than about 6 dB; this is the commonest impulse noise type found in industry and is typified by pneumatic chippers or hammers, e.g. in fettling and riveting.

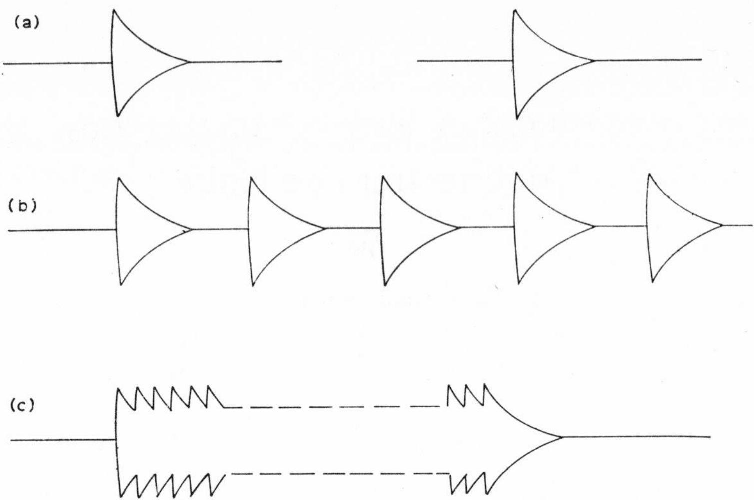

FIG. 32. Examples of wave envelope patterns of impulse noises.

USE OF SOUND LEVEL METERS

Conventional sound level meters can only cope adequately with Type (c) noises, using either the dB(A) scale or octave-band analysis. The results can be related to current damage-risk criteria with little or no correction for impulsive components (that is, where the striking rate is high, the ratio of peak-to-background level is low, or both).

However, in considering the use of a sound level meter, it should be noted that in standardization groups it has recently been suggested (International Organization for Standardization, 1970) that some impulsive noises (of rather undefined type) can be assessed by comparison with steady-state noise criteria, with the proviso that dB(A) values are obtained using the "slow" response characteristic of the meter and a figure of 10 dB(A) is added in respect of the impulsiveness of the noise. Whilst such a procedure may have its place with certain types of noise, perhaps Type (b), the 10-dB(A) correction and/or the measurement technique is apparently unvalidated and therefore quite unsuitable for other impulse noises. This will be discussed further.

It is not clear how this 10-dB(A) figure has been derived; whether this is because of a possible exceptional hazard of impulsive components in a noise—which is contrary to the evidence of Cohen, Kylin and LaBenz (1966)—whether it is to compensate for the inability of the meter to respond to the short-duration peaks of sound pressure (Dieroff, 1966), or whether it is a general safety factor covering both of these points. Whatever the rationale, 10 dB(A) must in fact be the wrong figure for many of the noises, because there is no sharp dividing line in degree of impulsiveness between Types (a), (b) and (c) noises; thus any correction factor should range over a continuum from 0 to 10 dB(A) (or perhaps more) between, respectively, an almost steady-state noise and a noise repeated, say, once per second.

As a matter of curiosity rather than scientific study, we have taken a superficial look at this technique with a few examples of impulses of Types (a) and (b). Using the 130-dB peak level, 15- and 50-ms duration, impact noises described by Walker (1970), it appeared that the "slow" meter response characteristic was necessary if the measurements were to give even a qualitative indication of increasing hazard as the impact rate rose from isolated impacts to 6·4 impacts per second. The meter readings with either "fast" or "slow" meter response settings were about 7 dB higher for the 50-ms duration impulses: this compares poorly with the 3·5-dB increase in hazard corresponding to a change of B-duration of 15 to 50 ms that would be predicted from the Coles *et al.* (1968) impulse noise criterion.

Thus, in spite of the fact that Walker measured TTS from these noises that was in the same general order of magnitude as that expected from steady-state noises having the same dB(A) values plus 10 dB(A), it seems probable that the sound level meter method has considerable quantitative limitations even for Type (b) impulse noises. Until more work has been done on this, the method seems so uncertain that, in our opinion, all it could be used for is as a preliminary rough estimate.

If the noise level, without the 10 dB(A) correction, is at least 15 dB(A) below the steady-state noise damage-risk criterion (corresponding to the summed durations of the noisy periods each day), then the noise can be regarded as safe; if 15 dB(A) above it, then the noise can be regarded as hazardous. If less than 15 dB(A) different from the steady-state noise criterion (that is, within ± 15 dB of it), then the interpretation is uncertain and it would be advisable to supplement it by a pressure/time measurement and analysis of the type applicable to Type (a) noises.

From both theoretical considerations and the International Electrotechnical Commission specifications (1961 and 1965) for sound level meters, it is obvious that these are unsuitable for measurement of Type (a) noises. Our own observation with noises of 300 μs duration and 136- and 160-dB peak levels confirmed this view.

In spite of this, it is interesting to note that the handbook of one of the sound level meters used quoted 100 to 120 dB as being "deafening'" and to be found in "gunfire"; in fact, the hazardous 160-dB peak-level noise gave maxima of 107 to 109 dB(A), whilst the safe 136-dB peak-level noise gave only 98 to 100 dB(A). Therefore, for some noises of Type (a) even, sound level meters of the types quoted appear to give results that may have some, though minimal, quantitative value, provided certain rules are applied as follows: (i) that the highest relevant 10-dB unit in the range selector should be used in order to minimize the effect of needle inertia; for example, the needle has to move through a shorter distance for $(100-2)$ dB than for $(90+8)$ dB; and (ii), that readings of 90 dB(A) or more should be regarded only as an indication of possible hazard needing more comprehensive analysis.

Moreover, as Type (a) noises are separated by intervals that do not allow any integration of energy between impulses and as the fast response gives results nearer to the actual noise level and is less dependent on the range selector setting, the fast response would now seem to be more appropriate. But, there being no sharp division between noise Types (a) and (b), no rule can be offered as to when a fast and when a slow response should be employed. In short, in the present state of knowledge, sound level meters cannot be regarded as suitable instruments for impulse noise assessment, except with those noises that are so rapidly repetitive (Type (c)) that correction factors for impulsiveness are barely needed anyway and would probably introduce rather than correct errors.

OSCILLOGRAPHIC MEASUREMENT

Coming now to the oscillographic measurement technique and method of auditory evaluation proposed by Coles *et al.* (1968), it would seem that this is the method of choice for noises of Type (a), helpful for Type (b), but inappropriate for Type (c). In this, the pressure/time history of the impulse, arriving at grazing incidence on the microphone, is analysed in terms of peak level and of A- or B-duration, as illustrated in Fig. 33. The potential hazard is then evaluated by reference to the graph shown in Fig. 34.

A number of adjustments may be applied, and indeed have been embodied in the CHABA (1968) version of our criterion, as follows:

(i) Where impulses arrive at normal incidence to the ear, a correction of 5 dB should be made to the peak level to allow for the greater auditory hazard involved.

(ii) The criterion is based on repetition rates in the order of 8–30 impulses per minute—the repetition rates with greatest hazard (Ward, 1962)—and exposures to around 100 impulses per occasion on perhaps 10 occasions per year. Precautions cannot safely be relaxed for even one occasion, however. When greater or lesser repetition rates are used, it is difficult to quantify the reduction in hazard, and it might be advisable to ignore this factor and thereby retain an inherent safety factor. Where exposure is to occasional single impulses only, an estimate of 10 dB has been made for the reduced hazard and the higher peak level therefore allowable (but see modifications to this, described below).

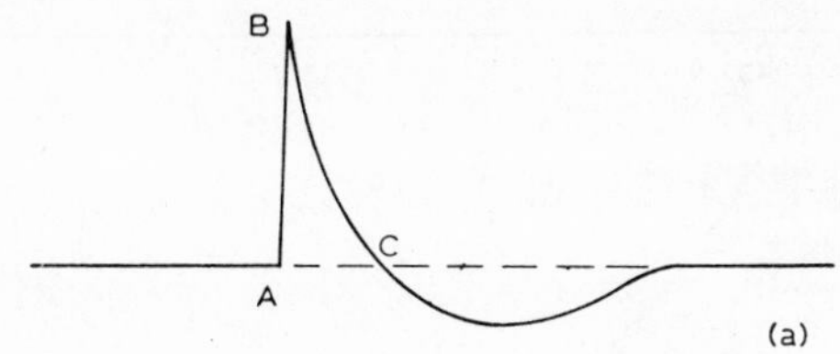

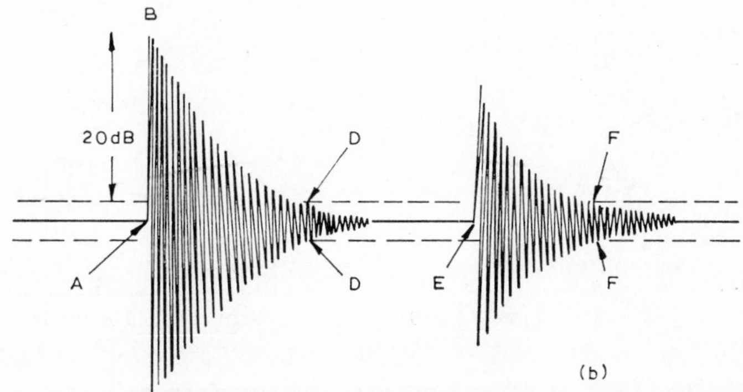

FIG. 33. Idealized evaluations of oscillographic waveforms of impulsive noises. Peak level = pressure difference AB. Rise time = time difference AB. (a) A—duration = time difference AC. (b) B—duration = time difference AD (plus EF for example in the case of a relatively long-time reflection).

(iii) If it is desired to cover more than 75% of persons, to which percentage the criterion of acceptable degree of auditory impairment is applicable, the specified peak levels might be lowered by about 5 dB or 10 dB to cover the 90th or 95th percentiles or even 15 dB for still higher percentiles.

(iv) When ear protectors are worn, allowances of about 20 dB for ear plugs (e.g. V.51R type) or 30 dB for circumaural ear-muffs may be applied.

Since the original paper in 1968, however, a modification has been proposed (Coles and Rice, 1970) with respect to the correction factor for number of impulses per exposure. Explanation of how the new proposal was arrived at will not be repeated here, but it is gratifying to note that this now leaves no major discrepancy between impulse-noise TTS studies and the auditory hazard predictable from analysis of the noise, or between impulse and steady-state noises with regard to specification of auditory hazard.

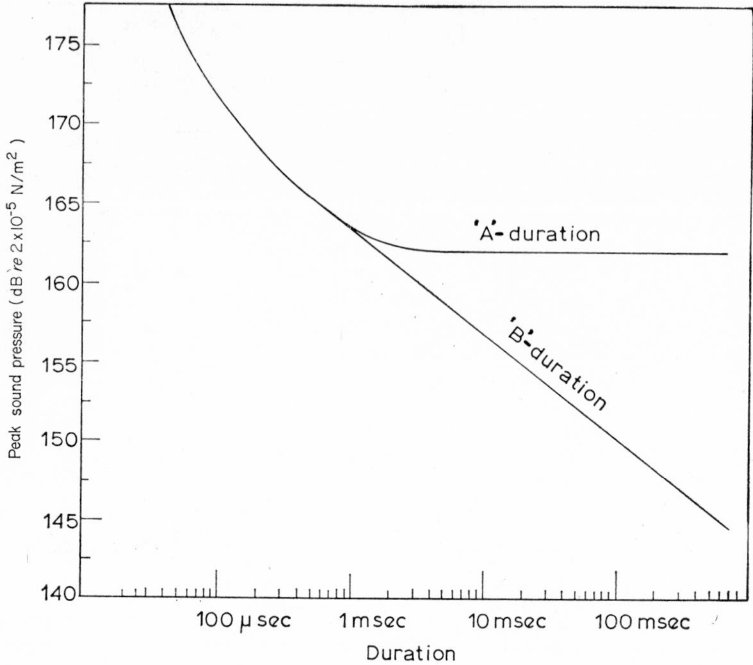

FIG. 34. Damage-risk criterion for impulse noise.

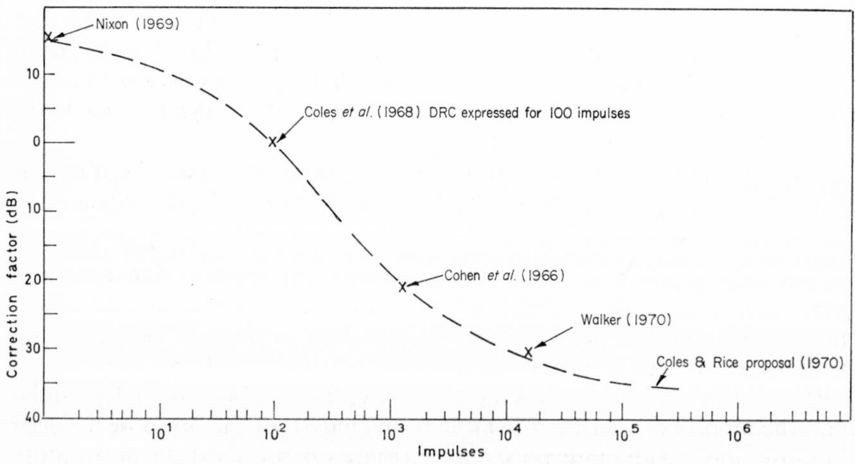

FIG. 35. Modified correction factor for number of impulses.

Probably, in course of time, the modification itself will prove to need some adjustment as, so far, it can only be claimed to be an approximation. Likewise, with respect to impulses having rise times that are substantially greater than the 0·3- to 0·5-ms upper limit referred to in the original paper, the permitted noise levels referred to in the Coles *et al.* damage-risk criterion may need elevating somewhat (by an estimated 0 to 8 dB in the rise-time range 0·5 to 5 ms). However, in the majority of industrial and experimental impulse noises the rise times come well within this upper limit.

Discussion on Papers in Section I

CHAIRMEN

D. E. Broadbent   J. D. Hood

PARTICIPANTS

D. E. Broadbent	P. F. King
M. E. Bryan	B. Kylin
W. Burns	A. Martin
R. R. A. Coles	Mrs. W. Passchier-Vermeer
H. Davis	P. Ransome-Wallis
A. Glorig	K. Ratcliffe
R. I. Higgins	D. W. Robinson
R. Hinchcliffe	W. D. Ward
J. D. Hood	

Dr. Ward: The papers by Dr. Kylin and Mrs. Passchier-Vermeer have both underscored the fact that if one has a steady noise that is interrupted (I am not referring to impact noise) the equal-energy hypothesis is somewhat over-protective. I wonder if either of the two authors have tried another type of calculation, one that seems to work for predicting the temporary hearing loss from intermittent noise; namely, that it is not the *energy* average over the period concerned that will determine how much temporary threshold shift will result, but the *level* average. It appears, in Dr. Kylin's data in particular, that the median exposure level, not the median exposure energy, was in the neighbourhood of 90 dB(A), which is what he found to be the effective level.

Mrs. Passchier: The results from the wood-working factory, with noise varying over the workday, show a good agreement between audiometric and noise measurements. In this case the noise has been rated according to the equal-energy principle. Therefore it is not correct to say that in this case the equal-energy principle is over-protective. Regarding Dr. Ward's suggestion, our noise was measured and rated automatically at the same time, so we are not able to do any other type of calculation.

Dr. Glorig: I think the conclusions in Dr. Kylin's paper are based on short-time energy summation over a few days and not on the basis of several years of exposure. Some of the data showing less hearing loss than one expects from the levels measured over a few days might be consistent with what happens over the long term: it is not reasonable to suppose that measurements made over a few days are representative of those that would be found over 5-year periods. It is very difficult to get an equivalent noise level L_{eq} for interrupted or intermittent noise over many years where the variations do not show up on the short term. Before we start discussing whether the equal-energy hypothesis is good, bad or indifferent, we need to learn a lot more about what those long-term exposures really consist of in terms of the total energy.

Dr. Kylin: Unfortunately, like Mrs. Passchier, I have not analysed the data in the way suggested by Dr. Ward. In reply to Dr. Glorig, I am aware of the difficulties and can only concede the point he makes. It is well known, as Dr. Glorig has also mentioned on previous occasions, that the noise has continually varied over the years and so we cannot obtain any good assessment of the noise in retrospective studies. This is a serious complication, but I can see no way out of it. The question has been asked why reference is made in our paper to measurements in both the dB(A) and dB(C) scales. For clarification I would explain that the noises were recorded with a flat-response tape recorder so that back in the laboratory we were able to obtain both measures. We used dB(C) only to give a rough idea of the noise levels of power saws and tractors. For transforming the data into the scheme proposed by ISO we went over to dB(A).

Dr. Ward: What Dr. Glorig said is true, but still the implication is that what was measured in these cases was a spuriously high equivalent level. In other words, the empirical fact is that we predict, from the L_{eq} determined by the equal-energy principle, more hearing loss than we actually observe. This could imply that things are more noisy now than they were in the past, and I do not think that is really the way things are. I might also point out that the mining industry is another case in which the exposure is very intermittent and where the observed hearing losses, according to some recent studies (Blaha and Slepicka, 1967; Jönsson, 1967; Sataloff *et al.*, 1969), are much less than predicted on the basis of the equal-energy L_{eq}.

Dr. Ransome-Wallis: I am interested to see how the assessment of hearing loss is now being treated as an exact science. In the Anti-Submarine Department of the Royal Navy during the last war, we carried out pure-tone audiometry on more than 3000 young and middle-aged males. The outstanding finding was the great variation in consecutive audiograms from the same subject due to an infinite variety of factors not directly connected with aural physiology, such as travel fatigue, alcohol, emotional conditions and anxiety states. In the investigation of presbycusis it is very hard to get an accurate assessment due, again, to many "outside" factors including general cardiovascular degeneration, upper respiratory infections and numerous other conditions which appear to influence the deafness of old age. It seems also that, to achieve any degree of exactitude in the assessment of hearing loss, comparative audiograms must be made under identical ambient conditions and using the same audiometer and the same operator throughout. In this connection we found, in the course of work carried out during the last war at the University of Toronto, that audiograms made in a dead silent room were often inaccurate owing to the tendency of the subject to hallucinate. More consistent results were obtained in a quiet, rather than in a silent room.

Dr. Broadbent: I think Dr. Wallis's last remarks are a salutary reminder of the importance of good audiometric conditions and of techniques of determination which take into account the sources of variance.

Dr. Hinchcliffe: Perhaps I could comment on Dr. Wallis's remarks regarding the influence of general medical conditions on hearing levels. Is there not the presumption, when we are dealing with the hearing levels of general or industrial populations, that only two factors influence the measures of central tendency, namely "age" and noise? Although other factors may, and do, influence individual hearing levels these factors are not—at least in Europe and North America—sufficiently prevalent to influence medians, averages or modal values.

Dr. Hood: May I put one question to Professor Burns? Supposing one could develop some means for detecting susceptibility to noise-induced hearing loss, how long-term is this likely to be? Is it possible, for example, that a person found to be susceptible at the time of testing may, some 2 or 3 years later, be found to be resistant and vice versa?

Professor Burns: It is well known that stability of performance in audiometry is far from absolute, and likewise there might be instability of the susceptibility condition. It would be rash to assume that an estimation of susceptibility, even though it were practical now, would be valid for an indefinite period, or at all times, even assuming otological normality. Dr. Hood has himself speculated on various possibilities, metabolic and so on, which might influence the degree of susceptibility. Various factors must be involved, but at the present stage we are trying to address ourselves to the more obvious and fundamental aspects of the problem.

Group Capt. King: I speak as a clinical otologist, so anything I say will have a medical bias. I was interested to see that Dr. Robinson's experimental work confirms what one sees in clinical practice. And that is that people with noise-induced deafness, if seen early enough in their careers, have a fair degree of loss early on during the course of their exposure which then, if they are followed up often for years, suffer no apparent change. One is always wondering if this is because their working conditions have changed or because they are particularly assiduous with protection, or whether it is in the audiometry; but it does seem to be an established physical fact. I was interested in Professor Burns's work in regard to a susceptibility test because this is the dream of everyone who is concerned with hearing conservation programmes. I think even so, despite the enormous amount of work that has gone into it, that this will still be a dream because on any given day, if a man comes to have his fitness for employment assessed, one may get him in a bad or a good phase. Nevertheless it might be an improvement on the present situation where one assesses men on the results of a pure-tone air-conduction audiogram and if they already show signs of loss at an early age they are perhaps considered unsuitable. If they have no signs of loss the only thing one can do is to employ them and check them relatively soon after start of employment, and if they then show signs of hearing loss somebody is going to be disappointed. In either event it can be an uneconomic process. The third point I would like to raise is the growing tendency among British otologists to regard the hearing range on the pure-tone audiogram as being 1, 2 and 3 kHz rather than 0·5, 1 and 2 kHz. It was probably the late Dr. T. S. Littler who started us thinking on this but certainly it is a notion which has grown. It is particularly applicable to this type of deafness where 500 Hz is only involved very late in the disorder and where, when the assessment of disability is being considered, we are in fact weighting the situation in favour of the claimant if we measure the average hearing loss at 1, 2 and 3 kHz, because in the average case there is more deterioration in the hearing higher up the range than there is lower down. Those who deal with the physics of the matter assure me that, in a general sense, for the purposes of reception of speech, the frequencies between 2 and 3 kHz are as important, if not more so, than those in the range between 500 and 1000 Hz.

Dr. Davis: The question about what frequencies ought to be considered and what constitutes a disability has been discussed back and forth in various committees and meetings. The criterion that was accepted in the Committee on Conservation of Hearing was the ability to understand everyday speech adequately. This does not mean monosyllables in the audiometric discrimination test, nor does it mean nonsense syllables in the psychoacoustic laboratory; the concept is everyday speech "as she is spoke", and this implies the value of contextual cues and also the careless way that people speak. There is a great deal of redundancy if we are talking about everyday speech and not about the unexpected message, the unfamiliar proper name or the important telephone number. With this qualification it is not necessary to hear particularly well above 3 kHz if 2 kHz is alright. Audiograms rarely take a nose-dive at that particular point. Efforts to show a failure in the understanding of speech by available tests—tests that do not involve nonsense syllables but real sentence intelligibility—do not show any great impairment for the kind of audiograms under discussion here, even some of those with severe 4 kHz dips.

Personally, if we were starting all over again with no established preferred frequencies built into audiometers simply because they are round numbers, I would opt for 750, 1500 and 3000 Hz as providing the best simple average, but our audiometers are not built that way. In the American Medical Association rule, which did try to take account of the higher frequencies, 4 kHz was valued only at 15%. That was the maximum contribution that could be made by that frequency, whereas 2 kHz was valued at 40%. I agree that one can do a little better with four frequencies than with three, or by weighting the frequencies if one wishes to confine these to three. But I caution against rules that are too complicated to be practical, and I hold now for continuing with 0·5, 1 and 2 kHz as a realistic measure when one is concerned with sentence intelligibility of familiar material in everyday speech.

Dr. Glorig: This problem is certainly not new to me nor to Dr. Davis; it has come up in the U.S.A. many times. I would like to tell a story about it that happened in California where I was a member of a technical committee (advising the Commission) that consisted of representatives from Management and Labour. We were deciding what formula California should use. Management went along with the medical profession and said they wanted 500, 1000 and 2000 Hz used; but Labour, seeing the large losses at 4000, wanted 4000 Hz included. The fight became so bitter they almost came to blows. The man who was sitting on the bench—the chairman of the group—didn't want to offend anybody, so when all the arguments were finished he said, "Apparently there is no way we can get together on this so I think we'll compromise, and take 3000 Hz which is halfway between 2000 and 4000, and we'll add it to the formula." That is how California got 3000 Hz in its formula: it had nothing to do with the scientific merits of the matter.

In reply to Group Capt. King, I would say that as I am also an otologist I have been in similar situations to him. But in our laboratory we have done a number of studies using different combinations of the three frequencies, including 3 kHz as a fourth frequency, and several other combinations. The first studies came out of the Wisconsin State Fair results where we looked at the data and tried to find which frequencies would best predict the speech reception threshold and the PB (phonetically-balanced word list) score. This is not the same test as discussed by Dr. Davis. We actually found that a person did not need hearing above 1500 Hz to get a good score—or a perfect score for that matter—using PB's as the criterion. We also found that if spondees were used—and this represents everyday speech better than PB's—one did not need much above 1000 Hz to hear everything that was said. In another of these studies, conducted by Dr. Ward to compare noise-induced hearing loss to gunfire loss, we had subjects with losses up to 200 dB per octave above 2 kHz.

Dr. Ward devised a very difficult multiple-choice test, determined by the consonant weighting of the words, and he found that as long as people had good hearing at 2 kHz they made just as good a score as the subjects who had normal hearing above 3 kHz. However, there is one variable in this that I must comment on. Does a person with good hearing at 3 kHz hear everyday speech better in a noisy situation? The criterion mentioned by Dr. Davis is based on everyday speech in quiet. That was because we never really knew what kind of a noise represents everyday noise, and we still do not really know. Research is in progress in the U.S.A. at several laboratories, and the Bell Laboratories have devised a noise which represents reasonably well everyday listening situations. I know that a lot of my otologist friends talk about patients with 3 kHz losses who are having trouble. I think if they were to consider the conditions under which the patients are having the problems, they would find that subjects with normal hearing at 3 kHz would probably have the same kind of difficulty. Going back to the Wisconsin State Fair study, we had the subject say if he thought his hearing was good, fair or poor. In no case did we encounter one who said his hearing was other than good if his hearing was good up to 2 kHz. It did not matter much what happened above 2 kHz. Those who had losses at 2 kHz, however, recorded fair and bad.

Dr. Hood: The frequency characteristic of the hearing loss in occupational deafness is not the only item deserving of attention when assessing disability. Earlier Dr. Davis made mention of the Sabine-Fowler method of computing percentage loss. This, as well as the Fletcher method, is based on the weighting of various frequencies with respect to their contribution to speech spectra. But this, surely, is true only in respect of conductive deafness and what we are concerned with here is a perceptive loss. The essential feature of all perceptive hearing losses that are cochlear in origin—and noise-induced hearing loss is such a case—is that they exhibit the phenomenon of loudness recruitment, and all available evidence suggests that in this respect cases of noise-induced hearing loss behave much the same as Ménière's disease. Loudness recruitment is a disorder in which loudness increases much more rapidly with intensity than it does in the normal subject. The common complaint of these patients is that they cannot hear you if you speak normally but if you shout they *tell* you that you are shouting. This phenomenon is strictly related to the degree of hearing loss: as the hearing loss increases this disorder of the loudness function gets progressively worse. This in turn has a reflection upon speech discrimination and, although the speech articulation curves of subjects with mild degrees of hearing loss may be normal in shape, with increasing hearing loss the speech discrimination progressively deteriorates. The articulation curve may rise to a maximum score of say 30% and then with further amplification it will decrease. This poor discrimination correlates remarkably well with the amount of loudness recruitment present. These are important considerations because it is not simply a question of the frequency characteristic that we have to be concerned with but this extra disability, which is much more serious than a straightforward conductive hearing loss.

Dr. Davis: I am sorry that Dr. Hood has brought Ménière's disease into the discussion. I think personally it has no place here whatsoever. The chronically-acquired kind of noise-induced hearing loss that is under discussion is certainly sensorineural in character and not conductive, but I think in many ways it more nearly resembles conductive impairments than it does the Ménière's type. I have been impressed by the lack of dysacusis, the retention of word discrimination, the lack of serious tinnitus. On the other hand recruitment is present and is very characteristic of this condition. This has led me in my teaching to distinguish between two kinds of recruitment, one of which I call benign recruitment. The other is the nasty kind (dysacusis) that goes with Ménière's disease. Benign recruitment is what we have in noise-induced hearing loss.

Let me amplify this. Dr. Fowler based his curve and weighting factors, not according to the Fletcher phonemes and nonsense syllables, but on his experience as an otologist, by studying his patients and the kind of complaints they brought to him. His view was that if there is recruitment the subject should be credited for recruitment at 4 kHz. I believe it was a 5-dB discount, so to speak, on his hearing loss. He would hear better, because most of his listening would be done at a level above threshold where his perception of loudness was more nearly normal. Some time ago (Davis *et al.*, 1950) we did some experiments in which I participated personally. We induced rather severe temporary threshold shifts in our own ears, and many of these were high-frequency dips because that kind of TTS is always at frequencies above that of the exposure tone. We had beautiful recruitment, so much so that the equal-loudness balances at the level of the exposure tone (at or above 100 dB) were substantially flat, in other words complete recruitment. Word discrimination was not perfect down at 40-dB loudness level, but it was fairly good at 70 and practically perfect at 100 dB. This was in aircraft noise with the message brought up loud enough to come through. The impairment from this high-frequency loss that was evident near threshold disappeared, which confirms the Fowler concept. We did on occasion get that nasty kind of recruitment, meaning that we had done things so severe to our ears that we had head noises, spontaneous tinnitus and greatly distorted tone quality, and the intelligibility function broke down badly. This was a more severe affair; fortunately it did not last with any of us and all the ears came back within normal limits, but we had in this experimental situation both the benign variety and the nasty kind, so we simply have to find out more about what kind of hearing losses people have. But don't be afraid of recruitment just because it has a bad name! I have recruitment at 3 kHz and an abrupt hearing loss just above 2500 Hz, but I was not aware that I had anything wrong with my hearing until I began to study hearing in 1942, and I think by that time I was really beginning to suffer from some presbycusis!

Mr. Higgins: When Dr. Glorig and Dr. Davis were discussing the interrelationship of frequency and loss of speech understanding or speech intelligibility, were they referring to two people conversing face to face, or were they also referring to the circumstance that arises socially—and possibly more important, industrially—where one person is standing behind another and trying to communicate?

Dr. Davis: All the tests of intelligibility that I had in mind used recorded speech, delivered through earphones, with no lip-reading involved. Lip-reading, of course, may be a practical help and an art at which people who suffer noise-induced hearing loss may become rather adept. But this is their good fortune.

Dr. Glorig: In reply to Mr. Higgins, I agree that lip-reading would be an aid to better the scores that I was referring to.

Dr. Hinchcliffe: I would like to make two comments, one regarding loudness and the other regarding the "low fence". First, may I enter a plea that loudness recruitment, speech discrimination loss and distortion of tone quality should not be considered as synonymous terms. On the other point, data obtained in a hearing survey that we conducted on a general population some years ago indicated that the low fence, that is the point where the subject begins to have difficulty in hearing, is age-dependent. Although people at the age of 70 begin to have difficulty in hearing at levels which correspond to speech hearing losses of 25 dB, Dr. Merluzzi's analysis of our data indicated that this value for the low fence is progressively smaller with increasingly younger ages. Thus, for young adults, this fence would correspond to no more than about 8 dB.

Dr. Bryan: I would like to ask Professor Burns and Dr. Robinson how they can be quite sure that they have excluded all cases of perceptive loss due to pathology from their non-pathological population. It seems to me that with perceptive deafness the aetiology is often uncertain, and in some cases unknown. Surely what their otological examination revealed was that there was a perceptive loss and in only a proportion of cases the probable cause? We can never be certain that this type of hearing loss is not due to some unknown factor or some incident which occurred in childhood. The results of a hearing survey that we have recently carried out upon the academic staff at the University of Salford are relevant to this point. Of the 503 subjects tested, 139 cases were classified as having pathological hearing. These 139 cases were re-tested and then examined by our otologist, Mr. I. A. Tumarkin, and their hearing losses categorized into:

conductive lesions	24	cases	(17%)
perceptive lesions	71		(52%)
mixed lesions	44		(31%).

The relevant medical history of each subject was elicited by means of a questionnaire. Using the criteria given by Burns and Robinson (1970) for the acceptance of normal ears, 54 of these 71 perceptive losses would have been mis-classified as normal. Even using a rather more rigorous set of criteria, 26 cases would still have been acceptable as normal in Burns and Robinson's survey as they had no known aetiology whatsoever. If our results are at all representative of the general industrial population they suggest that between 5 and 10% of Burns and Robinson's "normal ears" have a loss of hearing which should be attributed, at least in part, to unknown pathology and not to noise exposure alone. The results of our survey outline one of the dangers of making a diagnosis of noise-induced hearing loss in the absence of pre-employment audiograms. In 23 of our cases, exposure to high-level noise was reported but very often the same subjects had also been concussed or had acoustic trauma, or had had the usual range of childhood illnesses, or a combination of these. It would be a brave otologist who would be prepared to allocate the percentage of loss which was attributable to these various potential causes.

Dr. Robinson: It is impossible to be dogmatic as to whether one has successfully excluded all extraneous cases of hearing loss, but there are various indications on which one may rely. Firstly, after we had eliminated from our non-noise-exposed control group those cases which conformed to our working definition of "pathological", we ended up with a group whose hearing levels were distributed with nearly Gaussian statistics and in close agreement with the accepted international standard of normal hearing. This is evidence that the standards of exclusion were similar to those adopted by people concerned with standard determinations of the threshold of hearing; and in that field of study the experimenters can afford to be highly selective in case of the slightest doubt. Since the otologists in our survey followed the same precepts for the noise-exposed subjects as for the controls, this gives us some confidence that the noise-exposed groups were similarly expurgated. This is, of course, only circumstantial evidence—not proof. However, there is another factor which anyone who has looked at our results will have noticed, namely we found seemingly smaller hearing losses due to noise, that is smaller values of NIPTS, than in almost any other published study. Our viewpoint may be put in this way. Noise certainly does something to ears; therefore there exists a lower bound to the effect. One may always observe effects exceeding this lower bound by not being careful enough about exclusions, but the converse cannot apply. The evidence points to the fact that we have just about reached that bottom. If Dr. Bryan's suggestion is right that 5 to 10% of our ears classed as normal may have contained a component of unknown pathology I could not contradict this, but it would only mean that perhaps even we have not quite reached that lower bound. But as we are discussing here primarily the effects of noise, and not extraneous accretions of hearing loss, his evidence only underscores the point we have ourselves emphasized, namely that our basic understanding must start from the effects of noise alone.

Professor Burns: I would just mention that the otological procedure was laid down and, as far as we could ascertain, it was held reasonably constant throughout. The criteria to which Dr. Robinson referred of otological normality by the audiometric evidence are, I agree, important. In addition to the initial clinical examination the audiogram was examined by the otologist and if necessary the case was seen again subsequently if there was any suspicion that anything other than noise-induced hearing loss was present. These audiograms were scrutinized closely and we were fortunate enough to have Dr. Hinchcliffe to collaborate with us in this way. Perhaps he could assure us that we did not let the wheat get mixed up with the chaff?

Dr. Hinchcliffe: This comes back to my earlier comment that, in Europe and North America, only two factors, namely "age" and noise, significantly influence the measures of central tendency with respect to hearing levels determined on the general population (Glorig and Nixon, 1960). However, this does not hold for certain other parts of the world, for example Jamaica and Nigeria, where one or more general medical condition may be sufficiently prevalent to influence the central values also (Hinchcliffe, 1968).

Dr. Robinson: I should like to put forward a thought concerning the results of Dr. Coles, who is to be applauded for his efforts to embrace impulsive noise. This is something that Professor Burns and I had for the time being abandoned due to the difficulties. The question is whether his hearing loss measurements would in fact correlate closely with the sounds he studied if the latter were treated according to the same principles that Professor Burns and I used, and to which Mrs. Passchier-Vermeer and Dr. Kylin also referred, namely the idea of equivalent continuous sound level, L_{eq}. This amounts to asking whether the equal-energy principle would work right down to the extreme case of single impulses of Dr. Coles' type A, provided the noise-immission level were properly measured. Today that is quite a simple thing to do but, of course, it was not so simple at the time when we were embarking on our respective studies;

even now the arbitrariness with which the rating of impulse noise is surrounded is evident from the prevailing rule which instructs one to add 10 dB to a sound level meter reading if the sound is impulsive in character. This merely reflects the absence, hitherto, of anything more concrete to recommend short of leaving impulse noise out of the reckoning altogether. The position now, however, may be quite different. With the aid of digital signal analysis one could treat impulses of whatever waveform by calculating the *A*-weighted noise immission level and determining whether this measure correlates with the observed hearing threshold shifts. I hazard the opinion that this would be the case.

Dr. Coles: We had not thought of doing this but I agree that it is a thing we should do. I am not sure from what Dr. Robinson describes whether one will achieve this with portable equipment or not. What we all need is a small portable instrument for measurements on the factory floor instead of such cumbersome equipment as an oscilloscope and all the paraphernalia that goes with it. There is quite good agreement between the impulse criterion at the highly-repetitive long-duration end and the 85–90 dB(A) criterion for steady-state noise. Moreover, the slope of the B-duration line is extremely close to the equal-energy concept, although it was not drawn with this in mind but from experimental data, and it happened to come out close. This encourages one to think that there may be some future in the approach suggested and I should like to give it a trial in relation to further work which we are doing at Southampton.

Mr. Martin: Dr. Robinson's suggestion concerning the relationship between the equal-energy concept and hearing damage caused by impact noise is, I believe, a valid one. We have derived a formula which allows the equivalent A-weighted sound level of an impact noise (L_{Aeq}) to be calculated from a knowledge of the parameters of that noise, assuming that the noise waveform decays in an approximately exponential manner. Thus:

$$L_{Aeq} = 85{\cdot}3 + 20 \log p_h + 10 \log N - 10 \log k + 10 \log (1 - e^{-2k/N})$$

gives the equivalent level in dB(A), where p_h is the peak sound pressure in N/m^2, N is the repetition rate in impacts per second and k is the decay constant in sec^{-1}. We have applied this equation to impact noises encountered in industry. By substituting the derived values of L_{Aeq} into Dr. Robinson's predictive equation (see page 46), the persistent threshold shifts—or more specifically the "presumed noise-induced hearing losses"—which would be produced by such noises have been deduced. Comparisons of the predicted hearing levels and those actually observed in industry show a good agreement between the two. An example of these hearing levels is shown in Table XVII. This gives the median thresholds measured in 18 men, of median age 44·5 years, exposed to an L_{Aeq} value of 118 dB(A) for a median time of 18·5 years, and their predicted thresholds. From these figures it would appear that Dr. Robinson's predictive system, and hence the equal-energy concept, may be extended to include impact noise.

TABLE XVII. Comparison of observed hearing levels with values calculated for impulse noise according to the equal-energy principle (N = 18)

Audiometric frequency (kHz)	1	2	3	4	6
Observed (dB)	37·0	48·0	57·0	60·5	60·0
Predicted (dB)	41·3	48·5	55·3	58·7	58·5

The impact noises in these studies were produced by drop-forging processes and had repetition rates of the order of 0·5 impacts per second and peak sound pressures in the range 125 to 145 dB.

Dr. Coles: I thank Mr. Martin for this information and congratulate him on having achieved this correlation. I should like to return to Dr. Robinson's comment and ask what would be the minimum equipment requirements for using this technique in practice?

Dr. Robinson: For the field work only a high-quality tape recorder is necessary. Back in the laboratory one would need analogue-to-digital conversion equipment, the output of which would normally be in the form of punched paper tape for later processing. The digital computer can be programmed to determine any desired measure, such as the spectrum, and in particular the A-weighted integrated sound energy of the input waveform. Dr. Delany has such a system in operation in our laboratory and it is quite a practical proposition; it could not, however, be made portable. An alternative method is also functioning which in some ways is simpler. This uses operational amplifiers—weighting, squaring and integrating—driven directly from the analogue voltage signal at the tape recorder output.

Dr. Ward: The thing which now faces us is what to do about the "number of impulses" factor. It has occurred to me that if one accepts Dr. Walker's data, as shown in Fig. 35 of Dr. Coles' paper, as well as those of Cohen, Kylin and LaBenz (1966) and some data of C. W. Nixon (personal communication, 1969), the only point that needs moving to make this Figure an equal-energy relation is the original 100-impulse point (Coles *et al.*, 1968). If this is moved over horizontally to "10 impulses" a pretty good approximation to an equal-energy line is obtained.

Dr. Coles: An equal-energy line fitted to the rest of the data, as suggested by Dr. Ward, would actually change the zero correction point from 100 to 25 impulses, though we take his point in principle. Differences between this straight line and the relationship proposed by Mr. Rice and me amount to about 5 dB in the range 5–200 impulses and for over 50,000 impulses and if this were an error it would be on the side of safety. For simplicity of use or of instrumentation, the equal-energy correction factor would therefore seem to be an acceptable modification to our curve. On the other hand, the 100-impulse point was based on a best estimate derived from real data, and on theoretical grounds we consider that the curved line is likely to be the closer representation. Until Mr. Martin's full results are published we shall have reservations on the applicability of the equal-energy hypothesis and as to whether there is a linear continuity between steady-state and impulse-noise criteria.

Mr. Martin: I would like to ask Dr. Coles a question concerning his proposed correction curve for the damage-risk criterion for gunfire noise. The curve seems to extend the criterion to include a large number of impulses, which we know to occur in industrial situations. However, the pressure-time waveform of a gunshot impulse usually has an "*N*" configuration whereas the impact noises which occur in industry generally have a waveform with an exponentially-decaying type of envelope; the two are physically quite different. I therefore wonder if the two noises have similar effects on hearing.

Dr. Coles: I certainly do not have experimental data on the Friedlander-type waveform in great numbers, although this might occur in a few military situations. I cannot think of any industrial situation where it would occur, except perhaps on a proving range for heavy artillery or something similar. The data leading to the correction factors for the number of impulses were all based on the exponential type of waveform—even the gunfire data in this instance—measurable by B-duration. It is academic whether the correction factors would apply to large numbers of Friedlander-type waveforms since, for example, 10,000 impulses a day of this simple type do not occur in any industrial situation. Do these two waveforms have the same effects when one considers smaller numbers of impulses outside the industrial sphere? I think they probably do allowing, of course, for the fact that the noise level specifications are set differently for the two types of impulse. Certainly the data we had led us to draw the particular lines which are, to the best of our knowledge, equal-damage-risk lines.

Mr. Ratcliffe: Could one of the speakers say what is the connection between a noise spectrum which has a characteristic peak of say 2000 Hz and the dip in the audiometry curve which would result? I have an idea that if one were exposed to a peaky sort of spectrum from a particular machine, 8 hours a day and perhaps for 10 years, the loss in the hearing would be at a frequency which would be something like one and a half times the peak. Is this in fact true? If it is, is there a medical explanation for it?

Dr. Ward: There has been a lot of speculation about this sort of thing and it seems to be a combination of several factors. First of all the outer ear is resonant to about 2000 Hz, so more energy gets into the cochlea at about 2000 Hz than at other frequencies. In a broad-band noise—other things being equal—one therefore gets the most stimulation at about this point. Why stimulation at 2000 to 3000 Hz produces the most effect at 4000 Hz is still being argued, but I think it is mostly a question of the resonance of the outer ear. There is nothing intrinsically more fragile about the 4000-Hz receptor; that has been well established by Lehnhardt's (1967) research in Hamburg. There have been all sorts of theories in the past but the main effect, I think, is this resonance of the outer ear canal. In other experimental animals it is even more pronounced than in man. In the chinchilla, for instance, there is nearly 20 dB of amplification of 2000 Hz relative to the lowest frequencies.

Dr. Davis: There is little to add. We do not have any good idea as to why there should be this upward displacement of the frequency of greatest threshold shift. Most of our thinking turns on temporary threshold shift and it is still to be determined what the sharpness of the loss may be for the permanent shift that might come from working for a long time in the presence of a noise with a strong pure-tone component.

Professor Burns: Mr. Ratcliffe's question raises the hypothetical situation as to what would happen to a person who had worked virtually in a pure tone for a long time. If that is the correct interpretation, we cannot add anything specific from the field study which has just been completed, because we did not have any noises which resembled this situation. But I would go back to the remarks which Dr. Robinson made earlier to the effect that we were ourselves surprised that the variety of spectra we encountered, with slopes one way or the other, did not produce different audiometric results. I think it would be fair to say that the kind of industrial situation which is characterized by a pure tone at 2000 Hz is not something that one finds every day; we did not find it in 6 years.

Dr. Coles: I would like to comment on one aspect of this frequency effect. Admittedly Professor Burns and Dr. Robinson were dealing with broad-band industrial noises, but if one turns to impulsive noises it is not in the 4-kHz region that maximum permanent threshold shifts occur but higher, at 6 and 8 kHz. So there is *some* limitation on the seeming constancy of audiometric effect: there is something particular to this kind of noise, perhaps the very-high-frequency components and sharp rise times. I have also done two other studies that bear on the effect of frequency. In one, the noise was a pure tone and the frequency of the persistent effects was about half an octave higher; unfortunately the noise was such as to cause the maximum shift in the 4-kHz region anyhow, as with Burns and Robinson's industrial noises, but it was quite remarkable how narrowly defined the notch was when measured at frequencies in steps of 500 Hz. The other study was concerned with jet aircraft noise. The men wore ear-muffs but were only partly protected because the muffs were in rather bad condition, with broken fluid seals, so that there was a loss of low-frequency attenuation. These people got persistent threshold shifts in the 0·5- to 1-kHz range. The aftermath of that story, though, was that the shifts recovered after several years; so their frequency relationships can only be related to the persistent, rather than the permanent, type of threshold shift.

Professor Burns: Perhaps I might clear up a point that Dr. Coles mentioned about the effect of frequency found in our work. I emphasize that we did not deal with impulsive noises of the sort referred to by Dr. Coles. I do not want to give the impression that we feel there is no relationship between frequency of stimulus and pattern of loss—that is not the case—but for the continuous sort of noise that we were dealing with, there was this surprisingly insensitive reaction to frequency.

Dr. Hinchcliffe: Perhaps I could also comment on the plausible and implausible explanations for the preferential site of noise-induced hearing loss at 4 kHz. The fact that sudden blows to the head, which can be considered as bone-conducted transients, can produce a 4-kHz notch on the audiogram surely makes the "external acoustic meatus resonance" theory an implausible one. Amongst the plausible explanations, I would suggest that one consider those given by Littler (1965) and by Schuknecht and Tonndorf (1960). Littler pointed out that the basal part of the cochlear partition lies in the path of vibratory motion between the fenestra vestibuli and the fenestra cochleae. Schuknecht and Tonndorf pointed out that the most effective acoustic stress is that frequency which, in terms of its travelling bulge, has the fastest rise time. The frequency of 4 kHz probably represents a compromise between the decrease in sensitivity of the cochlea towards higher frequencies and the increasing rise time.

Dr. Ward: I do not regard the resonance argument as the least probable explanation of the 4-kHz notch. Of course all the other suggestions may play some part, including the one based on the fact that there are two blood supplies to the cochlea, so that the place where they just meet, corresponding to about 4000 Hz, may not be getting as much nourishment. But if this were the case then one would expect that 4000 Hz would recover more slowly than the 3000 or 1000 Hz fibres when given a fixed amount of initial TTS, say 20 dB. This is what Lehnhardt showed not to be the case. I would just like to add one thing with which I am sure

Dr. Coles will agree. It should not be assumed, just because a person who comes into one's office shows a tonal gap with a maximum at 6000 Hz, that it was necessarily caused by gunfire; nor, conversely, that if the peak is at 4000 Hz it was necessarily caused by steady noise. There is only a statistical relation and in the individual case it does not really give one much to go on as to aetiology.

Section II

Practical Aspects

Some Sources of Variance in the Determination of Hearing Level

By

M. E. Delany

National Physical Laboratory, Teddington, England

Summary

Errors in objective calibration of audiometers or shifts in reference threshold due to progress in standardization may involve systematic discrepancies between the mean value of hearing level as determined by different investigators. On the other hand, error variance associated with subjective uncertainty as regards auditory threshold, or errors due to shift in observed threshold level due to progressive familiarization with the technique on the part of the subjects concerned, are particularly significant in studies involving serial audiometry.

Such sources of variance are discussed and estimates of their probable magnitude are given.

VARIANCE DUE TO DIFFERENT REFERENCE THRESHOLDS

In this paper two quite different sources of potential error inherent in any determination of hearing level are considered. The first concerns the purely objective aspects of audiometer calibration. It is important that any user of an audiometer should be aware of which reference threshold was used in setting up the calibration of the instrument. Even if one is prepared to accept the manufacturer's calibration initially, it is essential in reliable audiometry that frequent checks of the calibration should be carried out. Moreover, the position as regards standardization of reference levels is not yet stable on a time-scale which compares with the necessary duration of prospective studies, and a user may therefore be faced with a change in the basic reference threshold of his instrument of which he may be unaware. It is only by paying careful attention to the different standards and recommendations as they are implemented that the introduction of unnecessary (and possibly large) variance into such studies can be avoided. Similar problems also arise when comparing one's own results with those published by other workers.

Some 10 years ago lack of standardization in the field of audiometry caused severe difficulties. In the U.S.A. the reference threshold specified in American Standard Z24.5: 1951 relating to the WE 705A earphone when calibrated on the NBS-9A coupler was used. In the U.K. the threshold specified in British Standard BS 2497: 1954 relating to the STC 4026A earphone on the artificial ear specified in BS 2042: 1953 was used, and in Germany the threshold determined by PTB (Mrass and Diestel, 1959) relating to the DT 48 earphone on the NBS-9A coupler was generally employed. As shown in Fig. 36, these reference thresholds

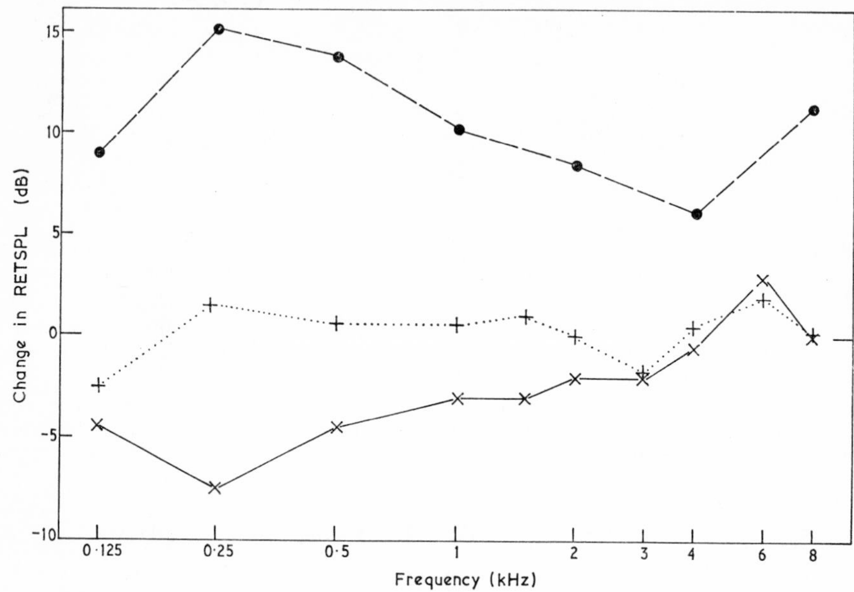

FIG. 36. Change in RETSPL associated with the adoption of ISO R389

—●— WE 705A/9A coupler (U.S.A.)
··+·· STC 4026A/BS 2042 (U.K.)
—×— DT 48/9A coupler (Germany)

differed by up to 22 dB, the American reference threshold averaging 10·5 dB higher than the British values and the German threshold 2·5 dB lower. The International Organization for Standardization (ISO) attempted to unify these threshold levels and their Recommendation R389 was published in 1964. This gives values of reference equivalent threshold sound pressure level (RETSPL) for five different combinations of reference type of earphone and artificial ear. The numerical manipulations behind the values contained in R389 have recently been disclosed (Weissler, 1968) and suggest an overall standard deviation for effective differences between the various entries of about 2 dB. However, error in the source material is of secondary importance, for R389 states that the reference levels shown in the various columns of the table all refer, as closely as could be ascertained from the available data, to the same auditory threshold. Carefully controlled tests have been carried out at NPL (Delany and Whittle, 1967) in which the threshold excitation voltages for several different types of earphone were determined using a group of 23 normal subjects and these values have been compared with those implied by R389 for three of the five combinations of earphone and artificial ear. Figure 37 shows that the maximum differences varied from 5 dB at 125 Hz to 9 dB at 8 kHz, and as the 95% confidence limit was 2 dB or less over most of the frequency range, these errors must be implicit in R389.

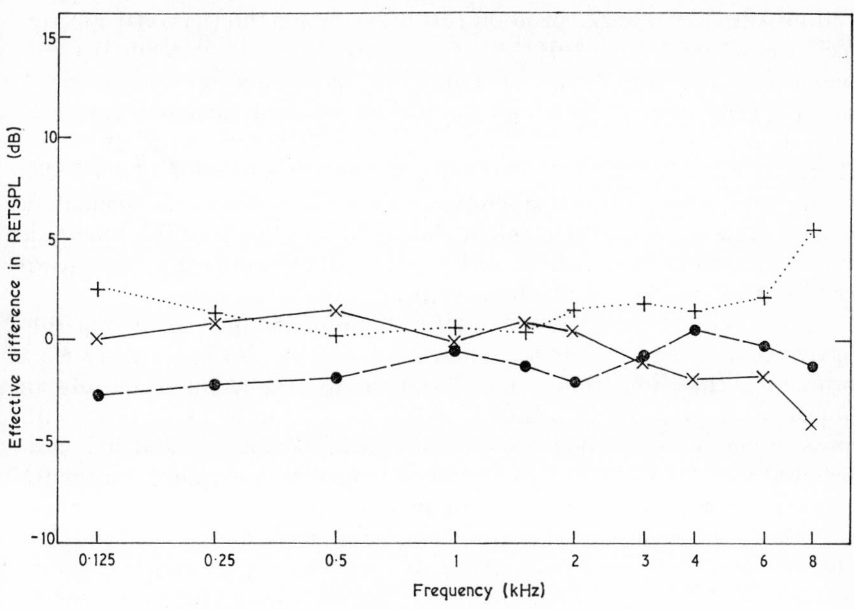

FIG. 37. Estimated difference in RETSPL inherent in R389

—●—	WE 705A/9A coupler	(U.S.A.)
··+··	STC 4026A/BS 2042	(U.K.)
—×—	DT 48/9A coupler	(Germany)

Further difficulties arise in that this specification relates only to the so-called reference earphone types (in Great Britain this is the 4026A), but these are hardly ever used on practical audiometers. To calibrate other types it would still be necessary to make a subjective comparison with a reference earphone. A number of such transfers have been carried out and in 1969 a supplement to BS 2497 was published (British Standards Institution, 1969) which gives values of RETSPL for the TDH39 earphone and for various PDR types; the equivalent ISO document is expected shortly.

Multiple specification of the reference threshold will always present a problem which becomes more acute with each additional item specified. There is a basic objection to the use of more than one type of artificial ear or coupler, particularly as not one of those referred to in R389 reproduces the acoustical characteristics of the human ear at all closely. As an interim measure only, it was agreed within ISO that the 9A coupler would be used to facilitate international comparisons, and an IEC publication on this coupler now exists (International Electrotechnical Commission, 1970a).

A new artificial ear has been introduced (Delany and Whittle, 1966) and an IEC Recommendation on this is available (International Electrotechnical Commission, 1970b). Because this artificial ear loads the earphone with the same acoustical impedance as the average human ear, a single specification of threshold for various types of earphone currently used in audiometry becomes feasible in place of the present multiplicity. Certainly recent NPL work shows that a single specification of RETSPL could involve less inherent discrepancy than the present arrangement. It is most important that agreement should be reached quickly, otherwise National Committees will probably proceed to standardize their own values of RETSPL and confusion will be further increased.

Although the transfer from one earphone to another involves a subjective transfer and entails the inherent variability associated with such a procedure, changing from one artificial ear to another involves only an objective transfer and in principle should be able to be made easily with an accuracy of $\pm 0{\cdot}2$ dB. However, difficulties have arisen and it is now believed that the figures given in 1969 for the 4026A earphone on the 9A coupler (British Standards Institution, 1969) are inconsistent with those previously specified for the same earphone on the BS Artificial Ear (British Standards Institution, 1968). As shown in Fig. 38, the discrepancy amounts to 3 dB at 2 kHz but reduces to zero at low and high frequencies. Fortunately the 4026A is not much used for clinical audiometry outside research establishments, its main function being to serve as a reference type; nevertheless, this discrepancy needs to be removed. Several other inconsistencies in the Standard also exist. For example, it has yet to be explained how the Audio 15 earphone was fitted to the 9A coupler to obtain the figures given—our examples of this earphone cannot be fitted to the coupler as the diameter of its aperture is too large. Further, different values of RETSPL are given for different models of PDR earphone when these are fitted with the same earcap (MX41/AR); it is almost certain that the differences between the values given are merely manifestations of the residual error of that Standard, because there is no reason to expect different values for these acoustically identical earphones.

Existing standards are deficient in other respects. For example, to date no method of calibrating circumaural earphones has been found which is satisfactory over the whole audiometric frequency range. The flat-plate

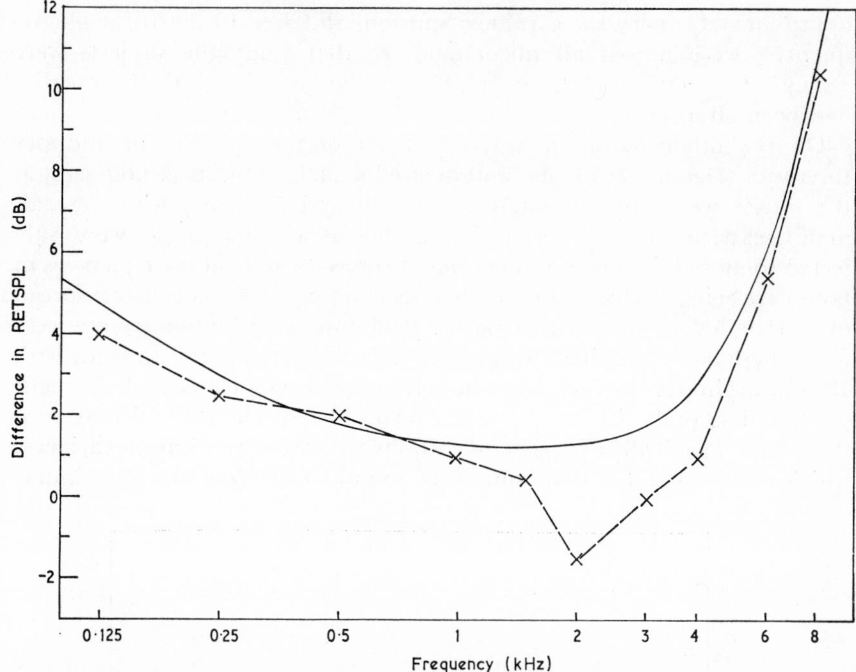

FIG. 38. Difference between values of RETSPL for the STC 4026A earphone on the British standard artificial ear (BS 2042) and on the 9A coupler:

—×— Implied by two parts of BS 2497 (Part 1:1968, Part 2:1969)
——— Recent NPL determination

coupler has proved acceptable only up to about 1 or 2 kHz and no real progress has yet been made on ways of adapting the IEC artificial ear to this type of earphone. Until a solution is found, the use of circumaural earphones in clinical audiometry is greatly inhibited.

VARIANCE DUE TO CERTAIN SUBJECTIVE FACTORS

We now consider one or two subjective factors which may enter into clinical measurements or into experiments involving determination of hearing level. If a person is subjected to repeated audiometry, the results obtained will not be identical on each and every occasion. If the subject is not well motivated, if pathology intervenes, or if he is exposed to intense noise levels, then the replication variance may well be very large indeed. Thus, Burns and Robinson (1970), from repeated tests on industrial control subjects not exposed to noise, found the replication variance was typically 20 dB^2 at 3 kHz and 76 dB^2 at 6 kHz, whilst subjects exposed to the highest noise levels showed a replication variance of approximately twice these values. Spurious shifts of 10–20 dB at all frequencies were not at all uncommon. In that study the subjects were somewhat selected and those with any obvious otological abnormality had been eliminated.

On the other hand, in a recent study of the stability of auditory threshold (Delany, 1970) the author used 4 male subjects (whose ages at the outset were approximately 20, 30, 40 and 50 years) who were all highly experienced in performing audiometric tests. They were subjected to 40 self-recorded audiograms, 4 complete tests at 6 frequencies in both ears being performed on each subject on each of 10 occasions spread over a period of about 27 months. Rudmose ARJ-4 audiometers were used, these being modified to produce pulsed test-tones and to work with 4026A earphones. In each case the left ear was tested first and the right ear tested second with no pause between. The results showed that with these audiometrically-experienced subjects the lowest replication variance, which occurred at 1–2 kHz, amounted to only 3 dB^2 (see Fig. 39). Similar

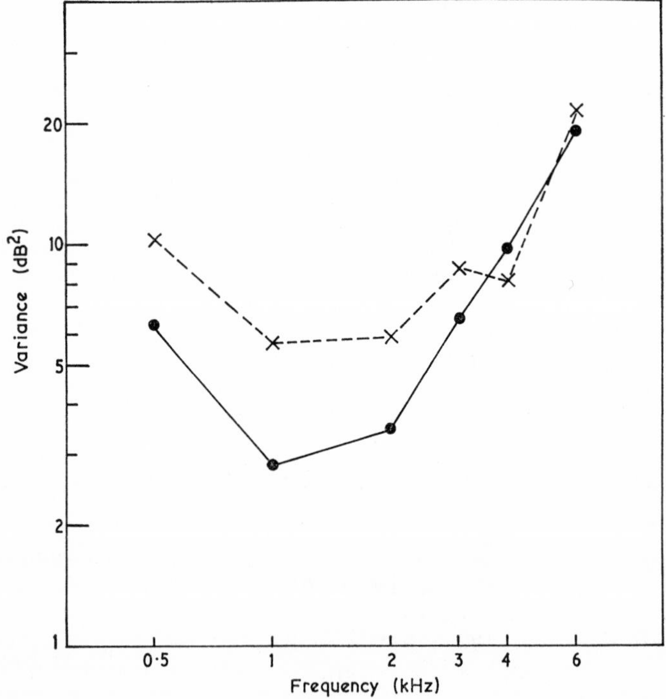

FIG. 39. Mean variance (between tests and between occasions) for 4 experienced subjects using self-recording technique.

—●— Left ears
-- × -- Right ears

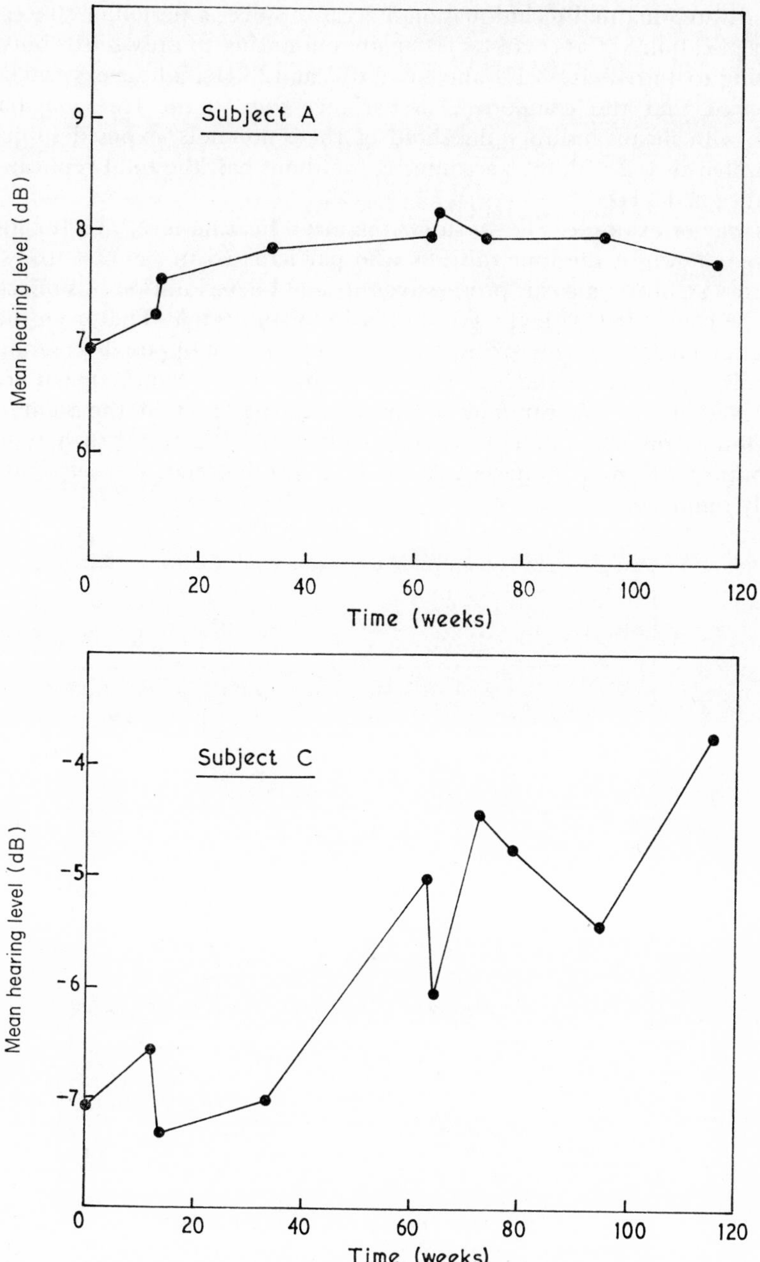

FIG. 40. Variation of mean hearing level with time for 2 subjects.

results were obtained with a further group of 8 subjects who were tested by 1 dB-step manual techniques on 5 occasions over a period of 30 weeks, the replication variance at 1 kHz again amounting to only 3 dB^2 but increasing to 15 dB^2 at 80 Hz and to 30 dB^2 at 12 kHz. These experiments suggested that the component of variance due to the true long-term changes in mean auditory threshold of these non-noise-exposed subjects amounted to 1–2 dB^2, thus accounting for about half the total replication variance at 1 kHz.

By way of example, Fig. 40 shows the mean hearing level as a function of time of two of the four subjects who participated in the first study of auditory stability; a clear, progressive threshold deterioration in subject C is to be contrasted with the great stability of subject A. That even these small long-term changes are real threshold shifts, as opposed to random error, is supported by the high correlation found between the mean hearing level in the left ear and the mean hearing level in the right ear determined on the different occasions. Figure 41 illustrates such results for one of the four subjects and, at 0·74, the correlation coefficient is highly significant.

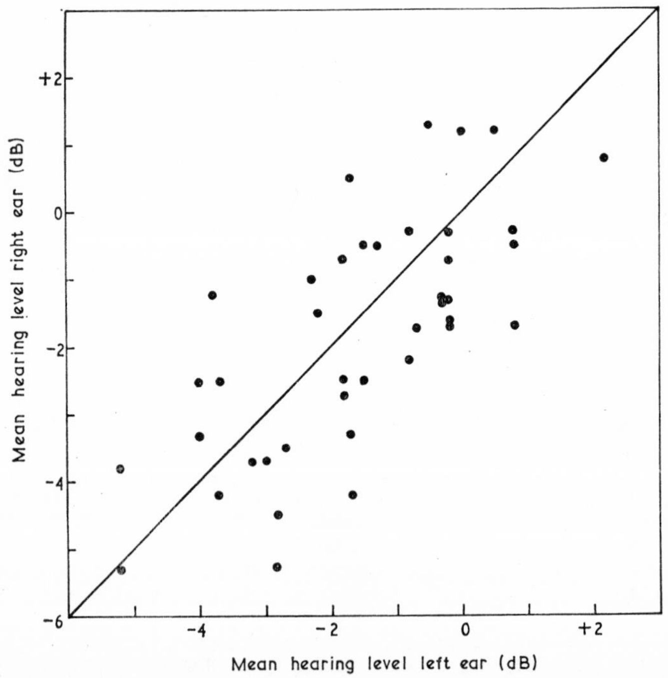

Fig. 41. Example of correlation between mean hearing level for the left and right ears (4 tests, 10 occasions, self-recording audiometry).

The type of earphone used to make measurements of auditory threshold can have a significant effect on the replication variance. Thus, whilst there is no significant difference in this respect between, say, the TDH39 earphone and the 4026A earphone, it is known that the liquid-seal circumaural earphone may exhibit a relatively greater replication variance. In tests carried out at NPL the replication variance for a typical liquid-seal circumaural device (Fig. 42) was comparable with, or

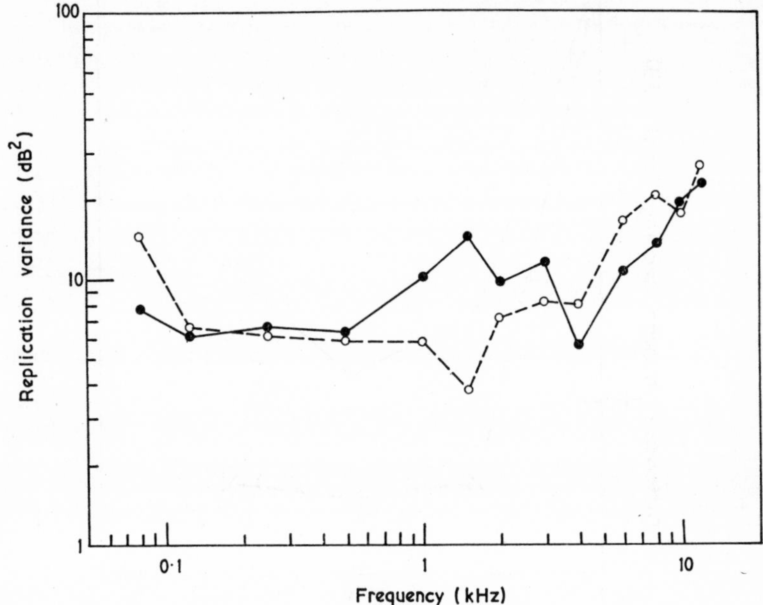

Fig. 42. Replication variance for threshold level determined using liquid-seal circumaural earphones.

—●— Circumaural earphones
- - ○ - - Mean for STC 4026A and TDH 39 earphones

even greater than, that obtained with STC 4026A earphones or with Telephonics TDH39 earphones over the audiometrically-important frequency range 0·5–3 kHz. Thus the merit of the liquid-seal circumaural earphone in conventional audiometry appears to reside mainly in its noise-excluding properties rather than in its reduced replication variance.

The use of different test methods can also introduce large additional variance. For example, it is known that self-recording techniques will generally yield lower values of hearing level than manual techniques. In an NPL study (Delany, Whittle and Knox, 1966) it was found that a regularly-pulsed self-recording technique gave mean values of hearing level up to 3·3 dB lower than 1-dB-step manual audiometry.

Even with the highly-experienced subjects, the second and subsequent tests on any one day indicated a hearing level approximately 1 dB lower (that is, more acute) than that given by the first audiometric test (see Fig. 43). With audiometrically naïve subjects a further apparent improve-

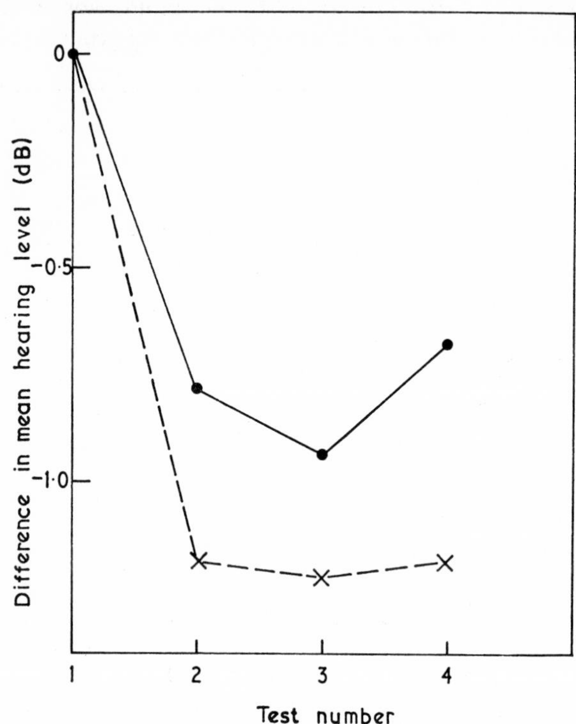

Fig. 43. Change in mean hearing level over 4 tests carried out on the same day. (Result obtained by averaging data obtained on 10 different occasions using self-recording audiometry.)

——●—— Left ears
– – × – – Right ears

ment in hearing level associated with familiarization with the technique is found and may continue over many tests, even though these are separated by days or weeks (Delany, 1970). A mean improvement of up to 9 dB averaged over 6 test frequencies in the range 0·5–6 kHz was observed with one group of schoolboys using self-recording audiometry, although from further experiments a value of 3 dB is probably more typical. This latter value is in accord with data extracted from unpublished work by J. J. Knight. Using self-recording audiometry, he tested each of 16 normally-hearing subjects twice a day for 5 consecutive days. As Fig. 44

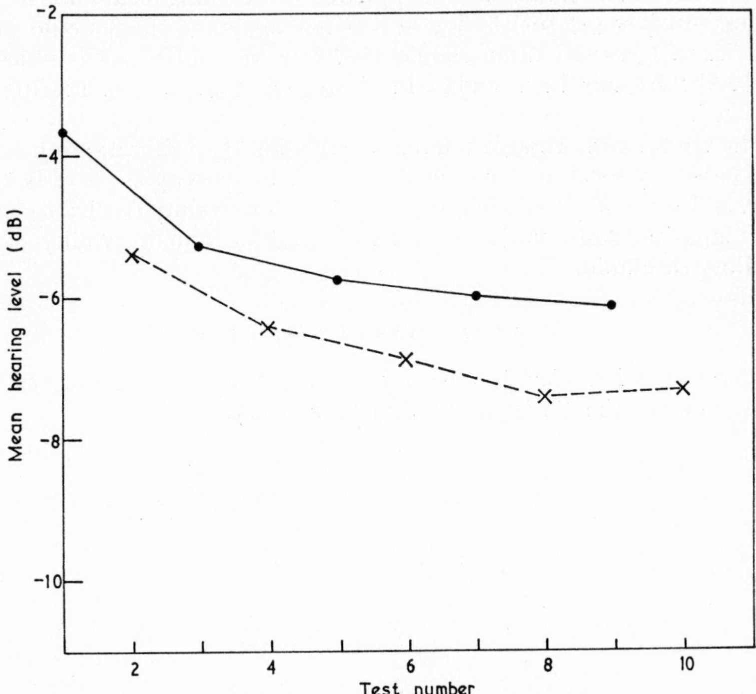

FIG. 44. Mean learning effects shown by 16 normally-hearing subjects with self-recording audiometry, performing 2 tests on each of 5 consecutive days (extracted from unpublished data obtained by J. J. KNIGHT).

——●—— First test on each day
– – × – – Second test on each day

shows, the second test on each day always indicated a significantly-improved hearing level compared with that of the first test. Moreover, even after 10 complete audiometric tests, the mean hearing level still appeared to be improving progressively.

CONCLUSIONS

Obviously a number of factors can operate together and combine to produce such a large residual variance that any genuine shifts in a particular experiment can be completely masked. For example, in serial audiometry the mean improvement in apparent hearing level due to familiarization effects could well more than outweigh any real deterioration due to exposure to moderate levels of industrial noise. On the other hand, if an experiment were, or could be, designed so that such effects were randomized, shifts due to practice or learning could inflate the residual variance to such a degree that few measured shifts would prove significant. Close attention should therefore be paid to such subjective factors before any field studies involving repeated tests of hearing are initiated.

The situation as regards reference levels for the calibration of audiometers is very much better than it was, say, 15 years ago. There is, however, still some way to go before calibration uncertainty can be neglected in comparison with subjective variance or long-term instability of the auditory threshold.

ACKNOWLEDGEMENT

The work described has been carried out as part of the research programme of the National Physical Laboratory.

Some Individual Factors influencing Audiometric Performance

By

S. D. G. Stephens

Medical Research Council, Cambridge and Teddington, England

Summary

Previous studies of the effects of tester and testee differences on auditory threshold measures are discussed. Two experiments are described. The first compared the variance of the "absolute" threshold with that of noise-masked thresholds, using Békésy audiometry. In this study, the variance for the frequencies 250 to 4000 Hz for the threshold in noise was significantly greater for extraverts than for introverts. Extraverts also showed a smaller leaning effect than did introverts.

In the second experiment, which considered Békésy-manual differences in naïve subjects, neurotic-extraverts differed from the other subjects. In this group the Békésy thresholds for the first three frequencies of the first ear tested were less sensitive than the manual thresholds. For the first frequency tested, this group also showed significantly greater variability than other subjects. These differences disappeared on further testing.

INTRODUCTION

With the enormous increase in air travel and its resultant noise over the past few years, the existence of individual differences in response to what is essentially an auditory stimulus has become more generally apparent. Thus most people are now aware that loud noises may have very different quantitative effects on their tense neurotic friends and on their more placid acquaintances. In recent laboratory studies of loudness estimation and uncomfortable loudness level (Stephens, 1970a, 1970b), the subjects' anxiety level has been found to influence the results obtained, as was seen earlier in galvanic skin response (GSR) studies (Bitterman and Holtzman, 1952). It would thus not be surprising if some of the intersubject differences found in various threshold measures were related to aspects of the psychological make-up of the individual concerned.

It has been shown (Swets, 1961) that subjective thresholds are determined by two largely independent processes, the detection mechanism of the subject, and his judgemental criterion. Consequently it would appear that there is sufficient potential for threshold measures of an individual subject to be affected by both his own personality, and also to a lesser extent, that of the tester, with the concomitant interaction of the two. These factors will obviously attain varying degrees of importance according to the test procedure used, and the population tested, whether naïve or experienced, of normal or impaired hearing.

THE INFLUENCE OF THE TESTER ON AUDIOMETRIC MEASURES

The bias arising from the audiometrician in manual audiometry stems mainly from his judgemental decision in the selection of a criterion for the threshold. This assumes particular significance when he is testing subjects who make large numbers of false positive responses (that is, they respond that they hear a signal when none is in fact present) which, as workers applying signal detection theory (Swets, 1961) have shown, may considerably influence the apparent threshold. This is more important in normal hearing subjects than in those with recruitment, who have a steeper psychophysical function relating intensity to detectability, at least for short durations (Counter and Tobin, 1969). Lesser influences of the tester's personality are mediated through his instructions and encouragement to the subject, and his care and accuracy in recording the threshold measures.

A number of studies (Jackson *et al.*, 1962; Rapin and Costa, 1969) refer, with somewhat conflicting findings, to the effect of various testers on the results obtained in manual audiometry. There appears to be no work that has set out to investigate this point systematically and there would surely be scope to apply a rigorous study on the lines of that used by Delany (1970) in his detailed investigation of the sources of variance in Békésy audiometry. This study could entail a number of repeated threshold measures made on a small group of experienced subjects by a range of audiometricians of varying experience and motivation. The fact that the expectancy of the tester under these conditions can affect the outcome of the test has been shown in various psychological experiments recently summarized by Rosenthal (1969).

It might be assumed that Békésy audiometry would obviate any observer effects. This is certainly true of major effects, but minor effects may stem from the enthusiasm which the tester imbues in the subject, an effect which may be partly overcome by issuing the subject with standard written instructions. A further source of observer bias comes in the reading of the Békésy tracings, but this may be easily overcome by two observers reading the cards independently, with a further observer checking in the case of discrepant results. This was the procedure followed in the recent MRC–NPL survey on industrial hearing loss (Burns and Robinson, 1970).

The development of techniques of "objective" audiometry, based on the average evoked electroencephalographic response (ERA) to repeated auditory stimuli, led to the pious hope that the results would be independent of both tester and subject. With this technique, repeated identical auditory stimuli are presented to the subject and the averaged change in the EEG evoked by these stimuli is found by use of an analogue computer. Unfortunately the results of this complicated and expensive technique are not as simple as might have been expected. The measure is objective in that it does not require any physical response from the subject, but Wilkinson *et al.* (1966) have shown that the size of the $P_1 - N_1$ complex may be related to the subject's level of arousal. As this complex is the main constituent of the waveform taken as an assessment of the auditory response, this could have important consequences on any measures obtained. Apart from any gross effects caused by sleep deprivation, temperature or drugs, the subject's level of arousal may be influenced by the tester and his attitude and enthusiasm towards the test.

In many ways a more important effect of the attitudes and personality of the tester lies in his interpretation of the waveform tracings. At and around threshold level it is often very difficult to distinguish whether or not a response is present, and it seems certain that the interpretation of results in this region will vary quite considerably from individual to individual. No study has been made of this effect nor even of the effect of the personality of the subject on the results obtained, where one might predict that the interrelation between introversion–extraversion and level of arousal, shown by Corcoran (1965) in vigilance studies, might have some bearing.

THE SUBJECT AND AUDIOMETRIC RESULTS

There is obviously rather more potential for the audiometric measures to be influenced by the personality of the subject than by that of the tester. It has long been postulated by Teplov and other disciples of Pavlov working in Russia (Gray, 1964) that individuals with a "strong" nervous system will have less sensitive thresholds than those with a "weak" nervous system, in which there is less inhibitory activity. These concepts of strong and weak nervous systems have been equated by some workers to the extraverts and introverts of Eysenck's terminology. Thus Eysenck (1967) has advanced the concept that introverts should have a more sensitive absolute auditory threshold then extraverts, and refers to an experiment by Smith (1968) as support for his hypothesis. Unfortunately, the number of subjects in that study was small and the methodology rather different from orthodox audiometric practice. A subsequent study on 38 naval ratings at Cambridge (Stephens, 1969) using both Hughson-Westlake (1944) and two-alternative forced-choice techniques failed to confirm this finding. Further studies using both Békésy and manual audiometry on various groups of audiometrically naïve housewives at Teddington by Whittle and a large study by Bryan *et al.* at Salford on 178 members of the university staff using manual audiometry have likewise failed to confirm this finding. These studies are not yet published.

The author's study (Stephens, 1969) used a combination of the standard Hughson–Westlake technique and a two-interval temporal forced-choice technique in order to separate the components of variance caused by variations in the sensitivity of the detection mechanism from those caused by variations in the judgemental criterion. The detection threshold was measured by taking as the threshold an arbitrary level of $d' = 1{\cdot}00$, and finding the intensity required to produce this level of detectability. The two-method approach showed that the level of neuroticism of the subjects was related to their judgemental variance, neurotic subjects having significantly more variance than stable subjects. It also showed that extraverts had larger variance in their detection mechanisms than introverts, a concept which could be explained in terms of fluctuations in the efferent tonus. Thus with manual audiometry the smallest overall variance was found in the stable introverts and the largest in the neurotic extraverts.

As the subject has complete control over the stimulus level in Békésy audiometry, personal differences might be expected to play an even more important role than in manual audiometry. Shepherd and Goldstein (1966, 1968) have shown the size of the excursion of Békésy tracings to be related to measures of anxiety, depression and defensiveness as assessed by the Minnesota multiphasic personality inventory (MMPI) (Dahlstrom and Welsh, 1960). They found, however, that small day-to-day fluctuations in the excursion amplitude of individual subjects could not be explained in the daily anxiety fluctuations as assessed by the Cattell IPAT 8-Parallel-Form anxiety battery (Cattell, 1962). Some of the variability in excursion size may be related to the subject's reaction time, which both Reason (1968) and Russian workers (Gray, 1964) have shown to be influenced by the personality of the subject.

Apart from these two studies on the influence of the subject's personality on the Békésy-excursion amplitude, possible influences on Békésy variance have not been considered. This is true for both Békésy determinations at "true" threshold and for noise-masked thresholds. Furthermore no study appears to have been made on the possibility of personality effects on the difference between the Békésy-determined thresholds and standard manually-determined thresholds. I present below the findings of a small experiment on the influence of personality, more particularly introversion on Békésy audiometry, and also data extracted from a larger study on the influence of the subjects' neuroticism and introversion on Békésy-manual differences.

A SMALL STUDY ON BÉKÉSY AUDIOMETRY

The main purpose of this study was to compare the variance found in determinations of the absolute threshold with that found in determinations of a noise-masked threshold, using a controlled external noise source.

(*a*) Subjects and equipment

Thirteen members of the staff of MRC and NPL were used as subjects. All had previous experience of auditory testing. The testing was performed with the subject in an audiometric test booth within the audiometry laboratory in NPL.

The stimuli were produced using a Rudmose ARJ-5 audiometer which included a noise source and mixing facilities. The earphones used were type TDH39 in MX41/AR cushions. The sound pressure levels were checked at the beginning and end of the experiment using a Brüel and Kjær 9A coupler and type 2112 audio-frequency spectrometer. The frequencies were checked and found to be within British Standard specifications.

(*b*) Method

The left-ear thresholds of each subject were determined at the same time of day on 4 days of 1 week. These thresholds were determined for the frequencies 250, 500, 750, 1000, 1500, 2000, 3000, 4000, 5000, 6000, 7000 and 8000 Hz. In each case the absolute threshold was determined first to obviate any TTS effects from the masking noise used in the noise-masked threshold determinations. Masking by 60 dB SPL of white noise was used. The Heron (1956) inventory of introversion and neuroticism was completed by each subject.

(*c*) Results

I. VARIANCE

Figure 45 gives the variance for the absolute threshold and for the noise-masked threshold, and shows a considerably smaller variance in the latter condition. The increased variance above 4000 Hz was found in both methods and may be attributable to earphone positioning; so, in further considerations of the data, the frequencies 5000 to 8000 Hz will be omitted. In the threshold-in-noise study where the overall variance is reduced, due presumably to the replacement of fluctuant internal noise with relatively constant external noise as a basis of the task, the judgemental component of variance will presumably be less, so that the test becomes more of a detection task. Thus the finding that the mean variance at the frequencies 250–4000 Hz was significantly ($P < 0{\cdot}01$) less in introverts than in extraverts is compatible with the previous study. This difference in variance was significant at five of the eight frequencies studied, and is shown in Fig. 46.

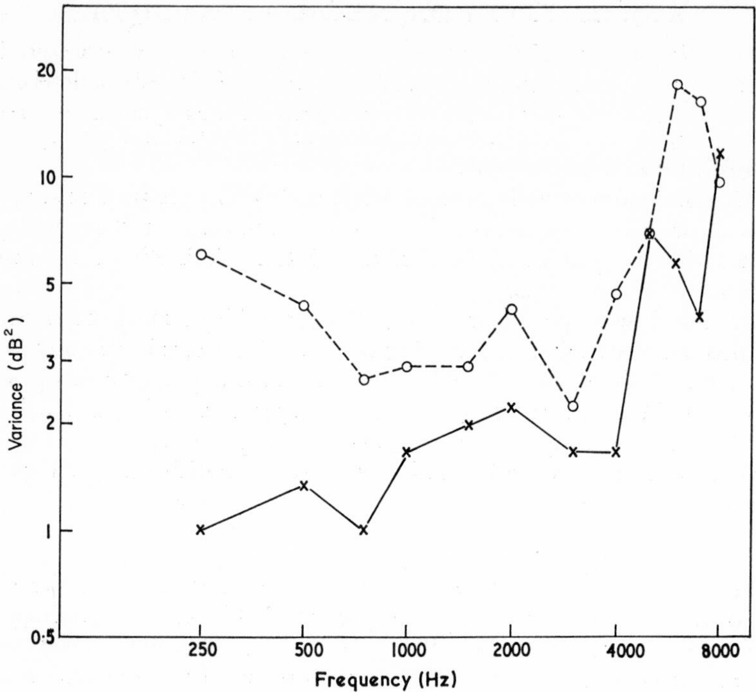

FIG. 45. Median intrasubject variance with Békésy audiometry; $N = 13$.
– – ○ – – Threshold variance
——×—— Threshold-in-noise variance

II. LEARNING EFFECT

Delany (1970) has shown that in Békésy audiometry there appears to be a peculiar learning effect which may be shown when the first absolute threshold measure obtained at any frequency is compared with the mean of any subsequent measures at that frequency. Thus there appears to be an increasing learning effect as one passes through the first three frequencies, followed by a gradual lessening of this until the sixth frequency shows no improvement, and sometimes less sensitive thresholds are found on retesting. Although different frequencies were used, a similar pattern of results was found independently in the present experiment. Figure 47 shows that introverts and extraverts showed different degrees of learning while conforming to the same overall pattern of results. The differences at 1000 Hz were significant ($P < 0{\cdot}05$) despite the small numbers involved, and an analysis of variance showed introversion to be a significant component of variance ($P < 0{\cdot}02$). These differences were in line with the relatively more rapid decline in performance found in extraverts in a rather uninteresting task.

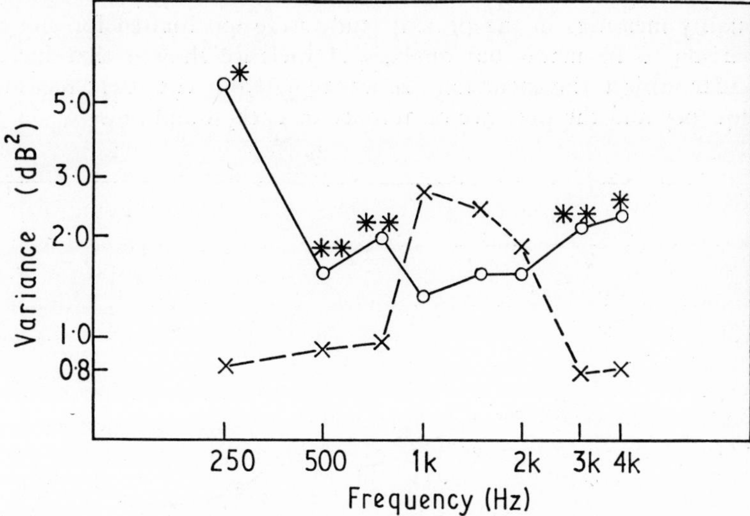

FIG. 46. Median threshold-in-noise variance.

– – × – – Introverts
——○—— Extraverts
Significance levels: *$p < 0·05$; **$p < 0·01$.

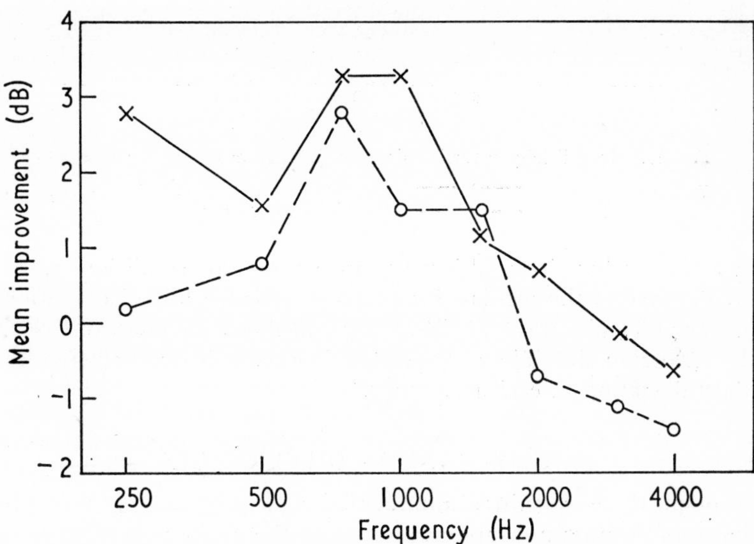

FIG. 47. Mean learning effect in Békésy audiometry.

——×—— Introverts
– – ○ – – Extraverts

Finally in regard to Shepherd and Goldstein's findings (1966, 1968) the personality measures in the present study were too limited for any real comparison to be made, but analysis of variance showed that for any particular subject, the excursion size was remarkably consistent regardless of frequency and the presence or absence of background noise.

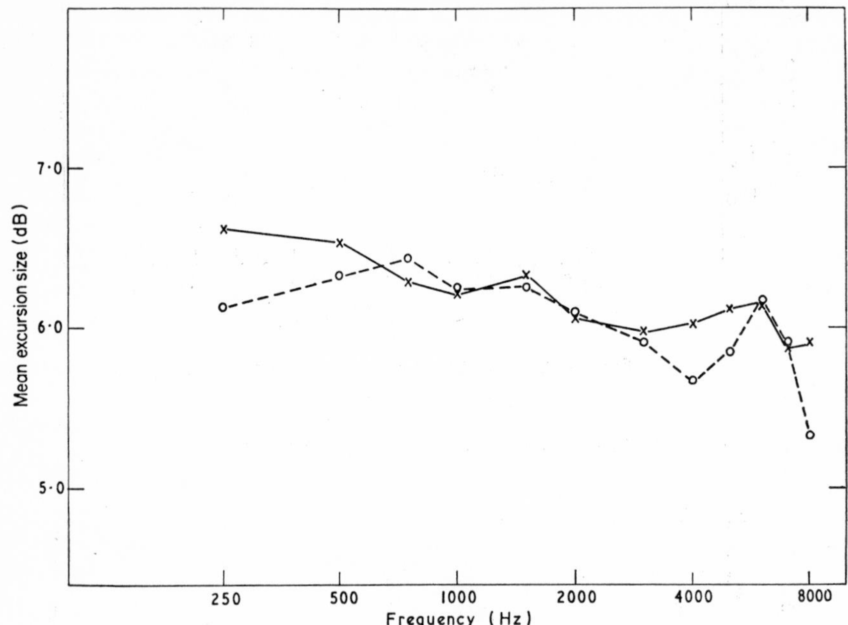

FIG. 48. Mean Békésy excursion size as a function of frequency; $N = 39$.
—x— Threshold
- - o - - Threshold in noise

Thus the median intrasubject variance across all conditions was only 1·13 dB², whereas the median intersubject variance for all conditions of frequency and noise was 3·01 dB². Figure 48 shows the effect of frequency on the excursion size. The change with frequency is small relative to the standard deviation at each frequency.

BÉKÉSY-MANUAL DIFFERENCES

Although there remain a number of dissenting voices, the general consensus of opinion now appears to favour the use of Békésy audiometry in large-scale surveys. However, much of the work on which the international standard is based is derived from studies using manual audiometry, and thus any differences between the results obtained with the two methods is of obvious relevance. Burns and Hinchcliffe (1957) and a number of subsequent workers have compared the results obtained using the two methods, but the majority of these studies have used relatively sophisticated subjects. Most subjects involved in any large-scale survey would be audiometrically naïve, and in order to remedy the lack of data for such subjects, a study was carried out by Whittle at the National Physical Laboratory on a large group of naïve suburban housewives. From these data (not yet published) it was possible to extract a group of 38 normal hearing subjects who were subdivided into four groups on the basis of their Heron (1956) scores of introversion and neuroticism.

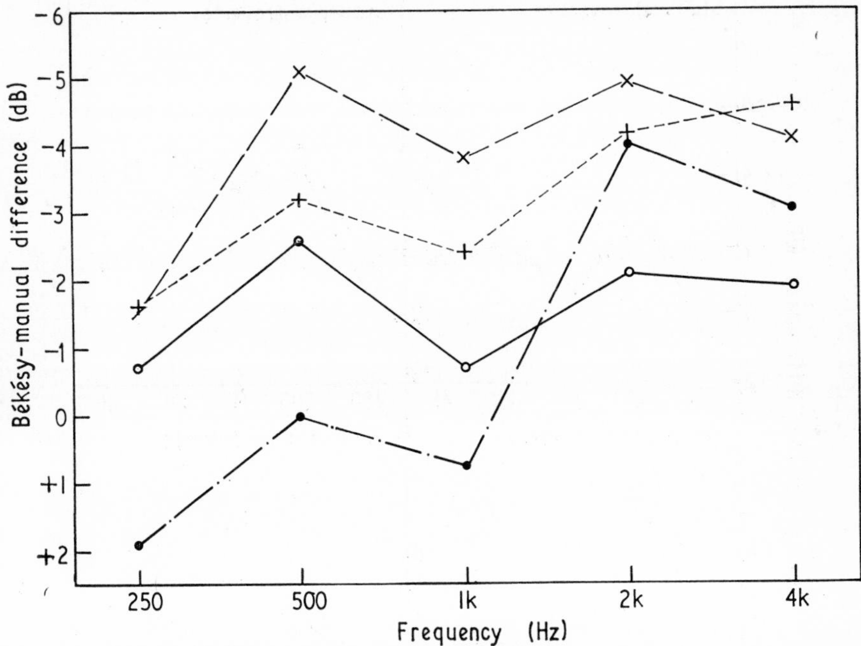

FIG. 49. Mean Békésy-manual difference for the first ear tested, for four groups of subjects.

——×—— Stable introverts; $N = 6$
– – + – – Neurotic introverts: $N = 11$
——○—— Stable extraverts: $N = 13$
•——●——• Neurotic extraverts; $N = 8$

The study was conducted in a systematic way using the Rudmose ARJ-5 audiometer which can be used for either Békésy or manual audiometry. In half the subjects the thresholds were determined by Békésy audiometry first and in the other half by manual audiometry first. The frequencies 250, 500, 1000, 2000, 4000, 6000 and 8000 Hz were used. All manual determinations within this group were performed by the same audiometrician. As in the previous experiment, the equipment was calibrated before and after testing.

Figure 49 shows the mean Békésy-manual differences in the four groups of subjects for the first ear tested. A positive value indicates that the Békésy measure implied less sensitive hearing than the manual measure. It will be seen that in the neurotic extraverts the Békésy threshold is relatively less sensitive than the manual threshold for the first three frequencies tested ($P < 0{\cdot}05$). This difference disappears with the second ear tested. Figure 50 shows the Békésy-manual differences for the first ear

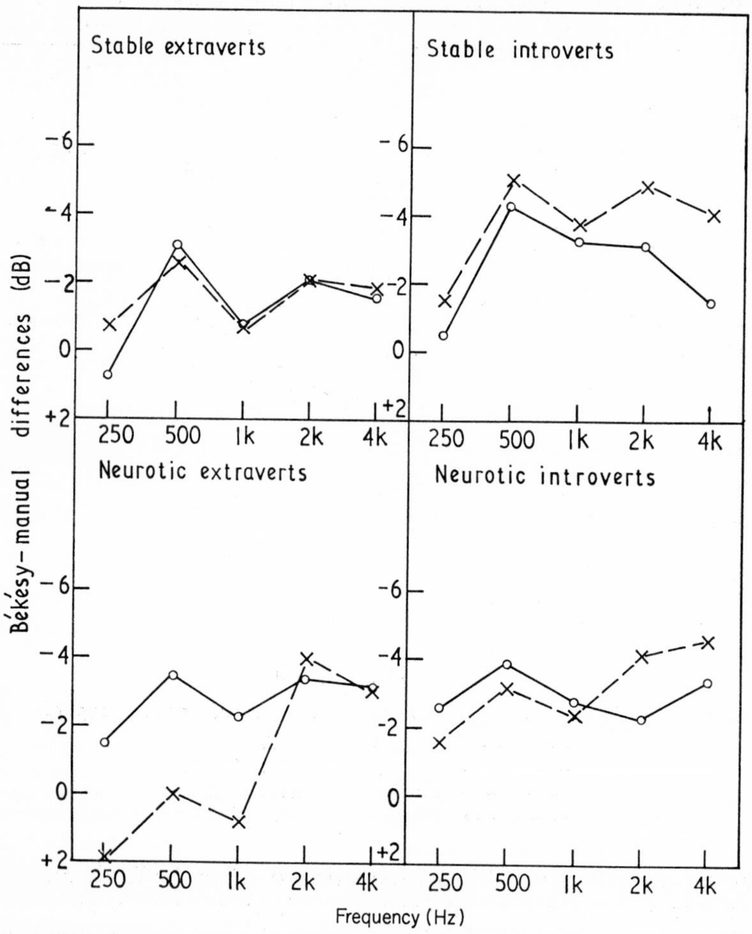

Fig. 50. Békésy-manual differences for 4 groups of subjects (Fig. 49) comparing the first and second ears tested.

– – × – – First ear
——○—— Second ear

compared with the second ear in each of the four personality groups, the difference in the neurotic extraverts for the first three frequencies being significant ($P < 0{\cdot}01$). These results would tend to suggest that the difference is essentially a learning effect and that these hysterics (neurotic extraverts) take longer to settle down to the idea of Békésy audiometry than do other subjects. This is borne out by two indirect measures of variability of the results which show that neurotic extraverts have significantly more variability for the first frequency tested than do the other groups of subject. This difference disappears with subsequent frequencies and is not seen in the second ear tested.

As it was impossible to obtain any direct variance measures on these subjects, two indirect measures which are independent of each other were devised. Comparing the left–right ear differences for Békésy and manual thresholds gave one measure of variance and the second took the overall Békésy-manual differences regardless of sign, for each ear separately. The first measure shows a significantly increased difference ($P < 0{\cdot}05$) at 250 Hz among the neurotic extraverts and the second shows the same for the first ear tested ($P < 0{\cdot}001$), but not for the second ear tested. This study would thus further serve to emphasize the importance of repeated determinations in the assessment of hearing level.

DISCUSSION AND CONCLUSIONS

The picture presented above is essentially that for normal-hearing subjects. This may become further complicated when considering subjects with various forms of hearing defect, which may have a higher incidence of abnormal personalities associated with them. Chaiklin and Ventry (1963), reviewing the literature of patients with non-organic hearing loss, found a predominance of neurotic and psychosomatic personalities. Perhaps of more importance, even in more organic causes of hearing loss such as Ménière's disease and, more surprisingly, otosclerosis, Hinchcliffe (1965, 1967c) has found a higher incidence of neuroticism than in the normal-hearing population. In view of the findings of Ingham (1966) and others, that patients become less neurotic as their physical or psychiatric condition improves, it would be interesting to know whether this difference found in otosclerotics disappears after stapedectomy.

The overall results of this study suggest that individual differences appear to affect the variability of audiometric results rather than their absolute sensitivity. It would thus emphasize the importance of obtaining repeated determinations of threshold on any one occasion in order to obtain a true measure of the subject's hearing level. Thus if time is limited it would appear to be more valuable to measure the hearing several times at a few frequencies rather than to try to cover a wide range of frequencies just once. The only qualification of this effect lies in the domain of the learning effect but here the effect is small and the results presented are based on such a small study that any conclusions must be tentative until further studies on this effect are completed.

ACKNOWLEDGEMENT

I would like to thank Mr. L. S. Whittle for allowing me access to the raw data of his study on Békésy-manual difference. The experiments described were carried out by the author at the National Physical Laboratory while working as a detached member of the staff of the MRC Applied Psychology Unit, Cambridge.

Hearing Conservation and Noise Control in Industry Organized and Performed by the Accident Branch of the Austrian Social Security Board

By

A. Surböck

Allgemeine Unfallversicherungsanstalt, Vienna, Austria

In Austria, as in many other European countries, special insurance against the consequences of industrial accidents and occupational diseases comes within the scope of statutory social security. The main responsibilities of the accident insurance institutions, which are the competent organizations, are

(a) prevention of industrial accidents and occupational diseases
(b) therapeutic treatment
(c) compensation in respect of industrial accidents and occupational diseases.

Compulsory industrial accident insurance has existed in Austria since 1889. In 1928 a decree was issued concerning occupational diseases, certain scheduled diseases being treated as industrial accidents as from 1st March of that year. In the course of time the schedule has been supplemented several times so that it comprises at present 39 diseases.

Along with silicosis, industrial skin diseases and infectious diseases of hospital staff, noise-induced hearing impairment ranks among the most-commonly occurring of occupational diseases. Our institution, the Allgemeine Unfallversicherungsanstalt, is the social security branch for all employees except those in agriculture, forestry or on the railways.

Up to 1961 occupational hearing loss caused by noise had no particular numerical importance within the scope of social security accident insurance, because noise-induced deafness attracted compensation only if it had been acquired in certain enterprises specified by law. These limitations were abolished in 1962 by an amendment of the legal provisions. Hence the necessity to give more attention to preventive measures.

We began organizing technical and medical measures to abate industrial noise in 1962. The medical aspects include the periodical checking of the auditory status of work people, the making of recommendations regarding hearing protection devices, and the assessment of fitness for work under noise exposure. Technical activities include noise measurements and the preparation of expert appraisals on measures for noise abatement in workshops.

Audiometric investigations and technical measurements are carried out for industry free of charge. The regular examinations of employees are guaranteed by systematic serial examinations. Serial audiometry is conducted on site in the factories, using vehicles specially constructed for the purpose. Those used for the medical examinations consist of three compartments. One of these is a waiting room from which the employee proceeds to an office where he is questioned in detail as to his occupational history and possible ear affections, head injuries, acute acoustic traumata, etc. After that he enters the examination room containing an audiometric booth, for the audiometric investigations. The whole facility, including heating and ventilation, can be operated either from the mains supply or from a battery installed on the vehicle. In our opinion the equipment of the vehicles is very important as the speed of carrying out the examinations depends upon it.

The object of these examinations is the quick recording of many employees: after exploring the medical history and occupational anamnesis, testing is confined to checking the pure-tone air-conduction audiogram at frequencies from 128 to 8192 Hz, supplemented by bone-conduction if necessary. Naturally it is not feasible in this mass examination to test each employee after a prolonged interval away from work, but this is not necessary for serial examinations of a purely screening character. The results of serial examinations are classified by a method that we have developed which selects appropriate cases for referral to an otologist for further examination. The results of the serial examinations, as well as the medical data, are fed into a computer, the following data being coded:

MEDICAL DATA FOR COMPUTER

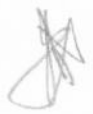

(1) Family name
(2) First name
(3) Maiden name
(4) Sex
(5) Factory
(6) Occupation
(7) Ear affections
(8) Head injuries
(9) Acute noise exposure
(10) Commencement of hearing loss (year)
(11) Commencement of tinnitus (year)

(12) Commencement of headache (year)
(13) Type of hearing protection and
(14) Length of time used
(15) Length of exposure
(16) Length of military service
(17) Branch of armed services
(18) Date of examination
(19) Examiner
(20) Noise level
(21) Number of the point of measurement
(22) Damage-risk criteria
(23) Air-conduction (128–11,584 Hz)
(24) Bone-conduction if necessary.
(25) Audiological diagnosis.

In order to perform a rapid classification of large numbers of audiograms we have evolved threshold templates relating tolerable hearing losses to age and length of exposure to noise. These thresholds are computer-processed and serve to eliminate all cases requiring no further action. If the curve of an audiogram shows an inconspicuous course and does not surpass the appropriate template, the case is classified ∅ by the computer. Other cases, including all those with bone-conduction curves, are assessed by our medical adviser. To facilitate visual assessment, the computer draws the audiogram curves by means of a plotter, and prints out all the important anamnestic data. Next the classification of the printed cases by the medical specialist is added to the other data in the computer. Subsequently the computer prints out lists of names of persons examined and also indicates what further action is needed in each case. Reports on the audiometric investigations are sent to the factory management and to the Factory Inspectorate. The measures indicated in the report, primarily examinations by a medical consultant, are arranged by another department of our institute, this department being responsible for handling individual cases right through to an eventual grant of compensation. The results of all the medical examinations obtained on individual cases in the course of the compensation process are, as already mentioned, stored in the computer. The medical data from all audiometric examinations of individuals are available at any time, and the rapidly growing number of our examinations has led to a steady improvement in the observation of the course of the affections.

Before adopting our threshold templates their validity was checked in the light of hundreds of cases. No defects have been discovered by subsequent checks.

Between November 1962 and December 1969 we conducted a total of 91,016 examinations in our vehicles, as shown in Table XVIII. In 5% of

TABLE XVIII. Serial investigations: breakdown by industry (in descending order)

Industry	Number of examinations	Industry	Number of examinations
Metals	43,548	Paper	3492
Textiles	12,869	Power	2115
Stone	7726	Transport	1187
Mining	6254	Leather	823
Chemicals	4285	Printing	467
Wood	4115	Building	307
Foodstuffs	3797	Other	31
	Total 91,016		

cases, an advanced hearing loss due to noise has been found. In 10% of cases a medical check has been necessary in order to clarify the hearing status, and 1% of all persons examined received compensation on account of loss of earning capacity; in order to qualify, the noise-induced hearing loss has to be assessed at 20% or more. Compensation is, of course, only granted on an otologist's opinion, based on the otological examination and on audiometric measurements using pure tones and speech. The assessment of loss of earning capacity is carried out in conformity with the recommendations of Boenninghaus and Röser (1958).

TABLE XIX. Compensation cases: breakdown by year of award

Granted in	Number of cases	Granted in	Number of cases
1947	1	1959	1
1948	—	1960	1
1949	—	1961	3
1950	1	1962	34
1951	1	1963	101
1952	1	1964	85
1953	1	1965	172
1954	3	1966	83
1955	1	1967	88
1956	1	1968	38[a]
1957	2	1969	17[a]
1958	1		

[a] Figures for 1968 and 1969 are provisional as not all the cases have yet been settled.

The number of cases in which compensation for occupational hearing loss was granted up to the end of 1969 amounts to 635. Up to the end of 1961 there had been only 18 cases. The growth of cases is shown in Table XIX.

Most of the compensation cases come from the metal industry. The breakdown of cases industry by industry is shown in Table XX and the age structure in Table XXI.

TABLE XX. Compensation cases: breakdown by industry (in descending order)

Industry	Number of cases	Industry	Number of cases
Metals	437	Chemicals	8
Textiles	53	Power	5
Stone	41	Transport	2
Wood	31	Foodstuffs	2
Mining	23	Leather	2
Paper	19	Other	2
Building	10		

TABLE XXI. Age structure of persons receiving compensation on 1st January 1970

Age class	Number of cases
1881–1885	1
1886–1890	1
1891–1895	9
1896–1900	33
1901–1905	142
1906–1910	210
1911–1915	146
1916–1920	31
1921–1925	38
1926–1930	14
1931–1935	6
1936–1940	4
Total	635

We also developed a standardized procedure for the technical measures. At each factory visited the noise levels in dB(A), dB(B), dB(C) and LIN are measured in all noisy departments. If the dB(A) value exceeds 80, we measure the sound pressure level in octave bands. This analysis furnishes a general view of noise conditions in the whole factory and facilitates a schematic assessment of the hearing loss risks at particular working places. To assess the admissibility of noise stress, we use the principles of the CHABA report (Kryter *et al.*, 1966), which in our experience best takes account of all the noise configurations occurring in the factories. From the tables in the CHABA Report, we obtain the permissible duration of the noise exposure. All these particulars are communicated to the factory in a report which includes diagrams of the measurements. The results of noise measurement are also processed by computer. For each factory we have the following data:

TECHNICAL DATA FOR COMPUTER, FOR EACH MEASURING POSITION

(1) Factory
(2) Type of factory
(3) Designation of measurement point
(4) Type of machine or device
(5) Type of measuring instrument
(6) Date of measurement
(7) Technician
(8) General description of the noise including permissible working time
(9) Noise level in dB(A), dB(B), dB(C) and LIN
(10) Sound pressure level in octave bands from 31·5 to 31,500 Hz.

In regard to the technical measurements, it is most important to adhere to a precise and uniform system, not only for the method of measurement but also for the selection of measuring positions. To characterize the latter, we compiled a large catalogue for all the machinery, equipment and working conditions involved, and at the present time this comprises 1000 items. The idea of this catalogue is to enable us in the future to extract information quickly, from computer, on the noise-level values of any given machine, etc. Compilation of the relevant data has not yet, in fact, been brought to a close.

Routine noise measurements and serial audiometry are repeated at intervals of 4 to 6 years. The results of control examinations and measurement are also processed by computer.

An advisory service to industry, provided by specialized engineers of our institution, also comes within the scope of technical noise abatement. This activity is manifold, ranging from short consultations on the spot to the elaboration of experts' reports on safety measures. Up to now 203 of these memoranda have been prepared, and further development in this field of activity is being particularly intensified in order to encourage as many factories as possible to adopt technical safety measures. As this positive service is given free of charge, a constantly rising number of factories is applying to us for information and advice. To this end, we maintain lists of firms producing or marketing sound-absorbing and soundproofing materials or which are engaged in other aspects of technical noise control.

In addition to the Management, both the Factory Inspectorate and the Works Council are informed of the results of medical examinations and technical measurements in order that they may co-operate in the enforcement of safety measures within the scope of their statutory functions.

Within the limits of our facilities, working groups are dealing with particular scientific problems. For instance, we assist candidates for academic degrees in carrying out experimental work, the results of which are of practical interest to us. As an example I may cite:

(a) does the recovery from TTS depend on its mode of origin?
(b) what is the influence of white noise of 75 and 85 dB on the rate of recovery from TTS?

To accomplish these tasks, the staff of our Department for Occupational Diseases and their Prevention consists currently of 21 people: 4 engineers, 3 measurement technicians, 6 audiometricians, 8 administrative staff and assistants. Add to this 1 medical and 1 technical consultant respectively. A further enlargement of the Department is envisaged within the next few years. This improvement in respect of personnel and equipment is essential to be able to cope in future with the rising volume of work. We want to attain a methodical listing of all noisy jobs and a periodical control of all employees exposed to noise. Our plan to eliminate progressively all sources of noise in plants, so far as it is technically feasible, will be pursued. According to our experience, it is of the utmost importance to tackle all problems by team work. Industrial noise abatement is an intricate problem and its success certainly depends on a well-functioning organization that mobilizes all the appropriate forces inside and outside the factories.

We intend in this way to replace individual efforts by developing an organization to maintain a complete register of and to supervise every noisy work-place and every exposed person. We have started the development of such an organization and are at the present time on the point of analysing the experience already gained. Our further organizational action will be subject to the results of this analysis; meanwhile the response to our activities proves that we have succeeded in getting off to a good start with industrial noise abatement in Austria.

Hearing Conservation through Regulation

By

F. A. Van Atta
Bureau of Labor Standards, U.S. Department of Labor, Washington, D.C.

I cannot claim to be an expert in noise control nor in any of the branches of acoustical engineering. I am, really, a sort of semi-scientific policeman somewhat accomplished in the writing of regulations. If I add anything to the state of the art it will be by way of getting other people's ideas applied on a sufficient scale that we will have a good chance to find out whether the proposer is a genius. If they do not succeed he is obviously not a genius. The opportunity to try out these ideas on a fairly large scale comes from some customs we have in the United States which I think are rather strange by British and European standards. One of those customs is that control of occupational safety and health conditions is traditionally a function of the individual States since it is not one of the functions specifically assigned to the Federal government by our Constitution.

We have, consequently, not had uniform regulations for the control of occupational noise exposures. Twelve of our fifty-two State jurisdictions had some sort of law or regulation on the subject by 1968 but there was no uniformity among them either as to permissible levels or as to enforcement practices.

The Federal government does have some responsibilities for employee safety through the Walsh–Healey Public Contracts Act which states about contracts for supplies sold to the government, "No part of such contract will be performed nor will any of the materials, supplies, articles, or equipment to be manufactured or furnished, under said contract be manufactured or fabricated in any plants, factories, buildings, or surroundings or under working conditions which are insanitary or hazardous or dangerous to the health and safety of employees engaged in the performance of said contract." These words are made an explicit part of each contract for supplies. The Department of Labor feels that these words mean exactly what they say: that the contractor has an obligation to provide an environment which does not present unusual hazards to the safety or health of his employees. The corollary belief that the Department has an obligation to consider all of the hazards of the occupational environment is reflected both in the "Green Book" of the 1940's which contained guide-lines for the first safety inspectors under the Act and in the more formal regulations which appeared in the Federal Register in December 1960. You will see that our regulations are not the ordinary sort of labour law of equal application to all workmen but an expression of a contractual obligation. Because the government is a large-scale consumer, they do apply to about 32 million of our approximately 48 million non-agricultural and non-governmental work force and to an additional 9 million through the McNamara–O'Hara Service Contract Act which concerns personal services to the government.

Our regulation of 1960 said, in full, "Noise shall be reasonably reduced or eliminated as a means of preventing fatigue or accident". In our amendment we wanted to make a statement that would be substantially more precise and, hopefully, more effective. We felt that we needed a definite threshold limit designed to prevent hearing loss. For ease of administration we preferred that the limit should be expressed as a single number and that it should be easily and quickly measurable with simple, portable equipment.

There has been little doubt for many years, and at least since the publication of the report of the Z24-X-2 Committee of the then American Standards Association (1954), now American National Standards Institute, that habitual exposure to excessive noise produces loss of hearing. The Committee did not choose to establish a standard for occupational noise exposure, largely because it could not decide what amount of hearing loss should be classified as significant or disabling. Since 1954 the medical profession, through its professional organizations, has defined disabling hearing loss as a loss which makes it difficult to understand speech in sentence form and, further, as starting at a loss in excess of 25 dB average (ISO 1964 scale) in the octaves centred on 500, 1000, and 2000 Hz.

On the basis of those definitions and of considerable data on hearing losses which have accumulated since 1953, the Intersociety Committee on Guide-lines for Noise Exposure and Control developed some criteria without setting a threshold value. These criteria will soon be updated but at this moment they state, in part,

> "The upper curve in Figure 1 indicates that of 100 persons exposed to 85 dB(A) . . . about 23 will have impaired hearing when they reach the age group of 50–59. This compares to about 20 persons out of 100 with no occupational noise exposure. This is an increase of three persons per 100 population for the noise-exposed group, or three percentage points. Because of the wide scatter of the data, so small a difference between groups cannot be attributed to differences in noise exposure with much certainty. . . ."

Probably the most significant thing about this statement is that the

Intersociety Commitee had settled on a single number—the *A*-weighted sound level—to represent the hazard of a noise. It is really not too surprising that it should be an index to the hazard since the *A*-weighting was designed to be the inverse of the loudness levels at 40 phons. That is, it represents the level of sensory response to the energy in the sound, which apparently has a direct relationship to the amount of damage which the energy can produce. The decision of the committee was based mainly on two studies, one in England by Robinson (1968) of the National Physical Laboratory and one in the United States by Baughn (1966). Robinson, in particular, presented strong evidence for the *A*-scale concept.

We accepted this evidence and adopted the *A*-scale noise level as the basis for hazard evaluation and took another look at the data on the percentage of the population impaired by long exposures to noise. It appeared to us to indicate that with 30 or 35 years' exposure the number showing impaired hearing would be 6 to 8% at 85 dB(A) and 15 to 17% at 90 dB(A).

We felt confident enough of our interpretation that we published the 85 dB(A) as a proposed threshold limit with some other provisions and held a public hearing. Following the hearing, the Department eventually settled on a level of 90 dB(A) as the limit for 8 hours per day habitual exposure and a permissible increase of 5 dB in intensity for each halving of exposure time up to a maximum of 115 dB(A). We are aware of the evidence that there should be some allowance for intermittency and some allowance is built into the 5-dB allowance since the equal-energy rule would allow only 3 dB for halving of the exposure time. This is also the rule both as to peak exposures and as to allowances for less than full-time exposure which was adopted at about the same time by the American Conference of Governmental Industrial Hygienists. The two actions were not interdependent but they also were not totally unrelated.

We also included requirements that impulse-type sounds should not exceed 140-dB peak sound pressure and that when engineering and administrative measures are not sufficient to bring the noise levels within the prescribed limits, hearing conservation programmes are mandatory. Our primary concern is the conservation of hearing but we feel very strongly that it must be done, in general, by noise abatement rather than by personal protection.

We now feel that we have a pretty good regulation but that is only the beginning of getting something done. The problem is motivating people to do something and the regulation, *per se,* does not do more than start the process. I think that the Department has some good ideas about how to motivate people in cases of this sort. At least we have some experience. We are responsible for the maritime safety programme under the Longshoremen's and Harbor Workers' Compensation Act. Our philosophy under this Act shows very plainly in the statistics of our activities. In a typical year we will make about 31,000 inspections and issue about 2700 orders for the correction of violations. We will also conduct training for about 12,000 people and have about 12,000 educational and enforcement conferences with high-level management. We will also bring a few enforcement actions.

We are convinced that you must have a large majority of your constituency convinced that the regulation you are trying to enforce is reasonable. We are equally convinced that convictions will not get compliance unless the constituency is also convinced that non-compliance will result in a quick and thorough clobbering. The results are seen in the figures. Figure 51 is for the longshoring programme and Figure 52 for the

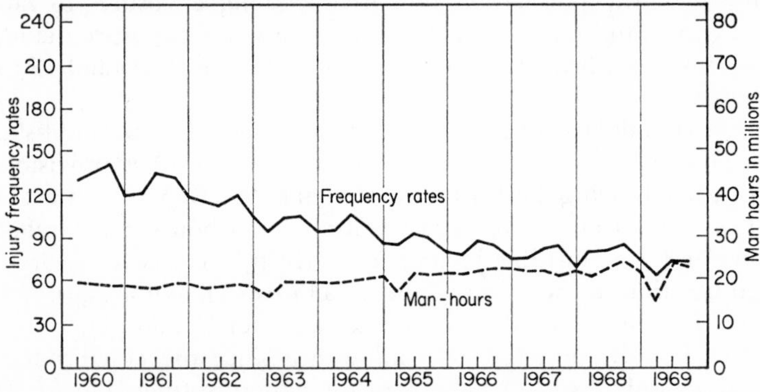

FIG. 51. Quarterly trend in longshoring work injury frequency rates, 1960 to 1970. (Reproduced by courtesy of U.S. Department of Labor, Wage and Labor Standards Administration; compiled by Bureau of Labor Statistics.)

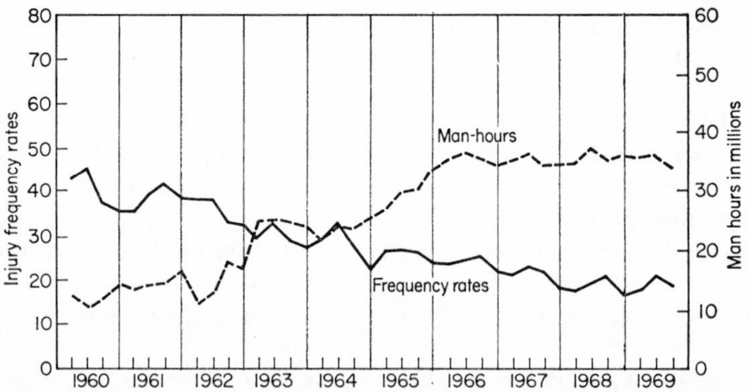

FIG. 52. Quarterly trend in shipyard work injury frequency rates, 1960 to 1970. (Reproduced by courtesy of U.S. Department of Labor, Wage and Labor Standards Administration; compiled by Bureau of Labor Statistics.)

shipbuilding programme. It will be seen that both programmes show a regular, consistent improvement of 7 to 8% annually in injury frequency rates.

It is still too early to have any solid statistical evidence as to what is being accomplished by this regulation. We do have some qualitative impressions. We know that there has been a notable increase in the demand for the services of both audiologists and of acoustical engineers over the past several months. There has also been a notable increase in the number of manufacturers of equipment who call us about reduction of noise in their equipment. We have had a very few companies which have included noise specifications in their new equipment orders for years—since 1956 in DuPont orders. Now we have many who are beginning to include such specifications. I do not expect miracles but I do think that we will see a rather prompt decrease in the production of noise-induced deafness and a gradual decrease in industrial noise.

As one indication of what has been happening, I might quote this excerpt from a letter to one of our regional directors:

> "(3) Our company has purchased Type 1565-A Sound Level Meter from General Electric Company and was the same type meter that your Mr. Brown took sound readings with in all areas of our plant on his recent visit. The readings that we took in our plant on January 13, 1970, and submitted to you in our letter of January 15, 1970 were comparable readings with what your Mr. Brown obtained in our plant.
>
> (4) A noise survey has been made in all areas of our plant. Hearing checks are being made of all employees by local physicians.
>
> (5) We are specifying the lowest noise levels available in new equipment purchases.
>
> (6) We have initiated a preventive maintenance program on all equipment in our plant.
>
> (7) We have put in effect a program where we are using only materials that will reduce noise such as flexible conduit, plastics, nylon and fiber, avoiding metal-to-metal contact and using sound-deadening materials wherever applicable and wherever such material is available.
>
> (8) We are working with our machinery and equipment suppliers in trying to obtain machinery parts that will reduce noise.
>
> (9) We have placed all machinery on resilient mountings.
>
> (10) Barriers have been installed between departments wherever practical.
>
> (11) Improved our quiet zone for lunch and rest areas.
>
> (12) Have the following personal protective equipment on trial at our plant and conducting educational sessions on ear protection:
>
> (a) Wilson Sound Silencers
>
> (b) Straightaway Hearing Protectors

(c) Billesholm Swedish Wool Dispenser has been installed in our weaving department.

(13) Plastic Faller Bars have been installed on all finishers in our pindrafting department.

(14) Sound filters and lint control bags have been installed on all equipment where applicable.

(15) Air lines throughout the plant are being checked once a month for leaks.

(16) Have replaced old type winders with 160 spindles of Autoconer at $1500 per spindle.

(17) Replaced three of our old type pindrafters with the newest equipment available.

(18) Replaced old type twisters with new Volkmann Twisters at a total cost of $50,000.

(19) In our highest noise area we have started an overhaul program on all of our looms where we are completely dismantling this machinery and rebuilding it from the ground up at a cost of $500 per loom.

Our plans for the coming year are to continue working in the above mentioned areas until we have reached our goal of complying with regulations as stated in the Walsh–Healey Act. We will also keep abreast of new items in sound reduction and with the aid of our insurance consultant and others work toward achieving our goal of noise reduction.

Sincerely,"

It is also worthy of note that the National Machine Tool Builders Association is in the process of producing its first standard procedure for determining the noise levels of machine tools and the Society of Automotive Engineers has just completed "A Study of Noise-Induced Hearing Damage Risk for Operators of Farm and Construction Equipment". This is also a first for that industry.

The Administration of a Hearing Conservation Programme

By

D. M. Bruton

Principal Medical Officer (Ground), Air Corporations Joint Medical Service, London Airport (Heathrow), England

At present there is increasing pressure on industry in the United Kingdom to pay attention to the problem of noise-induced hearing loss.

New safety, health and welfare legislation which is now under consideration indicates that it is intended to make provision for the protection of employees against the harmful effects of noise.

The Industrial Injuries Advisory Council has been asked by the Secretary of State for Social Services to consider "whether there are degrees of hearing loss attributable to exposure to noise in the course of employment which satisfy the conditions for prescription as an industrial disease".

In this climate of interest regarding noise-induced hearing loss it is possible that Common Law claims will become more common. A series of successful Common Law claims for noise-induced hearing loss would render industry vulnerable and no doubt further stimulate interest in the need for hearing conservation programmes.

For some years BEA and BOAC have run hearing conservation programmes which in the past 5 years have been conducted by the Air Corporations Joint Medical Service at London Airport. Our practical experience of running a hearing conservation programme indicates that there are various areas of difficulty and some of these problems will require careful consideration if such programmes are to become widespread and effective. Our programme has been run on orthodox lines. This means that we:

(i) conduct noise level measurements
(ii) provide hearing protection, and
(iii) perform pre-employment and periodic audiometric tests on noise-exposed staff.

It is my intention to enumerate some of the difficulties under the heading of each of these three requirements of a hearing conservation programme.

NOISE MEASUREMENT

First let us take noise-level measurement.

Noise-level measurement enables one to define those areas where the risk of noise-induced hearing loss exists. With rare exceptions, a single measurement on its own is of limited value and among the points that need to be considered are the following: the sound pressure level, the duration of exposure, the frequency spectrum, the area affected, the quality of the instrumentation, the location of the measuring instrument, and whether the noise is of sufficient duration to be measurable.

In some circumstances the noise sources may be mobile, for example motor vehicles or aircraft, and this further complicates the evaluation of the risk of hearing loss. Similarly, the factory layout may change frequently and repeated surveys could be required.

These points are mentioned to indicate that the evaluation of the risk of noise-induced hearing loss from noise level surveys is not a simple matter. Some idea of the complexity in the airport situation may be gained from technical reports such as that by Copeland and Robinson (1967).

The provision of hearing protection is not necessarily the correct remedial procedure when damaging noise levels have been established by a noise-level survey. In many cases it may be possible to establish noise-control measures to reduce noise emission at source or to prevent the transmission of noise, and it is better to do this where possible than to provide hearing protection. Additionally, experience of noise problems in one's own industry enables the specification of acceptable noise levels for new plant and machinery—a relevant matter in effective noise control.

In our medical service we have an occupational health engineer who is competent to advise on the purchase of suitable measuring instruments, who is competent to conduct noise-level measurement surveys, and who is competent to advise on matters of noise control.

This is the first practical obstacle to be surmounted in establishing a hearing conservation programme. For industries where the noise problem is of some magnitude it appears essential to have someone competent to undertake these tasks on the permanent staff. It is difficult to know if there are enough suitably qualified persons available to meet this requirement. Suitable persons have a habit of materializing to meet the need if the demand is great enough and this could occur in the field of noise-level measurement. Those practising in the fields of occupational hygiene, in acoustics, and in related engineering disciplines might well provide a suitable source of trained personnel if industry offers sufficiently attractive jobs in this type of work.

Even in large industries there may not be enough work to employ someone full time on noise measurement, and there is a great deal to commend the idea of employing an occupational hygienist, environmental engineer, call him what you will, to look after noise and other environmental problems. Some industries may have competent persons who could do this work in addition to their normal duties but, as already indicated, this is a specialized field with many pitfalls and it is difficult to feel that such a person would ever acquire the necessary degree of expertise.

If noise-level measurement is to be established throughout industry there appears to be a need for this facility to be supplied on a contract basis for many firms, either by independent companies or persons, university departments, institutes of occupational health, or governmental organizations. Even so, the changing circumstances of some industries imply that frequent surveys will be required. Subsequently, routine monitoring of noise levels may be necessary. This, however, is likely to be more within the competence of industry once the initial surveys are done.

HEARING PROTECTION 

Turning to the provision of hearing protection, one is faced with a bewildering array of equipment. The first requirement of a hearing protector is, of course, that it should provide satisfactory attenuation. Secondly, it should be capable of being worn. Both these points have certain associated problems.

Satisfactory attenuation is provided by many reputable devices available. Knowledge of the spectral composition of the noise to be guarded against, as well as the duration of exposure, will enable an intelligent choice of protector to be made. However, attenuation may make conversation difficult to understand or render inaudible certain warning sounds, such as the noise of an approaching vehicle, alarm bells or moving machine parts.

Satisfactory attenuation, therefore, may mean more than cutting out unwanted sound. It could also mean permitting the audibility of wanted sounds. These may be mutually exclusive requirements and make the choice of hearing protector a complex one.

Another point to watch is that the protection provided may not be as effective in the field as under ideal conditions. For example, some cup-type hearing protectors supplied with neck bands tend to slip so that the seal around the ear is broken and the attenuation lost. Again, with cup-type defenders the seal can get damaged, particularly if it is fluid-filled, and reduce the attenuation. It is a matter of experience that damaged seals are not always replaced.

As to the wearability of hearing protectors, there are several points worth mentioning. First there is a choice between plugs and muffs. Plugs are useful when protective headgear or uniform hats have to be worn. They are easily carried around and in this respect useful for occasional exposure. On the other hand, they are easily lost, may not be kept clean and are contra-indicated when the subject has discharging ears. Additionally, they need to be fitted and the subject instructed in their use.

Food manufacturing companies may be against the use of plugs in case they get lost in the product, and they can give rise to problems when used under conditions involving marked changes of barometric pressure, for example, in aircraft or pressure chambers, although this is not a general problem.

Ear muffs are usually clumsy—a point of some importance when working in confined spaces. They feel uncomfortable under hot working conditions. They are not readily portable or easily stored, and when required for intermittent use at different places tend to be left behind in the subject's locker. If the protector is produced with a headband only it cannot be worn with protective headgear or uniform caps. Combined protective helmets and ear muffs are available but appear to combine the disadvantage of both forms of protection. The use of an ear muff fitted with a neck band may resolve the problem of wear with a hat or helmet, but often at the expense of a perfect fit with resulting loss of attenuation.

Despite the foregoing remarks, a comfortable ear muff used for long periods of exposure to loud noise at a relatively fixed work-place, in otherwise good environmental conditions requiring no protective headgear, is quite acceptable to an employee. Unfortunately, these ideal conditions do not always occur and hearing protection is worn less often than one would wish. Nevertheless, hearing protection is an important line of defence against noise-induced hearing loss and efforts must be made to overcome these problems. Education can do much to improve wearer acceptability.

AUDIOMETRY

The provision of hearing protection and implementation of noise-level measurements cause less organizational difficulties than routine audiometry.

Pre-employment audiometry is not much of a problem. This can be readily fitted in to the pre-employment examination schedule. Routine periodic audiometry is, however, more difficult. Some system of recall must be organized and this will involve co-operation with departmental heads and personnel departments.

In our case, the audiometric unit is centralized, that is the booths and equipment are in one place. Unfortunately, this is not centrally situated —neither is it wholly practical to decentralize our facilities. Because of this, time is inevitably lost from work attending for audiometric recheck. This could be a major problem in factories spread over a fairly large area. It is a matter of practical importance that time loss be kept to a minimum if management co-operation is to be maintained.

The use of mobile audiometric units goes a long way to resolving this problem but the capital cost of such units, as well as running costs, can be considerable. In the past three years we have been able to hire the NPL Mobile Audiometric Unit (Burns and Robinson, 1970). This has enabled us to do large numbers of rechecks with the minimum time loss from work. Using this equipment we find it possible to check 4 men every 15 minutes. With the unit located close to the work place the time lost per man is of the order of 20 to 30 minutes. Thus audiometric rechecks of 2000 employees cause a time loss of about 700 to 1000 man hours.

Shift patterns also affect the availability of staff for recheck and audiometric staff may have to work at night or at other odd hours to cover shift workers.

An important technical point arises here. Ideally, audiometry should be carried out following a period free from noise exposure. This implies that subjects should be seen before they commence their shift. One has the choice of seeing a few persons each day prior to the start of shift or holding larger numbers off the shift until they have had their audiometric test performed. If large numbers are involved, neither method is practical.

The problem of temporary threshold shift occurring prior to the audiogram can be avoided if subjects wear hearing protection when noise-exposed before the test. Unfortunately, this cannot be guaranteed. Our assumption, of course, is that hearing protection has been worn. Additionally, if the recheck audiogram is regarded as a screening procedure it is possible to arrange recall of those with apparently significant hearing loss for a further audiogram following a period free from noise exposure.

In our large-scale surveys we have arranged that any person with a hearing loss in excess of 25 dB in either ear at 500, 1000 or 2000 Hz will be seen by the medical officer in attendance. This screening criterion results in a referral rate to the medical officer of between 1 in 4 or 1 in 5 of subjects under test.

The medical officer, exercising his clinical judgement, then decides whether a further audiogram is required. This results in approximately 1 in 20 of all subjects being referred for a further audiogram and more careful clinical evaluation. Of the cases seen at the time of the survey or at follow-up, a few will have clinical conditions requiring treatment from their family doctors and some may require referral to an otologist for investigation, diagnosis and treatment.

In our experience the numbers requiring onward referral at the time of periodic recheck have not been great, but one should bear in mind the fact that all subjects will have had a careful otological examination at pre-employment examination and some will have been seen prior to the survey for otological complaints which have developed in the interim. In other words, the diagnostic problems may already have been dealt with.

Widespread audiometric testing, particularly in companies without a medical service, could well result, initially, in many referrals to family doctors and consultants, and the facilities of the National Health Service severely overburdened as a result.

EVALUATION OF RESULTS

The validity of the screening criterion needs to be evaluated. It will be recognized that our criterion causes us to see only those who have a hearing loss in the speech frequencies. Marked deterioration in the high frequencies could go unnoticed and it is here that the first warnings of noise-induced hearing loss occur.

In fact, a check of all audiograms is carried out and the results of one such check may be of interest here. Of 1500 cards showing no losses greater than 25 dB in the speech frequencies, there were 600 cards with a loss exceeding 25 dB in the frequencies of 3000, 4000 and 6000 Hz. Here excuses must be made—no further evaluation of this point has been made to date and this information should be taken at its face value.

Obviously one would wish to know whether the losses were bilateral, whether a loss at 4000 Hz was as great or greater at 6000 Hz, and so on. Perhaps it is relevant to say that time is required to tap the mine of information provided by large-scale audiometric surveys and this time may not be readily available to an industrial medical officer who has to concern himself with many other matters. Nevertheless, in due course we hope to analyse the result of recent surveys in greater detail.

One such analysis was performed in 1964. Median noise-induced permanent threshold shifts at 500, 1000, 2000, 3000 and 4000 Hz were calculated for various exposed groups and the results showed no significant hearing losses for the groups as a whole. The simple conclusions to be drawn from this are that the hearing protection provided has been worn by these groups or that their particular noise exposure is not harmful.

Reliance on this sort of analysis is, however, not enough to protect the individual and we, of course, place greater reliance on seeing those with a 25-dB loss in the speech frequencies. This enables us to pay particular attention to those in whom auditory difficulties may be imminent.

In addition to conducting an examination to evaluate whether treatment or further investigation is required, we are able to give them, and management, specific advice regarding their need to wear hearing protection and to arrange frequent periodic audiometric tests to supervise their progress more closely. Our experience suggests that this is a satisfactory way of dealing with the individual and so far we have been able to rely on hearing protection as a means of preventing further hearing loss.

While much information of an epidemiological nature can be gathered from large-scale periodic audiometric testing of noise-exposed groups, the most important function of these tests is to enable one to find those who are at imminent risk of sustaining disabling hearing loss and to take necessary preventive action on behalf of the individual.

CONCLUSION

The problems of administering a hearing conservation programme in industry are in summary:

(1) Obtaining the co-operation of management and employees.

(2) Staffing. Technical, clerical and medical manpower will be required with the necessary level of skill.

(3) Equipment. Noise level meters, audiometers, audiometric booths and hearing protection are the principal requirement. The equipment must be of an acceptable standard and here the work of the International Organization for Standardization provides valuable guidance.

(4) Finance. One complete audiometric suite consisting of an automatic audiometer, a booth and associated equipment costs approximately £1700 exclusive of accommodation charges.

Staffing costs for such a single unit will be in the order of £1500 per annum, but if a comprehensive programme is undertaken by a large firm the cost of medical, clerical and technician manpower to meet the capacity of a two-booth unit and make regular noise-level measurements will be in excess of £5000 per annum.

A capital expenditure in the order of £15,000 can be anticipated for a firm with 2000 or so noise-exposed employees to be protected with annual running costs in the order of £5000.

(5) Organization. Noise-level measurement has to be organized on an initial and continuing basis. The information gained has to be evaluated and advice given on noise reduction and the provision of hearing protection.

Hearing protectors must be suitable, and routine purchase and distribution organized.

Advice must be given to staff regarding the risk of hearing loss and the protective measures available.

A programme of pre-employment and routine periodic audiometry must be established taking into account a number of factors which affect the success and validity of the programme.

The results of the programme need to be evaluated for the individual as well as the group and any necessary preventive measures instituted.

This short paper represents the view of a medical man who is, relatively speaking, a newcomer to the manifold problems of administering a hearing conservation programme, and it attempts therefore only to illuminate some of the broader issues from experience of the programme run by the ACJMS.

In our work we have had the benefit of valuable advice from experts in this field. The present trend towards comprehensive hearing conservation programmes throughout industry indicates that many more people are going to require advice. It is to be hoped that it will be available, authoritative and practical.

Noise Damage Liability—Evidence as to the State of Knowledge

By

M. E. Bryan and W. Tempest

Department of Electrical Engineering, University of Salford, England

Summary

The problem of deafness due to exposure to high-level noise at work has been with us from the beginning of the industrial revolution. Despite the fact that numerous countries have provided protection for workers at risk and made the employer liable for those deafened since the Second World War, this is not the case in Britain. In this country occupational deafness will eventually be compensatable under the Industrial Injuries Act, but what liability does an employer already have for the protection of his workers' hearing under the Common Law? In the only case for damages, as a result of noise exposure, to reach the courts, the plaintiff lost the case. One important feature of the case was that insufficient evidence had been presented to establish that there was general knowledge of the risk to hearing by exposure to that particular impulsive noise, which was due to a cartridge gun. On the other hand there is a considerable body of evidence that hearing loss due to impact and continuous noise has been well known since the early part of this century, and that it seems likely that employer liability for deafness, due to these types of noise, will almost certainly date from about 1950.

INTRODUCTION

Nine years ago in 1961, a conference entitled "The Control of Noise" was held, like the present one, at the National Physical Laboratory. This earlier meeting marks roughly the epoch when the Government began to take an interest in the question of compensation for occupational deafness. In the intervening years, there has been little overt evidence that this country as a whole has taken the problem of occupational deafness seriously; there is still no statutory protection or compensation for the worker at risk. However, last year the first signs of official intentions emerged (Department of Health and Social Security, 1969), and it is perhaps reasonable to hope that this signals a substantial amelioration of the workers' position before another 9 years have elapsed.

How big is the problem in economic terms? There has not, to our knowledge, been a survey in this country of the number of workers who are exposed to dangerous noise. Various estimates have been made as to the figure; Chadwick, at this conference, has suggested that "one-quarter of the working population labour in industrial noise environments potentially hazardous to hearing". Our own estimate is that one to two million workers are at risk. It has also been suggested that there are 100,000–200,000 noise-deafened people in this country at the present time. If all these afflicted people were to claim compensation from their employers successfully, the total bill the latter would be faced with might well be of the order of £50–£100 million. The cost of introducing noise control and noise-reduction procedures together with regular audiometric screening of employees at risk could well be anything up to £50 million each year.

Clearly then in economic terms industrial deafness is a problem of considerable magnitude. This may be one reason why this country is so slow in introducing noise-control legislation.

It seems highly probable that the Government will bring occupational deafness into the Industrial Injuries Act; however, the question we want to consider here is that of an employer's liability, at the moment, under Common Law. It is our intention to consider what evidence is available and relevant to a fair assessment of whether an employer is liable to pay compensation, and also from what date did he become liable.

THE CASE OF THOMAS ARTHUR DOWN *v.* DUDLEY, COLES, LONG LTD.

"Every medical man knows that noise causes deafness". This quotation is taken from a twenty-page article called "Noise in Industry" in the October 1953 issue of *Scope—a magazine for industry* (Anon., 1953). Few of us would disagree with the truth of that statement. However, in any assessment of an employer's liability for occupational deafness, the question of *when* the employer became aware of the causative relation between noise and deafness is of major importance.

In the only case for damages for noise-induced hearing loss to have reached the courts in this country, it was accepted by the medical experts for both the plaintiff and for the defendants that there was a probable causal relationship between the noise and the deafness (Coles, 1969). In this case, Thomas Arthur Down *v.* Dudley, Coles, Long Ltd., heard before Mr. Justice Browne at the Devon Assizes on 27th–31st January 1969, the plaintiff had been exposed to the impulsive noise of about 130 rounds per day fired in a "Tornado" rivet gun for some 14 days. To quote from the judgement,* the Judge said,

* Available from Hibbert and Sanders (official shorthand writers), 10 King's Bench Walk, Temple, London, E.C.4.

"The plaintiff's case was put in two ways. He says the defendants were negligent in failing to appreciate the risk of damage to the plaintiff's hearing by the work he was doing and failing to take any precautions to avert this risk. Secondly, he says the defendants are vicariously liable for the negligence of the general foreman—or the foreman carpenter—in failing either to take the plaintiff off the job he was doing or to provide proper ear plugs."

On the latter point there had been some conversation in which the plaintiff had asked for some cotton-wool for his ears.

The real point at issue in this case was whether or not the state of knowledge was such at that time (April 1966) that the employer was negligent. The plaintiff lost the case and the following remarks, by Mr. Justice Browne, taken from the judgement, are highly relevant to employers' liability: "Ought the defendants to have foreseen that the use of this gun might have caused injury to his (the plaintiff's) hearing?" He concluded on this point: "On all this evidence I am not satisfied in the light of scientific and technical knowledge available in 1966, that the defendants were guilty of any want of reasonable care in failing to appreciate and guard against the risk that the plaintiff's use of the 'Tornado' gun might cause injury to his hearing." In fact it was only from the end of 1966 onwards that the dangers of impulsive noise became generally known (British Standards Institution, 1966; Coles and Rice, 1967; Coles *et al.*, 1968).

On the other hand, when can it be said that an employer became guilty of want of reasonable care if he failed to guard against the risk that *continuous* or *impact* noise might cause injury to his workman's hearing? It is of prime importance that we should be fully aware of what evidence is available in order that, when the time comes, the courts arrive at a fully-informed assessment of the date when responsibility began.

A REASONABLE AND PRUDENT EMPLOYER

Before we consider the evidence which may well be used for assessing liability we ought to attempt definitions of what the words "liability" and "negligence" probably mean in this context. We could not do better than to return to the Devon case and to quote Mr. Justice Browne once more. He quoted, as the law on the subject, the views of Mr. Justice Swanwick in the case of Stokes *v.* Guest, Keen and Nettlefolds (Bolts and Nuts) Ltd. (1968, 1 Weekly Law Reports, 1776, at page 1783), who, having referred to a number of authorities said,

"From these authorities I deduce that the overall test of the reasonable and prudent employer, taking positive thought for the safety of his workers in the light of what he knows or ought to know, where there is a recognized and general practice which has been followed for a substantial period in similar circumstances without mishap, is that he is entitled to follow it, unless in the light of common sense or newer knowledge it is clearly bad; but where there is a developing knowledge, he must keep reasonably abreast of it and not be slow to apply it; and where he has in fact greater than the average knowledge of the risks, he may be thereby obliged to take more than the average or standard precautions. . . . If he is found to have fallen below the standard to be properly expected of a reasonable and prudent employer in these respects he is negligent."

It is with these criteria in mind that we proceed to an examination of the evidence as to the state of knowledge regarding occupational deafness.

MEDICAL AND TECHNICAL KNOWLEDGE REGARDING CONTINUOUS AND IMPACT NOISE DEAFNESS

Large firms employ medical officers or safety officers or both, part of whose function is that of keeping the management aware of new medical and technical knowledge concerning occupational diseases. It is therefore relevant to review briefly the specialized literature on occupational deafness.

The earliest reference to deafness and noise seems to be Ramazini (1713), who noted that millers and coppersmiths and those "dwelling near the Nile in Egypt" became hard of hearing due to noise exposure. The symptoms of noise-induced deafness in blacksmiths were accurately described by Fosbroke in the *Lancet* (1830–31). In 1886, Barr wrote that 75% of the boilermakers he had tested heard with difficulty, and that disturbance began immediately upon entering work. Labyrinthine deafness was discussed at the British Medical Association and reported in the *British Medical Journal* in 1925 (McKenzie, 1925), and we infer that noise was accepted by British otologists by that time as causing nervous deafness. In 1934, Sir Thomas Legge, at that time Senior Medical Inspector of Factories, described boilermakers' deafness and suggested "stopping the ears with cotton-waste or india rubber and plasticine mixed with cotton-wool", and gave directions for making ear plugs (Legge, 1934). McKelvie (1927) reported that 7% of 1101 cotton weavers suffered from nerve deafness and was of the opinion that the machinery was responsible and that quieter looms should be used to give protection. In 1952 the President of the Section of Otology of the Royal Society of Medicine gave his address on "Some effects of intense sound and ultrasound on the ear" (Dickson, 1953), so we can safely say that by this time all the factors of continuous and impact noise which induced loss of hearing were known and available in the medical literature (McKelvie, 1927; Dickson *et al.*, 1939; Bunch, 1937). A danger level of 90 dB for continuous noise had been proposed (Dickson, 1953) which is not so very different from the limit proposed in an unpublished Ministry of Labour consultative document 15 years later.

Throughout the 1950's there were several English text-books on occupational health published which dealt with the dangers of noise and advised the use of ear protection (Davies, 1957; Harvey and Murray, 1958; Schilling, 1960). American text-books were also available at that time (Sappington, 1943; Harris, 1957).

Ear plugs have been manufactured in this country since the 1914–18 war by Antiacoustic and Mallock Armstrong. This firm started making *ear defenders* during the Second World War at the request of the firm developing the first gas-turbine aero-engines, and these defenders have been on sale since that time. They were advertised in an authoritative top management journal having a circulation of 7000 in 1953 and have been on display at the Industrial Health and Safety Centre in London since 1954. Ear protection such as the Lee Sonic Ear-Valv was also available from the United States during the 1950's. Several firms started manufacturing ear defenders in this country from about 1959–60. These have been supplied to the Services, British Railways, the weaving industry, the aircraft industry, British European Airways, the forging industry and steel industry.

GENERAL KNOWLEDGE REGARDING CONTINUOUS AND IMPACT NOISE DEAFNESS

Not every foreman, works manager or company director, however, reads the *Lancet* or the *Proceedings of the Royal Society of Medicine*, so we must consider what information there is available in the non-specialist literature.

The earliest general reference we have so far found is of considerable interest. In Walter Greenwood's classic novel, *Love on the Dole* (1933), a story of working-class life in Salford in the depression years between the wars, a description is given of a local engineering works. In the forging shop "the thump caused giddiness"; in the riveting shop "every man was stone deaf after a six months' spell of work here". It is difficult to escape the conclusion it was well known by the public in 1933 that forgers (blacksmiths) and riveters suffered from the occupational disease of deafness. In 1947 *The Times Review of Industry* printed an article by E. J. Evans of the National Physical Laboratory called "Noise in the Factory" (Evans, 1947). In it he stated: "There are many industries where extremely noisy conditions prevail. In weaving sheds, for example, it is impossible to converse except by shouting at close range and boilermakers' deafness associated with the noise in boilerworks is well known." The article was mainly concerned with the sources of noise and noise reduction, the inference being that excessive noise was undesirable. For relief from very high noise levels found in such occupations as boilermaking and riveting he says it is necessary to use ear defenders to obtain relief. He mentions commercial ear plugs, the use of plasticine and cotton-wool, and that the British Services used soft-rubber ear defenders during the Second World War which had been designed by Knudsen.

In a book by V. L. Browd (1953), intended for the layman, it is stated: "Sound itself is one of the most effective damagers of the hearing: repeated or lengthy exposures to sound—in machine shops or in heavy industry—is bound to damage hearing."

We have already mentioned the article which appeared in *Scope* in 1953. This set out in unequivocal terms the dangers to hearing of exposure to noise in excess of 85 dB, that the damage was irreversible, that noise control was possible and that ear protection was available, as also was specialist advice. It says at one point: "Prolonged exposure to noise is a prolific cause of deafness throughout industry—this is an urgent social problem which management cannot ignore." It is interesting to speculate how many top management people saw this article.

The year 1953 was quite an eventful one as it seems it was the first time a question was asked in the House of Commons if the Government was taking steps to protect the hearing of men employed in the operations of chipping, riveting, stamping, plating and heading (Parliamentary Debates, 1953, **513**, 1101). The Government clearly was well aware of the problem and about noise control and personnel protection in the form of ear coverings. In 1955 there was a debate upon the motion of Sir Lionel Heald: "This House notes with concern the detrimental effect of noise and vibration on the health, well-being and efficiency of the nation, and urges H.M. Government to give careful attention to the importance of research and education in this field and the need for more effective measures for the protection of the public" (Parliamentary Debates, 1955, **546**, 2665). In this debate, reference was made to the 1953 article in *Scope* and to two articles in *The Times* (Anon., 1955a) with the title "The Curse of Noise" which appeared on 24th and 25th October 1955. In the first of these articles it is stated: "It is possible to specify fairly closely the noise levels that must not be exceeded if permanent deafness is to be avoided (such noises occur only in industry)." We would also refer to the following articles in *The Times* (Anon., 1955b, c, d), particularly "Noise Dangers in Industry" which appeared on 29th April where it was stated: "Acoustic trauma is perhaps the most frequent danger to ears in industry." Other parliamentary references were made in 1959 and 1960 (Parliamentary Debates, **600,** 49; **618,** 1571).

The Industrial Welfare Society (1961) carried out a survey of noise in industry which was aimed at "giving the industrial layman a picture of the problem (of industrial noise) as a whole". The questionnaire was sent to the Society's 700 member firms, of whom only 8% replied. Hence it covered 87,000 workers or 1% of the country's labour force. There were 25% of the firms replying who felt they had a case or cases of occupational deafness; and 70% felt they had a noise problem. Some firms had carried out noise surveys and 18 firms had taken action and introduced various noise-abatement procedures including the use of ear muffs.

In 1961 the conference on "The Control of Noise", mentioned at the beginning of this paper, took place. It was attended by some 350 representatives, largely from industry and industrial research organizations. The proceedings were published by H.M.S.O. (National Physical Laboratory, 1962) and have had a wide sale.

In 1962 Berry wrote in the *New Scientist* (Berry, 1962): "It has been established that prolonged exposure to noise at high levels may produce permanent hearing loss. This point, more than any other, is likely to define the industrial attitude to noise. A hearing loss which is severe enough to constitute a social handicap may come to be regarded as an industrial injury." The implications of this are far-reaching—prophetic words and a warning to the many industrialists who might have seen his article.

The year 1963 was an important one in the history of employer liability for noise-induced deafness. In that year the Wilson Committee report was published (Committee on the Problem of Noise, 1963). This committee was set up by the Government in April 1960 to "examine the nature, source and effect of the problem of noise and to advise what further measures can be taken to mitigate it". It recommended that the Ministry of Labour should:

(a) disseminate as widely as possible existing knowledge of the hazard of noise to hearing,
(b) impress on industry the need to take action to reduce the hazard as it is at present recognized,
(c) advise industry on practical measures to this end.

As a result, the Ministry of Labour published a four-page leaflet called "Noise and the Worker" (Form 2124) in 1963. This pointed out the dangers of loud persistent noise, gave some criteria for the assessment of risk, and suggested some courses of action. Apparently 20,000 such leaflets were printed and are understood to have been distributed "in a somewhat haphazard way" by the Factory Inspectorate offices to firms employing more than 250 persons. It also refers to the better-known 24-page pamphlet "Noise and the Worker" (Ministry of Labour, 1963) which is available from H.M.S.O. The general literature is clearly a rich and fertile, though somewhat difficult, field for research. We would not claim that the above list of references is complete.

EMPLOYER'S LIABILITY FOR OCCUPATIONAL DEAFNESS DUE TO CONTINUOUS OR IMPACT NOISE

The assessment of employer's liability for industrial deafness will clearly be the responsibility of the courts. However, it is our responsibility to make sure that all relevant evidence is available so that a fair assessment can be made. The following comments may have some relevance.

1. A large firm which employs specialists to look after the health of its employees must have its liability assessed against the background of the medical and technical knowledge available. In this case it would seem that such a firm should have become aware of the hazard and of its own responsibilities no later than the early 1950's. This would be particularly true of those firms in the traditionally noisy industries involving such operations as riveting, stamping, forging, chipping, and weaving. Indeed it seems very likely that deafness has always been regarded as an occupational hazard in noisy industries, although not until after the Second World War did noise abatement and hearing conservation procedures, together with specialist advice, become available.

2. Those firms with no medical officer or safety officer would seem to have to be judged against the background of general knowledge. It would seem to become increasingly difficult for an employer to put up a convincing defence of ignorance as the 1950's wore on. Indeed it seems very likely that by 1963 all but the smallest firms would have had the dangers brought to their notice. Again the traditionally noisy industries would seem to be more clearly liable as their operations were specifically mentioned in the general literature.

3. The small firm, perhaps with some new noisy process, might be able to put up a convincing defence into the 1960's. But credibility would be wearing rather thin in the last few years with the increased activity of the Factory Inspector, new factory regulations being considered, and with the activities of noise suppression salesmen.

Ear Protection and Hearing in High-intensity Impulsive Noise

By

M. R. Forrest

Army Personnel Research Establishment, Farnborough, Hampshire, England

High-intensity impulsive noise is less common in industry than "steady-state" continuous noise; consequently it has been much less intensively studied. The most common source of hazardous impulsive noise is gunfire, but several industrial processes will also give impulsive noise of sufficient intensity to damage hearing.

High-intensity impulsive noise, as its name implies, differs from continuous noise, firstly in the extremely high peak sound pressures encountered, generally above 140 dB (*re* 2×10^{-5} N/m^2) and sometimes exceeding 180 dB; and secondly, in its very short duration, often as little as a few milliseconds. Within these limits a wide variety of different pulse shapes is encountered. It is evident that high-intensity impulsive noise cannot be properly measured by the techniques used for continuous noise, and that the damage-risk criteria developed for continuous noise are not applicable. A damage-risk criterion for impulsive noise, taking into account peak pressure level, duration and number of impulses, has, however, been given (Coles *et al.*, 1968).

The types of ear defender normally used against continuous noise (Rice and Coles, 1966) are generally found to offer adequate protection against impulsive noise. Unfortunately, the problem of hearing low-level sounds, particularly speech, becomes acute if ordinary ear defenders are used; good hearing of speech or alarm signals is often essential for safety, and the effect of the ear defenders is especially noticeable during the quiet periods between impulses. Communication may be preserved by the use of a closed system using noise-cancelling microphones, and earphones mounted within the defender, together with a trailing wire or magnetic loop; but this solution is too expensive and too clumsy for many purposes.

The ideal would be an ear defender which attenuates noise far more than speech; this can be realized in practice if the noise and speech differ in some physical respect, and the obvious difference in this case is the very high level and short duration of the former. Speech during the quiet periods is then heard relatively normally while the peaks of the high-intensity impulsive noise are removed. Little speech intelligibility is lost, since the impulse duration is short. The ERDEfender, developed by the Explosives Research and Development Establishment, uses this principle; here a basically normal pair of ear muffs is equipped with a microphone, peak-limiting amplifier and earphone built into each ear cup so that sounds of up to about 95 dB SPL are heard almost normally but the amplifier limits transmission above this level.

While the ERDEfender is very efficient it is rather expensive, and a little cumbersome. A much simpler means of achieving the same result, but with a slightly less sharp cut-off, is provided by the increase in impedance of a small orifice at high levels (Ingard and Ising, 1967), where the originally laminar air flow becomes turbulent. With the great difference in peak level between high-intensity impulsive noise and the wanted sounds such as speech, the more gradual increase in attenuation should not be too serious in practice.

Several types of ear defender with some form of small orifice have been designed, usually to obtain a particular frequency response. The orifice, together with the volume of air enclosed by the defender, forms a Helmholtz resonator, giving negligible attenuation at low frequencies and a fairly good attenuation above, usually, about 2 kHz. If the damping is small the attenuation at intermediate frequencies is negative. A similar effect is obtained with normal ear defenders with an accidentally introduced leak. The object in this case is to exclude the more harmful high frequencies while admitting low and intermediate frequencies to ease communication; one of the most ingenious designs is Zwislocki's Selectone-K plug (Zwislocki, 1952; Rice and Coles, 1966), which incorporates a two-stage acoustic filter. By itself this frequency-selective effect offers only a relatively small improvement over conventional defenders, but the existence of an amplitude-sensitive effect from the increase in impedance can also be demonstrated and offers a potentially greater improvement.

To take advantage of this effect a modified V.51R ear plug has been designed. The core of the plug was removed and replaced by a disc of 0·13-mm (0·005-inch) steel skin pierced by a 0·64-mm (0·025-inch) diameter orifice, thus giving a very much lower attenuation than for the original V.51R. The speech attenuation of the modified plug is of the order of 5 dB as against about 20 dB for the unmodified plug (Rice and Coles, 1966). The increase in attenuation first becomes apparent at about 110 dB (*re* 2×10^{-5} N/m^2) but does not become useful until much higher levels are reached. For impulses above 140 dB the increase is quite steady at the rate of about 1 dB per 2 dB increase in incident impulse, until the limit set by the attenuation of the unmodified plug is approached; Fig. 53 shows this increase measured in a cadaver ear using microphones near the ear-drum and just outside the ear-canal entrance.

The modified plugs have undergone extensive testing in the field as well as in the laboratory and the results have proved very encouraging. They have been provisionally termed "Gundefenders" to emphasize their intended use against gunfire-type noise, as with their very small low-frequency attenuation they would evidently be of little use against many types of continuous industrial noise.

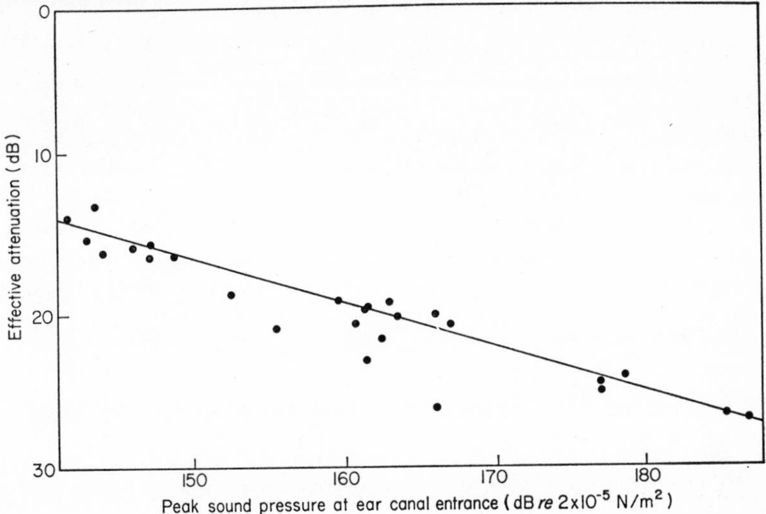

Fig. 53. Impulse attenuation from "Gundefender" ear plug as a function of peak sound pressure at the ear canal entrance.

It is possible that other mechanisms to attenuate the peaks of high-intensity impulsive noise may also be developed in the future. In any case, for high-intensity impulsive noise it is now possible to provide adequate ear protection for only a small loss in communication. The improvement over conventional defenders, welcome in itself, also means that adequate ear protection will be used more widely, and to that extent will be more effective, since one of the chief objections to its use will have been removed.

ACKNOWLEDGEMENTS

The author wishes to thank Surgeon Cdr. R. R. A. Coles, R.N., for his help and encouragement, and the Medical-Officer-in-Charge at the Institute of Naval Medicine, Alverstoke, where most of the work on the "Gundefender" ear plugs was carried out.

Discussion on Papers in Section II

CHAIRMAN: E. König

PARTICIPANTS

N. Ashworth	R. I. Higgins
H. A. Beagley	R. Hinchcliffe
C. H. B. Binns	W. J. Hunter
D. M. Bruton	E. König
M. E. Bryan	G. L. Lee
D. L. Chadwick	A. Raber
R. R. A. Coles	S. D. G. Stephens
H. Davis	F. A. Van Atta
M. E. Delany	C. Wakstein
E. D. D. Dickson	J. G. Walker
M. R. Forrest	W. D. Ward

Dr. Hinchcliffe: The papers by Dr. Delany and Dr. Stephens have certain similarities and I would first congratulate the speakers on their studies regarding the size of the variability in threshold determinations, and of the factors determining it. I remember that when I first went into this field 15 years ago at the Psycho-Acoustic Laboratory at Harvard, Dr. Zwislocki was then doing some studies on the effect not only of learning, but also of motivation, which has not so far been mentioned here (Zwislocki *et al.*, 1958). There is one particular question I would like to ask Dr. Delany. I was interested in the systematic trend in hearing level as a function of relatively long-term duration (120 weeks). Perhaps this is presbycusis. If so, one is in a position to see whether it is age-dependent, or whether the changes in hearing levels regress on initial hearing level. The relevance of this is indicated by Miall and Lovell's (1967) studies on blood pressure. These workers showed that age *per se* plays no direct part in determining the rate of change of blood pressure, even though average blood pressures are much higher in the old than in the young, and even though almost all old people have higher blood pressures. Age may appear to play a part solely because blood-pressure changes are on average positive, and increase with higher pressures. It is yet to be shown whether or not this applies to hearing levels also.

Dr. Delany: The variation of mean hearing level with time, of which examples for two subjects are shown in Fig. 40, gives the hearing level averaged over four tests in each of 2 ears at 6 frequencies. From analysis of the original data there was no obvious systematic difference between frequencies, although this would be expected if the shifts were presbycutic in origin, and it was for this reason that the results for different frequencies were combined. Of course, towards the higher frequencies the replication variance increases fairly rapidly so that, if a separate analysis at each frequency is carried out, these comparatively small shifts in hearing level may become less significant. Increasing the number of degrees of freedom by averaging over the 6 test frequencies does improve the matter considerably. Unfortunately, with only 4 subjects it is impossible to determine whether the systematic trend in hearing level regresses on age or on initial hearing level. It happens that subject C, who showed the greatest systematic trend, was the oldest (aged 50), but initially the same subject also had the most acute threshold. On the other hand, the subject (A) showing the most stable hearing was 40 years old and had the least acute initial hearing. All 4 subjects ended up with less acute hearing compared with the start of the experiment.

Dr. Stephens: In reply to Dr. Hinchcliffe's point concerning the effects of motivation, I looked at the results of my detection-threshold experiment in terms of the subject's direct achievement motivation and failure avoidance motivation. These were assessed by a personality inventory (Argyle and Robinson, 1962). I found no significant correlation of either of these measures with the variances or the thresholds at the 4 different frequencies 250, 1000, 4000 and 8000 Hz.

Air Vice-Marshal Dickson: We carried out tests at the RAF Central Medical Establishment, on some 25 otologically checked personnel, under standard conditions, and the only variants were the times of day when we were testing—morning or afternoon—and the different operator. We found differences of as much as 10 dB between the various times at which these tests were carried out (Brown, 1948). Could Dr. Delany say if there was any otological check on these subjects over the period of 2 years? All tests carried out for threshold variations should, at some time or other during the period of testing, also have otological examination to see that there is no obstruction in the auditory meatus, and I place no reliance on audiometric findings unless there is a clinical otological examination before the test is applied.

Dr. Delany: We are aware of the experiments described by Air Vice-Marshal Dickson and we know that other people have also claimed that hearing level appears to depend on the time of day at which the measurements were made. On the 10 different occasions spread over the 2-year period, our experiments were made at different times of the day between 10 a.m. and 4.30 p.m., and we have found no correlation at all between mean hearing level and time of day. Neither did we find any correlation of mean hearing level with the time of year. Moreover, the largest mean shift, with subject C, amounted to only 4 dB. All subjects in fact had had an otological examination at some point in time, and nothing untoward found, but certainly an examination was not carried out on each and every occasion on which measurements were made. Audiometric tests were not, however, carried out if any subject reported that he was feeling unwell. In view of the very small threshold trends observed it seems clear that any clinical symptoms present must have been irrelevant to their hearing. Indeed, it seems probable, for the purposes of this type of experiment, that audiometric normality and stability renders otological examination unnecessary.

Dr. Coles: Dr. Delany mentioned that Burns and Robinson found much higher replication variances—twice the size I believe—in their noise-exposed populations; and he said that when the subject is not well-motivated, when pathology intervenes, or when he has been exposed to intense noise levels, then the variance may be much larger still. Was the greater variance found simply because, with noise exposure, there were TTS or PTS, which of course has a much larger scatter? If there was no TTS or PTS one would have a measure of the test–retest variance alone. But as soon as there is a changed hearing level, then one has a variation in the amount of change of hearing level due to the noise. This is of great current relevance because of some enormously large variances in field work with which I have recently been concerned, the standard deviations being anything up to 13 dB. We were encouraged, though, to find that other workers in the military field—and "field" is here meant literally—found very similar results. We are trying to explain these effects. Maybe the answer is in Dr. Delany's statements, but I wonder whether real auditory threshold shifts were confounded with the ordinary audiometric test–retest variance.

Dr. Delany: The figures for replication variance for industrial control subjects were not actually taken from the reference cited but were obtained from analyses I myself carried out on raw data which were subsequently included in the report cited. The data relate to measurements taken approximately one year apart on a group of 33 young males who had been exposed in the interim to noise levels not greater than 82 dB(A). Tests were only carried out before the start of a shift so that any slight TTS due to noise exposure is likely to have completely disappeared overnight and otological examinations were carried out on all occasions with no obvious pathology present. This group could therefore be truly regarded as control subjects.

At each test the following sequence was used: left ear 0·5, 1, 2, 3, 4, 6; right ear 0·5, 1, 2, 3, 4, 6; left ear 0·5, 1, 2 kHz, so that a measure of replication in the left ear was built in. Although, as Fig. 39 shows, the sudden change of stimulus from left to right ear without interval or warning inflates the variance considerably at 0·5 and 1 kHz, nevertheless by 2 kHz the effect is not so important and the two independent determinations of hearing level in the left ear at 2 kHz can be used to obtain an estimate of replication variance. By either method the estimated replication variance for these industrial subjects exposed to minimal noise is very much greater than that for the laboratory subjects.

Dr. Walker: I would like to comment on a point that Dr. Delany mentioned in his paper regarding the use of circumaural earphones. I would agree with his comments in general, although some work which I have done with circumaural earphones, which were specifically designed to reduce the variance, gave very significant improvements in the test–retest variance at high frequencies. With ordinary supra-aural earphones, variances of about 20 dB^2 at 6 and 8 kHz are normal, whereas the circumaural earphone gave variances of 4 dB^2 at 6 kHz and 10 dB^2 at 8 kHz, which is a significant improvement.

Dr. Delany: The results presented in Fig. 42 relate to a type of liquid-seal circumaural earphone available commercially, a type which is currently being used for audiometry. In obtaining these values, normal audiometric procedures were followed with no special device to ensure accurate earphone replacement. They do not therefore represent the best possible performance from the particular point of view of replication variance. Thus it is quite possible that the device currently being investigated by Dr. Walker shows lower variance at high frequencies although the values he quotes do seem unrealistically low. Indeed, the value of replication variance for 6 kHz is smaller than that usually associated with the inherent uncertainty of audiometric threshold, even at the most favourable frequencies.

Dr. Beagley: Can Dr. Delany account for the difference in replication variance between right ear and left ear; is it perhaps an order effect which could be balanced out by alternating the starting order?

Dr. Delany: In this type of audiometric test it would seem likely that two effects might be expected to produce a difference between the replication variance associated with the two ears of the same person. On the one hand a lower replication variance might be expected for the right ear in view of the fact that it was always tested after the left ear and the subject would therefore have had practice with the technique. On the other hand the subject has been concentrating on tests at six frequencies in the left ear when suddenly, and without an interval for rest, the test stimulus switches to the right ear and some confusion is engendered. This apparently persists for two or three frequencies. Referring to Fig. 39, it would seem that the latter effect dominates, and this accords with my subjective impression of the test. The subjects involved were highly experienced at performing this type of audiometric test and an even greater effect is observed with inexperienced subjects, for example in the joint survey carried out by the Medical Research Council and the National Physical Laboratory (Burns and Robinson, 1970). I think it quite possible to balance out these effects by suitable design of experiment but I am not sure that this is necessarily a good thing to do. It may well be that randomizing the test sequence will so inflate the residual variance that the main effect being investigated will cease to be significant; it is probably better to reduce the effect by allowing a reasonable rest period between testing the two ears, to allow the subject to relax. Also it may be advisable to allow a longer test period at the first frequency tested in each ear so that the subject has a chance to practise.

Mr. Lee: Serial audiometry and related serial noise level measurements ought to produce some unique data. From the data by the Austrian Social Security Board it may be possible to abstract information of great value to industry in other countries. Could the Austrian experts say whether the data available indicate any rate of change of noise levels in factories, for example have they increased or reduced by so many decibels per annum in a particular factory or industry?

Dr. Raber: We have investigated most factories only once, but in some plants we have already made two or three serial audiometric tests. In many cases we have found deteriorations of hearing, clearly typical of classical noise-induced hearing loss, among workers who, at the time of first investigation, had already been exposed for 25 to 35 years to a steady-state noise and who had continued with the same level of exposure until the second, and sometimes the third, audiometric investigation 3 to 6 years later. I would stress that these changes were clearly distinguishable from progressive presbycusis and were not confined to frequencies below 4 kHz. I would also mention that we are now trying to simulate the work of Dr. Robinson (Robinson, 1968; Robinson and Cook, 1968). We were truly astonished to find, out of a bulk of nearly 30,000 mass audiometric data on workers exposed to continuous noise, only 600 cases without otological abnormalities, personal history of ear disease, gunfire experience, etc. When we examined the audiograms meeting these stipulations, we found relatively mild cases of noise-induced hearing loss. In our opinion this means that there are many other factors influencing the degree of hearing loss in noise-exposed people.

Dr. Davis: Is the information that is obtained by Dr. Raber on the individual audiograms used to protect the individual worker? When the individual reports abnormal hearing—something lying outside the boundary of the template—does the Organization move the worker into less noisy surroundings or provide personal protection in other ways? If this is not done at the present time, is it planned that this will be done in the future?

Dr. Raber: When a worker's noise-induced hearing loss is too great in relation to his time of exposure, our Institution tries to persuade him to change his job. If he does so, he can obtain a special compensation (Übergangsrente). If he refuses, we cannot compel him to give up his noisy work. Nevertheless, we strictly recommend the use of ear protectors which, however, we are in reality unable to enforce. When the hearing loss induced by occupational noise causes a loss of earning power of 20% or more, our Institution has to pay compensation even if the worker continues to work at the noisy place. If a worker leaves his noisy working place because of a marked noise-induced hearing loss but remains in the same factory, we follow up his hearing condition. All people receiving compensation on account of occupational "deafness" are submitted to monitoring tests. In most cases we see no further deterioration, apart from presbycusis. A few workers showed an improvement after retirement in spite of a previous noisy occupation for as much as 40 years.

Dr. Binns: Can the Austrian representatives give any information on the annual cost of their programme, how much is being paid out annually in compensation, and as to whether it is assumed that all noise-induced hearing losses are due to industrial conditions? One would imagine that with noise pollution being increasingly widespread and a great deal of noise being self-inflicted these days, particularly amongst young people, there is probably going to be, in future years, a large problem of noise-induced hearing loss quite extraneous to that produced in industry.

Dr. Raber: Mr. Surböck's department employs 22 engineers and clerical staff. Salaries, pension fund contributions and the inclusive costs of equipment amount on the average to A.S. 2 million per annum (£32,000). In December 1969 our Institution paid compensation in 573 cases of occupational noise-induced hearing loss, the average payment being A.S. 700 (£11). This amount is paid 14 times per annum, following the custom for salaries and pensions in Austria. In many cases we are aware that, in addition to the noise-induced hearing loss, we are also compensating for presbycusis and hearing loss from gunfire during the last two wars, especially when the persons concerned served in tank or flak units. Our arguments for compensating these cases are as follows. Before the age of retirement people do not usually suffer a social handicap from presbycusis but through an additional hearing loss caused by occupational noise a moderate degree of hearing impairment can develop. When we are of the opinion that the occupational noise exposure has materially influenced a multi-conditioned hearing damage, we suggest compensation to the relevant compensation boards.

Dr. Walker: There has been a great deal of discussion concerning the use of criteria for the assessment of hearing damage and compensation for the resulting social handicap in relation to the American State and Federal decisions and Mr. Surböck has mentioned the Austrian procedure which uses the loss of earning capacity as a basis for assessing the amount of compensation. How do the American and Austrian criteria for assessing compensation compare and, in particular, is the Austrian assessment the more liberal?

Dr. Wakstein: The figures given by Dr. Raber show that the payment is something like 10% of a typical salary and it goes on for the rest of a man's life. American workmen's compensation awards cover a very wide range: $3700 for full loss in Virginia and $33,000 for full loss in Hawaii. That is all a man gets; after that is used up there is no more. The average production worker earns about $5000 per annum. For say 50% loss and an above-average award, say the third quartile figure of about $10,000, the award is $5000, or about 1 year's pay. So it seems that the Austrian scheme is more liberal: a man can get 10% of his salary for the rest of his life. I think one can safely assume that Austrian workers will live at least 10 years beyond the age, say 40, at which they start to get compensation for noise-induced hearing loss.

Dr. Raber: May I give a very simplified example of our compensation procedure. A man earned in the last year A.S. 6000 per month (£97). If he becomes totally disabled as a result of an accident at work or through a registered occupational disease, his compensation will be two-thirds of his previous earnings, A.S. 4000 (£65) fourteen times a year. Total disablement means that the loss of earning capacity is 100%. In case of total deafness, for example through an explosion, the hearing loss is 100% and we consider the loss of earning capacity to be 50%. In the above-mentioned case, the benefits would be A.S. 2000 (£32) fourteen times a year. But occupational noise mainly results in a moderate hearing loss of about 40% of normal hearing. The compensation would thus be A.S. 800 (£13) with an assumed loss of earning capacity of 20% ($6000 \times 2/3 \times 20/100$). Since noise-induced hearing loss is irreversible the compensation is to be paid for life. A moderate degree of hearing loss means, in clinical otology, that conversational speech is understood up to a distance of 4 m, and whispering is heard up to 25 cm. To evaluate the degree of hearing loss in compensation cases we use the results of speech audiometry.

Dr. Coles: I would like to ask a question about the speech audiometry as used by Dr. Raber. Presumably, if he is relating speech audiometry to hearing ability as measured by the distance at which a person can hear a whisper or conversational voice, the speech audiometry refers to the 50% or 40% intelligibility level, sometimes called the speech reception threshold level. Does Dr. Raber also use the percentage of words which the person fails to hear, that is the discrimination loss; does he relate this at all to the amount of noise exposure or to the pure-tone audiogram; and does he use this in calculating the amount of compensation?

Dr. Raber: We use the German version of speech audiometry according to Hahlbrock (1957), which consists of two tests. In the first, polysyllabic numerals are tested, such as "dreiunddreissig" or "vierundachtzig". In the second test, monosyllabic nouns are offered. The second test is performed in order to evaluate the discrimination loss. Dr. König is known to be an expert on this matter and the methods of Boenninghaus and Röser (1958) are also used in Basel, so perhaps he would be able to explain the details.

Dr. König: According to the table which was established in Germany by Boenninghaus and Röser, the assessment of the degree of hearing disability is based on speech audiometry. This table, which may be compared with the chart of Social Adequacy Index as published by Davis (1948), permits one to obtain the percentage of hearing loss from two measures: first the *hearing loss for speech* measured in decibels, and second the *discrimination loss* or the maximum articulation score subtracted from 100%. In this connection it should, however, be mentioned that, for the assessment of the hearing loss for speech, numbers are used in Germany instead of two-syllable spondee words, whereas the discrimination loss is measured, as in the U.S.A., with the phonetically-balanced (PB) lists of one-syllable words (Hahlbrock, 1957). Boenninghaus and Röser have elaborated a further table which permits one to obtain the loss in earning capacity (Minderung der Erwerbsfähigkeit) from the percentage of unilateral or bilateral hearing loss. However, I would like to stress that in Basel we are not quite happy with the use of the two above-mentioned tables, which do not take account of hearing in noise. Furthermore we do not employ the same lists of words as used in Germany. In fact, because of certain language difficulties, we have ourselves developed phonetically-balanced lists of disyllabic spondees as well as of monosyllables (König, 1966). With regard to the experience found in Germany, the results of our measurements usually show a better correlation with the results obtained in the U.S.A.

Dr. Coles: I have one point which really refers to Dr. Hood's earlier comments. Is there, generally speaking, any correlation found between the discrimination loss and the pure-tone loss on the audiogram?

Dr. Raber: Röser (1963) published a rather simple relation between the degree of loss of speech intelligibility (for numbers) and the hearing loss at 500, 1000 and 2000 Hz from the pure-tone audiogram. In the case of noise-induced hearing loss his rule is as follows:

$$\text{Hearing loss for numbers (in dB)} = \tfrac{1}{6}\{3H_{500} + 2H_{1000} + H_{2000}\}$$

Some years ago we investigated this matter by regression analysis and we also tried to estimate the above-mentioned discrimination loss for monosyllables from the pure-tone hearing levels. For these regression analyses it was very important to consider the data from each otologist separately.

The standardization of speech audiometry appears to be very difficult. As a matter of fact, there exists a great variability in the tapes used in speech audiometry even if they come from the same factory. We had data from an otologist in which the difference between the true hearing loss for numbers and that estimated by regression formulae was 10 dB or less in 96% of the cases. For monosyllables the discrimination loss actually found in patients differed by more than 10% from the value given by our formulae in 30% of the cases.

Dr. Hinchcliffe: For clarification, could Mr. Surböck and Dr. Raber say whether or not, according to Austrian law, a person who has suffered an occupational noise-induced hearing loss can be compensated only if there has been actual loss of earning capacity? This is important because English law has seen a change in this matter. The Departmental Committee on Compensation for Industrial Diseases (The Samuel Committee) reported, in 1907, that boilermakers' deafness was unquestionably an injury due to employment. It did not, however, prevent a man from continuing his trade and could not, therefore, at that time give him a right to claim under the Workman's Compensation Acts for compensation on the ground of incapacitation. However, under Section 55 of the National Insurance (Industrial Injuries) Act of 1946, which replaced the Workman's Compensation Act, a disease which causes loss of faculty and not necessarily loss of wages may be prescribed under this Act and then the affected worker may be entitled to benefit. Also could the Austrian representatives clarify whether Austrian law distinguishes between industrial accident and occupational disease?

Dr. Raber: If the manager of a big factory loses a leg because of an accident at work, his loss of earning capacity from this will be practically zero. Nevertheless he will be compensated. Amputation of a leg is considered to cause a loss of 40% of what is called earning power, irrespective of profession. In the case of noise-induced hearing loss, we theoretically compensate for the loss of earning power but actually we compensate for the degree of hearing impairment. Furthermore if a worker receives benefit for suffering from occupational hearing loss, he is not automatically removed from the noisy working place. Austrian law embraces hearing loss by accident during work or on the way to or from work, as well as occupational hearing loss.

Dr. Davis: I should like to make a comment and also ask a question. The comment is that the development in the United States of the occupational workmen's compensation has been exactly parallel to the situation in Austria. It started, at first based clearly on the concept of loss of earning capacity, but it gradually developed, through custom and court decisions, to the concept of Scheduled Injuries for which certain definite agreed amounts would be paid. The amount depends on the wage of the individual at the time of accident or of separation from employment. We differ in not making payment during continued occupation. My question concerns the payment for partial hearing impairment. Is there any gradation, and on what kind of scale? Is it related to decibels or determined as a function of some measure of impairment?

Dr. Raber: For this we use the tables of Boenninghaus and Röser (1958), in which there is a sliding scale for the relation between percentage hearing loss and percentage impairment or handicap. Occupational noise produces, on the average, a loss of 40% of normal hearing and since total hearing loss is equated to 50% loss of earning power, this means that the resulting impairment is 20%. Cases with pure noise-induced hearing loss of 60 to 80% are very rare, but of course the benefits would be correspondingly higher.

Dr. Wakstein: With reference to Dr. Van Atta's paper, there would seem to be two possibilities for regulating noise by the Federal Government. One is the way that it adopts with the sale of cigarettes, by requiring that a notice of the danger to health be put on each package. The second way would be through the Interstate Commerce Commission since I understand that the Federal Government can make requirements about goods that are sold in interstate commerce. Is there any likelihood that these methods will be used? The various laws that Dr. Van Atta described presumably have some teeth in them, but have they bitten yet and to what extent?

Dr. Van Atta: The short answer to Dr. Wakstein's first question is no. The control of noise would not be within the authority of the Interstate Commerce Commission and regulation could not be that way under our Statutes. As for labelling, I do not see how it would work. There is, however, a possibility within the five Bills in the Congress at the present session of which the Congressional prophets are saying that one or more are bound to pass. These Bills vary only in detail and are all aimed at Federal regulation as a matter of occupational safety and health in all industry which *affects* interstate commerce. This is a substantial constitutional change from what we have had before, namely that the Federal Government may regulate industries which *engage* in interstate commerce. When and if any of these Bills, or any likely modification of any of them, go into effect, the Federal Government will have substantial regulatory authority over at least 72 or 73 million out of our total labour force of 75 million. They all provide for control by regulations but it remains to be seen what will actually happen after the law is on the Book. It is one thing to have a law and another to have some money for the enforcement of that law. Under the Walsh–Healey Act, which is the one we use most, and the Service Contract Act, we do not regulate as a matter of law but as a matter of contract. The only sanction which we have is to cancel the present contract or to deny future contracts. We have very little use for enforcement under these laws. Our man-power is quite small. We go into about 3000 plants a year and out of those 3000 inspections we normally have about three legal actions which go to a hearing. One reason that we have only three is because we never lose a case: the penalty is always the same, denial of Federal contracts for three years. For a company in the supply business this is an unhappy thing.

Mr. Higgins: There is one custom which you have in America that we might do well to emulate in the United Kingdom, and that is the practice of companies granting employers' liability insurance not to guess when they can measure. In other words, they employ trained industrial hygienists to evaluate the working environment. Could Dr. Van Atta comment on the extent to which these activities of the employers' liability insurance companies help the hearing conservation programme in the United States?

Dr. Van Atta: This is rather a dubious question because how much these activities help is not necessarily related to how many there are. We have a theory in the United States that when a problem arises, the insurance company will be the first to complain and the last to do anything about it, but this is not particularly unreasonable because they have no real sanction except to withdraw the contract and that is an unhappy thing for the insurer to do as well as for the company. However, a number of companies, and three of the largest in particular, have excellent acoustical consultants and, to the extent that they wish to have the service, their insureds are entitled to have it. A considerable number of them use it, and I should not draw too black a picture of the situation. A number of companies have their own acoustical staff who do excellent work. Bethlehem Steel has done so for many years. Dupont Company has had noise requirements in all purchase contracts for equipment since 1956 and have been trying, though without altogether succeeding, to get suppliers to supply what they want. Several other companies have started acoustical programmes between 1953 and the present time and are doing a great deal towards hearing conservation. Even some of the mining companies have quite good noise reduction and hearing conservation programmes.

Dr. Hunter: In Dr. Bruton's hearing conservation programme, if a hearing loss greater than 25 dB at a speech frequency is found in a pre-employment medical examination, are any special precautions taken about that person or is he treated in exactly the same way as would be the case if this loss were discovered at routine audiometry?

Dr. Bruton: Where a person has, at re-check audiometry, what one describes as significant hearing loss we would take steps to protect his hearing by first of all advising him that he is at some degree of risk, by ensuring that he is provided with hearing protection, and by arranging more frequent audiometric follow-up. If at pre-employment medical examination a person has a significant hearing loss—and I do not think 25 dB in one single speech frequency in either ear is a significant hearing loss on its own—and if he was coming into a noise-exposed job, we would again take steps to advise him to wear hearing protection. We would advise management that he must wear hearing protection when noise-exposed, and we would formally arrange more frequent periodic follow-up. Whether he actually wears hearing protection, of course, is very much up to him.

Dr. Hinchcliffe: I wish to congratulate Dr. Bryan on attempting an analysis of a very difficult subject, which might be termed forensic audiology. He has treated the subject as it is dealt with by the Common Law at the moment, that is under the law relating to negligence. However, the problem arising under the Common Law with regard to securing redress for someone suffering from occupational noise-induced hearing loss would be overcome if noise-induced hearing loss were a prescribed occupational disorder since, in that case, it would be covered by Statute Law. As I mentioned before it would appear that, although hearing loss is not at the moment recognized as an occupational disorder at English law, there is no reason why this should continue to be the case (Hinchcliffe, 1967b). It might be argued that the Devon Assizes case (T. A. Down *v.* Dudley, Coles, Long Ltd., 1969) is of no great interest since close scrutiny of the information relating to the medical status of the plaintiff indicates that he suffered not from an occupational noise-induced hearing loss but from a sensorineural hearing loss, due perhaps to vascular occlusive disease. Nevertheless, it would appear that the Judge accepted not only the expert's evidence but also the evidence regarding the usage of the gun and that this was not necessarily dangerous. Thus, in the scientific sense, it might be argued that the Judge reached the correct decision for the wrong reasons.

Mr. Chadwick: Dr. Bryan has given a very interesting account of the literature relating to occupational deafness. For the sake of historical accuracy I would like to go even further back. Ramazini's treatise (1713, 1740) is a fascinating early work on occupational medicine and in it he actually recommends aural protection, stating that "the continual action of the sound and noise . . . and the Repercussion of the internal Air on the sides of the auditory Passage greatly weakens and spoils the Organs of Hearing of those who happen to live near the Cataracts of the River Nile in Egypt, since they are all render'd deaf by the Noise of the falling Water". He goes on to say "The Ears may be fill'd with Cotton in order to hinder their internal Parts from being injur'd by the Noise." Glorig

(1958) in his monograph "Noise and Your Ear" draws attention to the advice given over a century ago to a correspondent in the *Lancet* who requested a remedy for preventing the hearing loss caused by rifle shooting. The answer was to use cotton in the ears. Comparatively speaking, however, these are modern references. The Book of Ecclesiasticus (38, 28) gives a vivid description of "the smith, ... sitting by the anvil ... the noise of the hammer and the anvil ever in his ears". There is, moreover, a description of aural protection extending back a thousand or so years before this. In the works of Homer, whose precise date of existence is lost in the mists of time, but who is considered to have lived somewhere between 850 and 1200 B.C. (Monro, 1926), are recorded the wanderings of Odysseus. Many ships had come to grief when sailors lured by the seductive songs of the Sirens had been wrecked on the rocks surrounding their island. To avoid this, Odysseus moulded wax to stop up his oarsmen's ears. His own ears were left free but in order that he should not be tempted by the singing and cast himself overboard, he ordered his men to lash him to the mast. When he heard the enchanting songs of the Sirens, he shouted to his sailors to untie him. Because their ears were plugged they paid no attention to him and rowed safely past the treacherous island and away from harm. Returning to the action for noise deafness which took place at the Devon Assizes, this was interesting not only in its legal aspects, but also from the otological standpoint. Coles (1969) has published a detailed commentary on the case which highlights one of the problems constantly besetting the otologist. This is the difficulty encountered when noise-induced deafness complicates a pre-existing hearing loss from other causes. In this particular instance the claimant was known to have prior perceptive deafness of considerable degree and during the course of his noise exposure he sustained severe vertigo with subsequent complete hearing loss in what had formerly been his better-hearing ear.

Dr. Ashworth: The gradually increasing awareness in industry and particularly among the workers themselves, of Common Law liability in cases of acoustic trauma, is going to put industrial medical officers in a very awkward position. One of the most useful features of serial audiometry is that of educating the workers, trying to get them interested themselves in protecting their own hearing, but if we are doing serial audiometry and encounter definite cases of increasing acoustic trauma, what do we say to our patient? Where do our loyalties lie?

Dr. Bryan: Mr. Chadwick makes a cogent point in regard to the difficulties which face the otologist in dealing with cases of pathological noise-exposed subjects. However, I must reiterate that in the Devon case both sides agreed there was a probable causal relationship between the noise and the deafness (Coles, 1969). The point at issue was whether or not the employer knew that this type of noise could produce deafness. Regarding the position of industrial medical officers, it is easy to see how questions of divided loyalties arise when they know quite well that noise causes deafness but are unable to convince their employers of the latters' liability. I should have thought that if employers had their responsibilities pointed out to them, as far as protecting their workers' hearing was concerned, then industrial safety officers would have fulfilled their obligations. In the last resort the responsibility must lie with the employer.

Dr. Wakstein: Dr. Bryan has done extremely valuable work in documenting the fact that there has been knowledge about the relation between noise and deafness for some time. It seems to me that we at this Conference know this: he is talking to the converted; but our responsibility is to make sure that other people know about the risk of hearing damage. Maybe some of the public have not read *Love on the Dole,* or Bell's W.H.O. monograph, nor looked at all Dr. Bryan's references. Indeed, in relation to the Devon Assize case one can go back as far as 1956 when there was some concern about the effect of impulsive noise on hearing, and if one refers to Kryter and Garinther (1963) there are some two dozen references going back into the '40s. This raises the question: maybe we know about these references, but if the public do not know I wonder whether an employer could in fact be held negligent. Dr. Bryan also raised a question that industry will consider very important: how much will it cost to quieten their machines? We have made a simple estimate of this cost for the U.S.A. (Bugliarello *et al.*, 1968) taking the number of workers to be 5·5 million in metal working and 16·2 million in manufacturing. We assumed that machines would have to be quietened between 10 and 30 dB, that between 10 and 100% of them would need to be quietened and that the life of a machine is 10 years. We used data kindly supplied by G. E. Parsons of Hercules, Inc., on the cost of noise control measures and the associated reductions in sound pressure levels during a 14-year programme of noise control; the figure was $70 per decibel per worker. We arrived at figures of $3400 million per year to quiet all machines in manufacturing by 30 dB, and $38·5 million per year to quieten 10% of machines in metal working by 10 dB. Even the large figure is only one-half of 1% of the gross national product of the U.S.A. Presumably a similar fraction would apply in Britain, so this estimate ought to be encouraging to industry. Obviously some companies will have greater expense than the average but these might take note that one compensation claim will buy a lot of machine quietening. Ear muffs are a lot cheaper but they are uncomfortable and are therefore often not worn in dangerously noisy areas or are sprung apart to make them more comfortable, with the result that the necessary protection is not provided. Thus machines have to be quietened too.

Dr. Ward: Describing the Gundefender ear plugs, Mr. Forrest said that for impulses above 140-dB peak sound pressure, the increase of attenuation was quite steady at the rate of about 1 dB per 2 dB increase in impulse level. This sounds right but I am curious how that was actually measured.

Mr. Forrest: The 1 dB increase in attenuation per 2 dB increase in incident impulse level was originally derived theoretically, but has also been confirmed experimentally using both artificial ears and cadaver ears. The intensity of the shot was varied by moving the source to different distances. Successive impulses from a starting pistol do vary in shape, and this is probably the main cause of the experimental scatter; but there did not appear to be any important systematic changes, which would have been detected by the microphone at the ear canal entrance. I should add that the plugs only become really effective above about 150 dB.

Mr. Chadwick: Problems associated with the use and abuse of ear protectors are frequently encountered in clinical practice. Hearing loss resulting from the high-intensity impulsive noise associated with spare-time rifle shooting or the firing of double-barrelled shotguns is a not uncommon form of recreational deafness. A case recently presenting was a 25-year-old member of an amateur rifle-shooting club who showed a sharp rise in hearing threshold of 60 dB at 1·5 kHz, increasing to a maximum loss of 75 dB at 4 kHz. The need for greater awareness of the auditory hazards of sports guns has been stressed both in this country (Coles and Rice, 1966) and in the U.S.A. (Taylor and Williams, 1966). In previous papers (Acton, Coles and Forrest, 1966; Acton and Forrest, 1968) Mr. Forrest has urged the necessity for protecting the hearing when firing such weapons. His present paper emphasizes the desirability of preserving communication whilst at the same time providing adequate protection for the cochlea. If the provisional Gundefenders he has described achieve this aim, this is indeed a great step forward in aural protection. Up till now, loss of the ability to understand speech has been one of the main stumbling blocks when trying to encourage individuals to wear suitable protectors. The following three cases illustrate both what can be achieved and how failure can arise when aural protection is prescribed.

1. The first example was a middle-aged man complaining of tinnitus and "woolly hearing" in the left ear. He had recently taken up clay-pigeon shooting with a 12-bore shotgun, wearing no protection. His audiogram showed a classical C^5 (4 kHz) dip, the threshold at this frequency being 55 dB. He was fitted with ear muffs and continued shooting. His loss at 4 kHz has been reduced to 25 dB and has remained steady at this level for several years. Here, comparative success from protection has been achieved.

2. Case number two was a 27-year-old engineer in a printing firm.

Following the installation of a new and noisier machine he had become aware of deafness. Mallock–Armstrong ear plugs were fitted and some hearing improvement resulted. He found, however, that whilst wearing them he was unable to distinguish the delicate changes in tone on which periodic adjustments of his machines depended. He discarded his plugs and his hearing again deteriorated. Initial success followed by failure when protection was abandoned.

3. The final case was the operator of an industrial gas-turbine generator which produced impulsive peaks of high-intensity noise. Although partial hearing protection was obtained by being enclosed in a sound-damped booth, his initial audiogram revealed an "acoustic dip" at 4 kHz in the right ear of 60 dB and in the left ear of 30 dB. Ear muffs were provided, and over a period of 2 years the dip in the right ear had improved to the 20-dB level. The left ear not only showed that the notch had deteriorated to 65 dB, but also that there was considerable perceptive loss at all other frequencies. It transpired that whenever he wanted to listen to someone speaking he was in the habit of lifting the cup away from his left ear "so that he could hear better"! Success on one side; failure on the other.

Just as one can lead a horse to water but cannot force it to drink, so with the provision of aural protection. My otological colleague Charles Smith at a Royal Society of Medicine meeting in March 1967, observing that "half a loaf is better than no bread", suggested that perhaps those who refuse to protect both ears might at least be encouraged to preserve the hearing in one.

Section III

Assessing Hearing Loss

Presbycusis in the Presence of Noise-induced Hearing Loss

By

R. Hinchcliffe

Institute of Laryngology and Otology, University of London, England

Summary

It would appear that attempts to attribute any hearing loss to noise exposure, and to apportion the loss to this factor, is not a simple exercise and is fraught with difficulties. Nevertheless, an audiological assessment is possible but conclusions must rest, as elsewhere in medical diagnosis, on a question of probabilities.

INTRODUCTION

An undoubted relationship between noise exposure level and hearing level now emerges in various reports. In particular, there is the report of the extensive investigation of hearing and of noise in industry which has just been completed in this country by a joint Medical Research Council and National Physical Laboratory team (Burns and Robinson, 1970). The data obtained now enable one to specify, with some precision, the proportion of people working in a given occupational noise environment who will attain, at a given frequency, a particular hearing level after a specified number of years' exposure.

Glorig and Nixon's (1960) assertion that ageing and noise exposure are the only factors that influence the measures of central tendency in the hearing levels of the general population is commonly subscribed to, and this is supported by the recent data obtained by Burns and Robinson in this country. However, as has been demonstrated from population studies in Jamaica (Hinchcliffe, 1968), this assumption may not be tenable for populations outside Europe or North America. Moreover, in assessing to what extent occupational noise is responsible for impaired hearing in a given individual as opposed to a population, many other factors must be considered. For example, Konigsmark (1968) lists at least sixty different types of hereditarily-determined hearing loss alone, without considering the plethora of non-hereditary types of hearing loss. Furthermore, where the question of compensation arises (and this is the very practical situation in which we find ourselves, or shall be confronted, in assessing noise-induced hearing loss), we shall have to determine how much of the hearing loss is functional (non-organic). Our experience indicates that, in cases where compensation is involved, it is not a question of whether or not there is a functional component, but to what extent there is a functional component. Finally, the multi-causality of presbycusis (Weston, 1964; Hinchcliffe, 1968), let alone the question of whether it exists as a separate entity (Schmidt, 1967), poses considerable problems for the physician who is confronted with an older person who has spent a lifetime working in one or more noisy industries.

Thus, the question "presbycusis or noise-induced hearing loss?" may not be a valid one or, at least, is too simple a question to entertain, despite the fact that, contrary to some beliefs, the audiometric picture of "presbycusis" is essentially different from that of noise-induced hearing loss. It therefore behoves us, in the present analysis, to consider first what is meant by the term "presbycusis", and then how an assessment is conducted on the individual case.

PRESBYCUSIS

Zwaardemaker (1893) coined the term "presbyacusia" to denote the poorer hearing of elderly people. Although Glorig and Nixon (1960) would restrict the use of the term to hearing losses due to physiological changes with age, others would apply the term to any sensorineural hearing loss occurring in old age. For example, Shambaugh (1960) considers that endolymphatic hydrops may be secondary to presbycusis, so that evidence for this otological disorder would not preclude a diagnosis of presbycusis. Schuknecht (1964) holds that a horizontal audiogram, which indicates the stria vascularis atrophy that Fleischer (1952) described in the aged cochlea, is compatible with the diagnosis of presbycusis. However, the audiogram in presbycusis characteristically shows a gradual fall-off of the hearing level with positive acceleration towards the higher frequencies. Population studies, for example in Britain (Hinchcliffe, 1959a) and in the U.S.A. (Glorig *et al.*, 1957), have consistently shown that, with increasing age, the hearing levels of negligibly noise-exposed and otherwise otologically normal people show a corresponding deterioration which is positively accelerated and is more marked for the higher frequencies. Thus average values are available for the purposes of making "presbycusis" corrections to data for noise-exposed populations. Robinson (1968) has indeed pointed out that analysis has indicated that subtraction of a standard "presbycusis" correction was beneficial to the data reduction.

Further analysis (Hinchcliffe, 1962a) of these average hearing levels on negligibly noise-exposed and otherwise otologically normal populations showed that, when the intensity of the threshold stimulus was expressed in terms of a quantity $(\phi - \phi_k)$, where ϕ is the physical intensity of the threshold stimulus and ϕ_k is the physical intensity of some reference level, an exponential decrement with age was exhibited. Moreover, a single curve seemed to fit the data for all frequencies from 250 Hz to 4000 Hz. Furthermore, all sensory threshold sensitivities appeared to exhibit this exponential decrement with age. Thus this ageing phenomenon of threshold sensitivity is not confined to hearing. However, not only do the majority of older people have poorer hearing levels than younger people, but they also have other auditory deficits, which have previously been listed (Hinchcliffe, 1962b). In particular, there may be a marked loss in the discrimination of both undistorted speech (Gaeth, 1948) and of distorted speech (Bocca, 1958). The latter condition, particularly, is indicative of impaired temporal lobe function so that, not unnaturally, it has been argued that many of the features of the auditory disorders with which the elderly are afflicted are primarily of central, rather than of peripheral origin (Hinchcliffe, 1962b). Nevertheless, degenerative changes have been described in various parts of the auditory mechanism so that a pathological basis for degenerative auditory disorders (perhaps a better, more descriptive, term than presbycusis) would appear to exist. Beginning peripherally and moving centrally, the following changes have been reported; changes in pinna size (Hsi-Kuei *et al.*, 1958); atrophy of the walls of the external acoustic meatus (Babbitt, 1947); calcification of the basilar membrane (Mayer, 1920); spiral organ degeneration—primary (Crowe *et al.*, 1934) or secondary (Fieandt and Saxén, 1937); stria vascularis atrophy (Fleischer, 1952); spiral ganglion degeneration (Crowe *et al.*, 1934); hyperostosis senilis progressiva meatus acoustici interni (Sercer and Krmpotić, 1958); degenerations in the auditory neurones in the brain stem (Kirikae *et al.*, 1964); and changes in the cerebral hemispheres (Hansen and Reske-Nielsen, 1965).

The question, however, arises as to whether these degenerative changes in the auditory subsystem are primary or secondary. Korenchevsky (1961) has endeavoured to discriminate between physiological and pathological processes of ageing and between physiological and pathological causes of ageing. He also points out that overwhelming evidence has accumulated to prove that present-day old age is an abnormal pathological syndrome in which physiological processes of ageing are complicated and aggravated by the various so-called degenerative diseases of old age. It could therefore be argued, with respect to hearing, that the principal causes of presbycusis, viewed as a clinical diagnosis, are pathological ones. Indeed Stein (1928) considered that arteriosclerosis was the principal aetiological factor in presbycusis and our analysis of Fabinyi's (1931) data indicates that the severity of the hearing loss in the elderly is related to the degree of degenerative arterial disease. Moreover, the importance of degenerative arterial disease in the aetiology of presbycusis was reasserted at the last

(IX) International Congress of Audiology in Mexico City both by Rosen (1969a) and by Bochenek and Jachowska (1969). Furthermore, Rosen and Olin (1965) stated that a longitudinal study in Finland had shown that institution of a non-atherogenic diet is associated with better hearing levels, and these trends are reversed when the diets of the control and the experimental groups are interchanged (Rosen, 1969b). Notwithstanding the assertion of Loeper and his associates (1961) that lipid infiltration is the consequence and not the cause of the vascular degenerative changes in atherosclerosis, Stamler (1960) points out that, almost without exception, experimental atherosclerosis closely resembling that in man has been associated with hypercholesterolaemia. Although it is possible to measure and to quantify the level of cholesterol in the blood, and to measure arteriosclerosis by external recordings (Cooper *et al.*, 1967), it is still questionable to what extent one can apportion a person's hearing loss to vascular degenerative changes, acting either directly on the auditory apparatus or indirectly by accelerating the physiological ageing. However, as Robinson (1968) has shown, utilizing data on essentially non-noise exposed populations, it is possible to use "presbycusis" corrections and, with the knowledge of the dispersion of the data, it is possible to assess the probability with which a given hearing loss is likely to be due to the "ageing process", having, of course, adequately assessed the person's audiological status and being cognizant that presbycusis-type curves are not characterized by notching. The pathological basis of presbycusis—as a degenerative disorder which generally involves the whole auditory subsystem, but with variable emphasis in different people, including non-involvement of the spiral organ (Hallpike, 1962)—probably affords an explanation for the simple additivity of threshold shifts in "presbycusis" and noise-induced hearing loss, the lesions of which are typically and discretely located in the basal turn of the spiral organ.

ASSESSMENT

The audiological assessment of an individual where noise-induced hearing loss is suspected is very much the same as that where any other hearing loss is under investigation, with the exception that a non-organic component in the hearing loss must be excluded where compensation is involved. Since malingerers usually follow equal-loudness contours for their simulated auditory thresholds, a sharp high-tone notch or an abrupt cut-off in the threshold audiogram almost certainly precludes a functional component, which would, however, be indicated by a type V Békésy audiogram (Jerger and Herer, 1961). In such an event, evoked response audiometry would be the next logical step in attempting to quantify the non-organic component (Beagley and Knight, 1968).

Abnormal curves of compliance versus excess intrameatal pressure on tympanometry indicate a conductive component in the hearing loss which can only be quantified by combined air- and bone-conduction audiometry.

The occurrence of temporary threshold drift (TTD), either as Carhart's (1957) tone decay on manual audiometry, or as a disparity between pulsed test-tone and continuous test-tone recordings on Békésy audiometry, indicates a neuronal lesion. Since noise-induced hearing loss is essentially a spiral-organ lesion (Igarashi *et al.*, 1964), demonstration of any of the previously cited phenomena indicates that factors other than noise have been, or are being, responsible for the hearing loss. Noise damage preferentially produces hair-cell damage at a point located 10 mm distant from the basal end of the spiral organ, so that audiograms showing other than a high-tone notch or an abrupt cut-off at high frequencies, for example low-tone notches or predominantly low-frequency hearing loss (as in endolymphatic hydrops), again indicate factors other than noise in the aetiology of the hearing loss. Even when one has found that a person who has been exposed to occupational noise has, after a "presbycusis" correction, a high-frequency loss with no conductive or non-organic component, and no evidence of a neuronal lesion, one is still not necessarily justified in attributing the loss to the noise since there are again many factors which can produce degeneration of the basal turn of the spiral organ (assuming that the more specialized audiometric tests indicate that this is the locus of the lesion). Apart from congenital aplasias (Scheibe's cochleo-saccular arrest), there is the possibility of infections, tumours of the stato-acoustic nerve (admittedly rare), or a consequence of ototoxic drugs. Gannon's (1969) study is particularly relevant to the latter factor. Even though noise-exposure levels or drug blood levels may, in the absence of the other factor, be insufficient to cause a hearing loss, the two together may summate to produce hearing loss in what otherwise would have been a condition where no appreciable hearing loss would have resulted. Hearing loss due to head injury is a special case of stimulation hearing loss and is attributed to generation of a high-intensity transient that reaches the cochlea by bone conduction (Schuknecht and Tonndorf, 1960).

Even when we find that a man, who has been working for an appreciable length of time in a noisy industry, has a classical high-tone "traumatic" notch, it may not be justifiable to attribute this to the noise. The majority of these people would have used fireworks in childhood or fired guns, in connection with military service or as a hobby, or both, prior to engaging in the occupation. Although, in random samples of the general population, it was found that measured hearing levels correlated with both the number of rounds of 0·303 ammunition fired (Hinchcliffe, 1959b) and the number of times a 12-bore gun was used (Hinchcliffe, 1961), Atherley and Noble (1969) failed to demonstrate, in a number of occupational groups, a relationship between a history of previous exposure to military gunfire and present hearing level. This discrepancy is yet to be resolved. Otopathologists would, however, be loath to attribute the latter finding to complete recovery of the hearing from the effects of acoustic trauma. It is possible that, in these samples, the effects of gunfire have been obscured by the many other factors which influence hearing level. This would also probably explain the finding that, in an unselected sample of patients attending a neuro-otology clinic, a history of previous, or contemporary, exposure to acoustic trauma or occupational noise or both is not correlated with the occurrence of high-tone notches in the auditory threshold. Or must we conclude that not only gunfire but also occupational noise does not have any long-term effects on hearing?

CONCLUSIONS

Because of the uncertainty of the degree to which other factors, whether they be in the nature of noises, noise-equivalents or otherwise, have influenced a hearing level before a person enters a given occupation, one can only say, with any reasonable degree of certainty, that occupational noise has influenced a man's hearing by being in possession of both pre- and post-employment audiograms. Even this safeguard does not enable us to exclude other factors which might damage hearing and have operated during the period of the man's employment.

Social Effects of Hearing Loss due to Weaving Noise

By

R. L. Kell, J. C. G. Pearson, W. I. Acton* and W. Taylor

Department of Social and Occupational Medicine, University of Dundee, Scotland

INTRODUCTION

The existence of a female weaving population employed in the jute industry in Dundee and surrounding towns should prove ideal for the assessment of the relationship between hearing loss due to occupational noise exposure and the resultant social handicap. Female jute weavers were chosen for this work for the following reasons:

(a) They have a long and continuous employment in the same industry, often with the same firm, and unaffected by breaks for military service. Subjects with up to 58 years of continuous work, broken only by annual holidays, were found.

(b) The present weaving looms were installed in the 1890's and it is estimated that the noise levels have not changed significantly during this period. The change from belt drive to individual electric power had little effect on the noise levels, which were measured by Taylor *et al.* (1965) and shown to be in the range 95–102 dB overall sound pressure level. A mean occupational noise level of 100 dB(A), for a minimum of 8 hours per day, may be taken as characteristic of jute weaving.

(c) Leisure pursuits and incidental noise exposure, for example rifle shooting and wild-fowling, which may cause permanent hearing loss, were minimal or non-existent.

Taylor *et al.* (1965) studied, retrospectively, progressive deterioration of the pure-tone threshold audiogram, for periods of up to 50 years' exposure to loom noise for a group of female jute weavers, using the results for 493 ears. Comparison of hearing levels with those of age-matched but non-noise-exposed populations, Hinchcliffe (1959a), Taylor *et al.* (1967) and Kell *et al.* (1970), show considerable losses, especially at frequencies of 2 kHz and above.

* Institute of Sound and Vibration Research, University of Southampton, England.

The pure-tone audiogram may not prove to be a good measure of the ability to understand speech, and thus a direct measure of this ability was thought to be desirable. In collaboration with the University of Southampton, two methods of speech audiometry were used in this study. The first was free-field speech audiometry performed against a noise background. The second was the established method of speech audiometry using headphones.

The female jute weavers thus appeared to be a suitable, homogeneous population to ascertain if the pure-tone threshold audiogram, by any combination of frequencies, will give a valid measure of social impairment. A control group of non-noise-exposed female subjects, matched for age and residence, was also investigated.

The object of Part I of this study was to assess the extent to which a known occupational noise contributed to social disability, pure-tone hearing levels and speech audiograms. Hearing levels, speech audiograms, and answers to a hearing questionnaire were compared for the female jute weavers and an age-, sex-matched control group.

METHOD

Measurement of threshold hearing level

Pure-tone air-conduction audiometry was performed at frequencies 0·125, 0·25, 0·5, 1, 2, 3, 4, 6 and 8 kHz in $2\frac{1}{2}$-dB steps, using a manually operated Peters SPD/2 clinical audiometer. After all weavers and half the control group had been measured, this audiometer was replaced by an Amplivox Model 83 audiometer incorporating 5-dB steps. Both audiometers were equipped with TDH39 earphones and MX41/AR cushions. For a small number of subjects an Amplivox Model 90 portable audiometer was used which did not incorporate 0·125 kHz but was otherwise of similar specification. The same test procedure was used with each test subject, that of Hinchcliffe and Littler (1958), Littler (1962), alternating right and left ears.

CALIBRATION OF AUDIOMETERS

As in previous studies, Taylor *et al.* (1965), Taylor *et al.* (1967), Kell *et al.* (1970), hearing level to British Standard 2497 (1954) was adopted and the departure from the calibration standard of Whittle and Robinson (1961) determined by an independent laboratory.

All results are based upon the following sound pressure level figures for zero dB for TDH39 earphones on a NBS 9A coupler.

Frequency (kHz)	0·125	0·25	0·5	1	2	3	4	6	8
SPL (dB)	50·5	30·5	15	10	9	10	10	23	15·5

The acoustic output of the audiometers was thereafter monitored weekly using Brüel and Kjær equipment. Audiometer frequencies were also checked during the survey period and, with the exception of 0.125 kHz on the SPD/2 audiometer (actual 115–120 Hz) and 4 kHz on the model 83 audiometer (actual 3·87 kHz), were within the ±3% allowance given in British Standard 2980 (1958).

AUDIOMETRIC ENVIRONMENT

A constant audiometric test environment was provided by bringing the subjects to the Department of Social and Occupational Medicine, in which a quiet room with double doors has been constructed in the basement. Measurements of the ambient noise level inside the quiet room with a Brüel and Kjær sound level meter type 2203 and octave-band filter type 1613 (Table XXII) are below those recommended for audiometric testing at 0 dB hearing level by Burns (1968).

TABLE XXII. Ambient noise level in quiet room

Octave band centre frequency (kHz)	0.125	0·25	0·5	1	2	4	8
Band pressure level in quiet room (dB)	17–22	9–14	(< 10, below internal noise level of sound level meter)				
Maximum permissible level (dB)	22	16	18	26	36	38·5	34·5

Measurement of speech audiogram

A pilot study (Taylor *et al.*, 1967) showed that the most common feature of hearing impairment was difficulty of communication against a background of noise or other voices. It thus was relevant to measure, on a controlled basis, the ability to distinguish speech from an interfering noise background. Semi-reverberant conditions were chosen since they approximate to normal domestic or work-place environments. The design and calibration of this method was carried out by the Institute of Sound and Vibration Research in Southampton University.

Speech audiometry was conducted against a background of 60-dB(A) low-frequency random noise in a sparsely-furnished room 4·5 m × 4·2 m × 2·1 m (15 feet × 14 feet × 7 feet), the subject sitting 1·8 m (6 feet) from the speech loudspeaker, situated directly in front, with two noise loudspeakers situated at either side of the subject (Fig. 54). A Ferrograph Series V tape recorder was used as a word source (frequency response ±3 dB from 40 Hz to 15 kHz at 7½ in/sec), feeding a Startronic type 113S 600-ohm variable attenuator (0–60 dB in 1-dB steps), Leak "TL/12 Plus" amplifier (±0·5 dB from 20 Hz to 20 kHz) and Wharfedale Super 8/RS/DD loudspeaker (±5 dB from 40 Hz to 20 kHz).

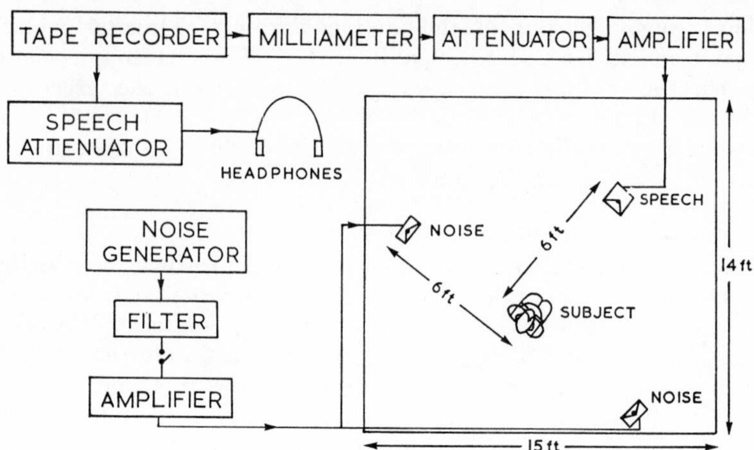

FIG. 54. Apparatus and layout for speech audiometry.

Background noise was generated by a pink-noise generator, filtered to give a predominantly low-frequency spectrum, feeding a Leak "TL/12 Plus" amplifier and two KEF Celeste loudspeakers (±5 dB from 65 Hz to 15 kHz). One-third octave-band analysis of this noise is given in Fig. 55. Following experimental work at Southampton, the decision was taken to use low-frequency random noise shaped to give a spectrum similar to that of babble, rather than recorded speech babble itself or pink noise.

The speech material used was phonetically-balanced monosyllabic word lists (Fry, 1961) which consisted of 10 word lists each of 35 words

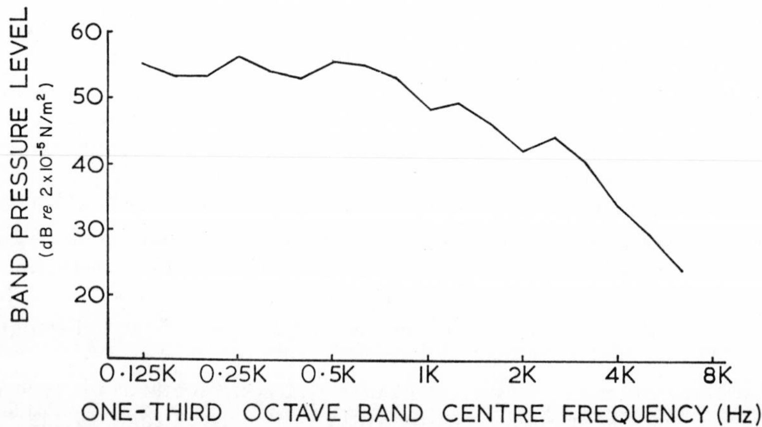

FIG. 55. One-third octave band spectrum of 60 dB(A) masking noise used in speech audiometry; measured at subject's head position.

(100 phonemes) spoken in a neutral "BBC accent". The 10 lists allowed a range of signal-to-noise ratios from 35 dB to −5 dB inclusive to be covered in 5-dB steps, with a practice list in addition. In practice, each word list was assigned to a specific speech level.

It was decided that the background (masking) noise level should be set so that young subjects with normal audiograms gave approximately 50% word score at normal voice level, that is, approximately 65-dB(A) peak level at the ear for face-to-face conversation. Setting the noise level to 60 dB(A) fulfilled this condition and the level of masking noise was kept constant in the study. A 50% phoneme score was achieved at a peak speech level of 60 dB. Twenty young persons (age range 17 to 35) with normal hearing verified this in Dundee for Scottish speakers, in addition to the Southampton test groups.

The procedure was to explain the nature and purpose of the test and then to introduce the subject to practice words at a relatively high level. By reducing the speech level in steps of 5 dB against the constant masking noise, speech audiometry was conducted from a high speech level clearly understood (although, for many weavers with hearing impairment, speech was not clearly understood at any level), to a low level at which a phoneme score of less than 50% was recorded. The noise level and speech level were checked, by sound level meter, in the subject head position daily.

Speech audiometry in the conventional manner by tape recorder and headphone was also undertaken. The output from the Ferrograph V tape recorder was fed into an Amplivox speech audiometer attachment type 14950, incorporating 120-dB attenuator and thence into Telephonics TDH39 earphones with MX41/AR cushions. The speech audiogram, without any masking noise, was then recorded in a similar manner to that of the masked speech.

Questionnaire

The questionnaire used was designed in the Department of Social and Occupational Medicine in Dundee, and subsequently modified after a pilot study (Taylor *et al.*, 1967). In addition to the basic demographic data, the questionnaire covered the following areas:

(1) Occupational history (with special reference to noise)
(2) Difficulties in communication
(3) Use of telephone
(4) Use of radio and television
(5) Difficulties at public meetings
(6) Use of hearing aid.

A complete list of the questions used is given in the appendix (p. 190).

Procedure

The hearing questionnaire was completed and followed by the taking of a medical history, including details of head injuries, ear pathology and exposure to drugs likely to affect hearing. A clinical otological examination was then made, including examination of the tympanic membrane and a Rinne test. Threshold pure-tone air-conduction audiometry was then conducted, followed by two methods of speech audiometry. The whole procedure, including breaks between tests, took approximately 1 hour.

Only the results from those subjects meeting the following requirements were accepted: (a) normal eardrums on otological examination, (b) external meatus free of cerumen, (c) no history of aural disease, past or present, (d) no upper respiratory tract infection at time of test, (e) no history of exposure to excessive noise (occupational, war service and leisure), other than weaving noise only, for the weavers.

Any subject with an abnormality in one ear was rejected from the study.

Selection of subjects

A minimum working life of 20 years' exposure to weaving noise was considered to be a basic requirement for the study. The work of Taylor *et al.* (1965) showed that after this time noise-induced hearing loss at 2 kHz increases more rapidly and, thus, difficulty in speech discrimination may also increase. Therefore, efforts were concentrated on identifying and interviewing long-service and retired weavers.

In selecting controls it was considered necessary that each came from the same town as the matched weaver, since the social activities in small towns differ from those in cities. The age-matching was done so that there was less than 5 years' difference in age between the members of each pair.

The study was conducted in Dundee and the surrounding Angus towns of Kirriemuir, Forfar and Carnoustie. In the country towns both weavers and controls were selected from the lists of the local general practitioners. In Dundee, weavers were selected from the factory lists of retired and long-service employees. Two sources of controls were required in Dundee, where there was considerable difficulty due to the high proportion of the population which had previously been employed in the jute industry. Cleaners in the University and randomly-selected patients from general practitioners' lists were chosen. In both groups many were rejected immediately because of noise exposure in the jute industry and are not shown in the tables.

Population studied

Details of the numbers of subjects examined are shown in Table XXIII. In all, 190 weavers and 218 controls were selected. Twenty-four weavers

(13%) and four controls (2%) could not be traced. The relatively large numbers of weavers in this category is due to the fact that the factory lists gave the last known address when employed, and extensive re-housing in the city in recent years meant that these lists were out-of-date.

TABLE XXIII. Populations. Response rates

	WEAVERS			CONTROLS		
Category	Dundee	Country Towns	Total	Dundee	Country Towns	Total
Number Selected	132	58	190	128	90	218
Not traced	22	2	24 (13%)	3	1	4 (2%)
Refusals	22	2	24 (13%)	25	25	50 (23%)
Rejected (medical reasons or noise exposure)	21	13	34 (18%)	30	13	43 (20%)
Less than 20 years' weaving	6	6	12 (6%)	—	—	—
Accepted for study[a]	61	35	96 (51%)	70	51	121 (55%)

[a] In this paper, the data on only 96 controls, matched to the 96 weavers, are presented.

Rejection rates in the weaver and control groups were similar, 18 and 20%. A total of 96 weavers satisfied the criteria for the study. They were compared with 96 matched controls selected from the 121 who also satisfied the criteria.

TABLE XXIV. Age structure

Age	Weavers	Controls
<55	10	11
55–64	33	31
65–74	42	42
75+	11	12
Total	96	96
Mean age	64·7	64·5

The mean time working in the jute industry and, hence, the mean exposure time to 100-dB(A) weaving noise for the group of 96 weavers was 41·6 years. The age structure of the two groups is shown in Table XXIV, the mean age of the weavers being 64·7 years and that of the controls 64·5 years.

RESULTS AND DISCUSSION

Social

The two groups contained similar proportions of married persons (30% weavers, 32% controls) and of people who lived alone (41% weavers, 36% controls). Thus, the factor of loneliness at home should have a similar effect on the social activities of both groups.

The main handicap found concerns difficulties in communication. The largest differences between the two groups occurred at public meetings, followed by talking with strangers, or family and friends, and in using the telephone. The numbers and percentages in the groups having difficulty in these areas are shown in Table XXV.

TABLE XXV. Hearing difficulty and communication

	Weavers	Controls
Difficulty at public meetings, church, theatre	69 (72%)	6 (6%)
Talking with strangers	77 (80%)	16 (16%)
Talking with friends	74 (77%)	15 (15%)
Understanding telephone conversation[a]	57 (64%)	5 (5%)

[a] 7 weavers and 1 control declared that they never used the telephone and could not answer the question regarding telephone conversation, and are thus not included.

Although only three of the weavers had stopped attending public meetings, church, etc., many of the remainder heard little despite moving to front seats. Habit appeared to be a factor in this continued attendance.

The results found for communication with strangers and with family and friends were similar. With known voices, difficulties occurred mainly against a noise background (47% in noise only; 30% at all times) whereas with strangers more weavers had difficulty at all times (32% in noise only; 48% at all times). The controls mainly experienced difficulty in noise, only one having difficulty at all times.

The very low ownership of telephones amongst the weavers (8%) compared with controls (58%) must reflect some dissatisfaction with the instrument as a means of communication.

The preferred volume of radio and television receivers also showed differences between the groups. Fifty-four weavers (56%) and four controls (4%) admitted that they liked the volume "high" but, because of the numbers living alone, there was no standard for comparison. Only three weavers and no controls had stopped listening to radio and television because of hearing difficulties.

Differences were also found between the groups in the subjective assessments of hearing made by the persons themselves, Table XXVI. Despite the high proportion of weavers who considered their hearing worse than normal (81%) compared with the controls (5%), only 9% of the weavers had a hearing aid and only 5% used an aid regularly. This must reflect the poor performance of current hearing aids for a noise-

TABLE XXVI. Subject's own assessment of hearing

	Weavers	Controls
Normal	18	91
Slightly hard of hearing	49	5
Hard of hearing	27	—
Very hard of hearing	2	—
Total	96	96

induced hearing loss, as well as the effect of the gradual deterioration of hearing over many years which may inhibit the weavers from taking action at any specific time. Furthermore, there was evident a natural disinclination to wear any form of artificial aid.

Pure-tone audiogram

The mean audiograms of the two groups are shown in Fig. 56. The average loss at 0·5, 1 and 2 kHz is 36·6 dB for the weavers compared with 12·8 dB for the controls.

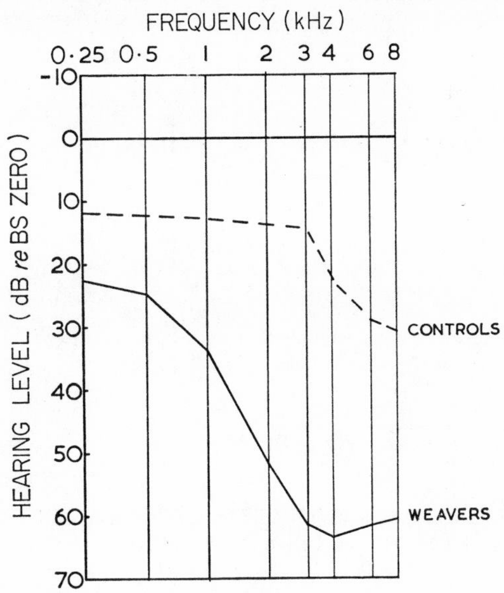

FIG. 56. Mean pure-tone audiograms of 96 weavers and age-matched controls.

Speech audiogram

The results for speech audiometry are presented in terms of the level, in dB, at which a 50% word score or phoneme score was achieved. The mean level at different ages is shown for the two groups, in Fig. 57 against a 60-dB(A) background noise, and in Fig. 58 with headphones. Also included in these diagrams for comparative purposes are the mean levels for 20 young persons with normal hearing.

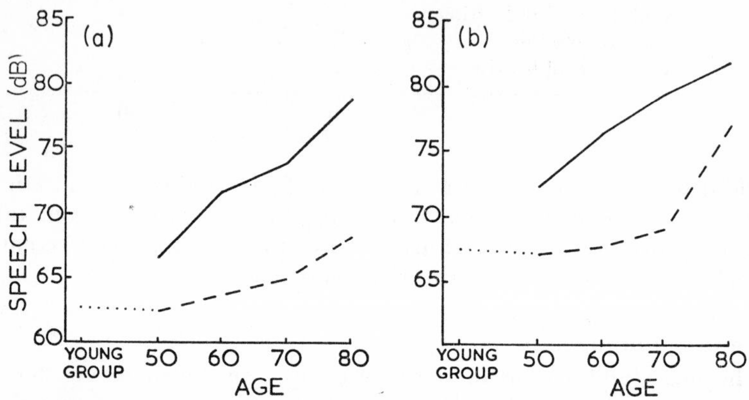

FIG. 57. Mean speech audiograms with masking noise, showing mean level at which 50% score was achieved for (a) phonemes and (b) words, at different ages in weavers, age-matched controls and young control group.

——— Weavers
- - - - Age-matched controls

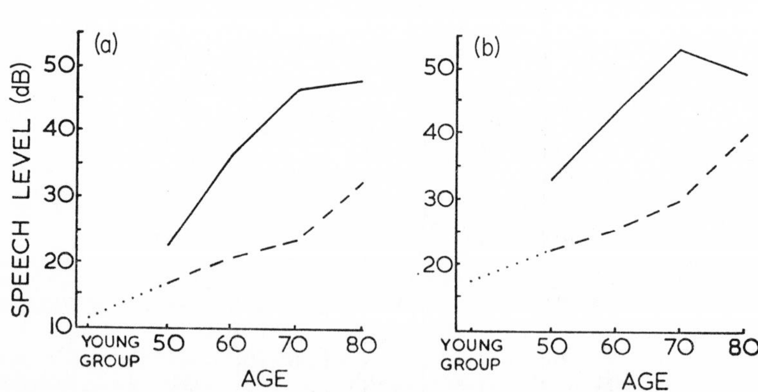

FIG. 58. Mean speech audiograms with headphones, showing mean level at which 50% score was achieved for (a) phonemes and (b) words, at different ages in weavers, age-matched controls and young control group.

——— Weavers
- - - - Age-matched controls

In all cases the weaving group requires higher sound levels to attain the same level of understanding of speech as the control group. Larger differences are found in the speech audiograms using headphones, where the subjects are listening to speech at or near threshold. Using this method the control group shows increased thresholds at all ages, although in the real-life situation their hearing is comparable to that of the young control group. Speech audiometry against a noise background provides a closer approximation to the real situation in both method and results, and for this reason is preferred to the headphone method.

CONCLUSIONS

The mean measured hearing levels of a group of 96 female weavers of mean age 64·7 years were greater than those of a group of 96 non-noise-exposed female controls of mean age 64·5 years. The average loss at 0·5, 1 and 2 kHz was 36·6 dB for the weavers compared with 12·8 dB for the controls.

Speech audiometry showed that the weavers, at all ages, had a poorer understanding of speech than the controls.

The social consequences of this impaired hearing ability were:

(a) difficulty at public meetings (weavers 72%, controls 6%)
(b) difficulty talking with strangers (weavers 80%, controls 16%)
(c) difficulty talking with friends (weavers 77%, controls 15%)
(d) difficulty understanding telephone conversation (weavers 64%, controls 5%)
(e) 81% of all weavers considered that their hearing was impaired (5% controls)
(f) 9% of weavers and no controls owned hearing aids
(g) 53% of weavers and no controls used a form of lip-reading.

The study has established the areas of social impairment due to noise-induced hearing loss. An attempt will be made in a later paper to relate these to pure-tone and speech audiograms.

ACKNOWLEDGEMENTS

This study was carried out under grants from the Advisory Committee for Medical Research (Research Fellow—Mr. R. L. Kell). We are indebted to the Medical Research Council for Grants to the University of Dundee (W.T.) and to the University of Southampton (W.I.A.).

We are indebted to local general practitioners, Dr. M. C. Hogg, of Dundee, Dr. W. Dodd, of Kirriemuir, Dr. J. G. Burgess, of Forfar, and Dr. D. A. McConnell, of Carnoustie, for their active assistance in the project. Our thanks are due to Mr. Douglas of the University of Dundee who arranged for University cleaners to be seen. We are also indebted to

Miss E. C. Knox of the Royal National Institute for the Deaf in Glasgow for audiometer calibration, to Mrs. M. McLaggan, Miss P. Knight, Miss C. Kane and Mrs. C. Gall who provided valuable interviewing and secretarial assistance, and to the members of the general population of Dundee, Kirriemuir, Forfar and Carnoustie, for their voluntary co-operation in the study. Lastly, we pay tribute to the jute weavers who represent a generation, now rapidly disappearing, of stable, long-service, industrious, happy and loyal people.

APPENDIX

QUESTIONS USED IN HEARING QUESTIONNAIRE

1. *Occupational history*

(a) Age started work .... Age retired...........
"Working life" ....

(b) Time at main job...........
Time off:
War.............. Other jobs.............. Children...............
(Check that total working life accounted for)

(c) Retirement
(i) Time in retirement..............
(ii) Part-time work during retirement?
Is it a noisy job?

2. *Extraneous noise exposure*

(weaving)

(a) Have you ever worked in a noisy job, other than ....?
Which?..............
How long were you in this job?

(b) Have you ever used a shotgun or rifle?
How often and for what length of time?

(c) Were you involved with gunfire, bombing, explosions, etc., during war service or as a civilian?

3. *Social*

(a) Members of household..............

(b) Do the people at home complain that you are deaf?

(c) Do you have difficulty talking with family and friends:
(i) in a quiet place?
(ii) when other people are talking?
(iii) in a noisy place?

(d) Do you have difficulty talking with strangers:
  (i) in a quiet place?
  (ii) when other people are talking?
  (iii) in a noisy place?

(e) Do people annoy you by shouting to make you hear?

(f) Do you lip-read?

(g) Do you use sign language?

(h) Do you have a telephone?

(i) Can you easily understand people on the telephone?

(j) Radio—
  Do you like the volume high?
  Do you like the volume higher than other members of the household?
  Do they ever turn the volume down?

(k) Television—
  Do you like the volume high?
  Do you like the volume higher than other members of the household?
  Do they ever turn the volume down?

(l) At meetings, church, cinema, theatre, bingo, etc., do you hear clearly if you have to sit at the back?
  Where do you normally like to sit?
  Have you changed your usual seat?

4. *General*

(a) How is your hearing at present?

(b) Do you have a hearing aid?
  Type..............
  Do you use it?

Clinical Picture of Occupational Hearing Loss obtained with the Hearing Measurement Scale

By

G. R. C. Atherley

Department of Pure and Applied Physics, University of Salford, Lancs.

and

W. G. Noble*

Department of Occupational Health, University of Manchester, Lancs.

Summary

The Hearing Measurement Scale is briefly described. It is a questionnaire which has been developed for use among people suffering from occupational hearing loss and its purpose is the assessment of disability in those with sensorineural lesions. It is used here to reveal the clinical picture of occupational hearing loss in men employed as drop-forgers. Results from two men are presented in detail together with their audiograms. It is shown that, despite similarity in terms of audiograms, the two men differ materially in terms of the clinical picture which they present. Two systems of assessment that depend on averages of pure-tone thresholds at 0·5, 1·0 and 2·0 kHz fail to show correctly which of the two men is the worse affected.

Results from the group of drop-forgers show, as would be expected, that the relationship is good between the various audiometric averages, for example, at 0·5, 1·0 and 2·0 kHz; 0·5, 1·0, 2·0 and 3·0 kHz. On the other hand the relationships between these averages and questionnaire scores is incomplete. It is argued on these grounds that pure-tone audiograms are an inadequate basis for the assessment of hearing disorder.

Questionnaire scores are compared among patients attending a hearing-aid clinic and occupational samples of metal dressers (chippers), weavers and drop-forgers. It is concluded that the clinical picture of occupational hearing loss for drop-forgers is not unusual for people in their sixth decade who have spent at least half of their working lifetimes in high levels of noise. The median clinical picture for these men is of an essentially trivial disorder of hearing. For those at and beyond the 75th centile of scores the picture is more serious.

* Present address: Department of Psychology, University of New England, Armidale, N.S.W., Australia.

INTRODUCTION

The purpose of this paper is to present results from a study of occupational hearing loss in men employed as drop-forgers. The study was made with the Hearing Measurement Scale, developed by Noble (1969) and described here in summary. The original purpose of the Hearing Measurement Scale was to provide a method for assessing auditory disability. The concept of auditory disability is described below. The purpose of the present study was to use the scale to gain an understanding of the clinical picture presented by men known to be suffering from occupational hearing loss.

Occupational hearing loss is a term used to describe persistent loss of sensitivity for pure tones brought about by noise encountered in the course of employment. The degree of such injury is related to the level of and total period of exposure to the noise. The usual audiometric picture is of an injury which develops relatively rapidly at first and later more slowly.

At some stage the injury reaches a point where the individual experiences disability. In terms of threshold of hearing, measured with pure tones, the point of onset of disability varies considerably between individuals and for this and other reasons assessment of disablement cannot be based wholly on pure-tone threshold determination. Disability arises not only because an individual suffers loss of hearing function but also because he experiences dysfunction of auditory ability. We mean by this that disability is experienced by an individual when the total disorder involves one or more of the following: difficulty in the perception of speech; difficulty in the perception of direction of sound; tinnitus; distortion of sound; and failure to hear the everyday sounds of life. In addition it includes hearing handicap which we define as the response of the person sustaining a hearing loss to that loss. People cope differently with similar degrees of disorder and the final disability is a complex of loss and adjustment to loss.

THE HEARING MEASUREMENT SCALE

A questionnaire is the most effective design for a multilateral method of assessment of hearing in a clinical context. This is not a novel idea; Silverman *et al.* (1948) and High *et al.* (1964) devised questionnaires for measuring hearing loss. Both studies used subjects with predominantly conductive lesions and we are doubtful, therefore, whether the instruments are appropriate for the assessment of hearing in people with cochlear sensorineural lesions such as occupational hearing loss. Blumenfeld *et al.* (1969) used the questionnaire of High and colleagues, called the Hearing Handicap Scale, among subjects suffering from presbycusis.

The results showed that the Hearing Handicap Scale was a less certain measure in that type of population than in the original test sample.

It was clear that a new instrument had to be compiled and tested in people with sensorineural lesions in order to provide a valid assessment of disability in such a population and that aside from sampling techniques was the issue of content. The previously reported questionnaires concentrated on speech hearing and we saw this as too narrow a coverage of hearing loss. Furthermore, neither of the existing scales incorporated "hearing handicap" as part of the assessment and we considered this an essential inclusion if a complete clinical picture was to be portrayed and a valid estimate of disability was to be obtained.

The final form of the Hearing Measurement Scale comprises 42 scoring items in seven subsections. These are:

(1) Speech hearing
(2) Acuity for non-speech sound
(3) Localization
(4) Emotional response to hearing loss
(5) Distortion of speech
(6) Tinnitus
(7) Personal opinion of hearing

Sections 1, 2, 3 and 5 deal principally with hearing loss; sections 4, 6 and 7 with hearing handicap. Tinnitus (section 6) is included under the latter heading because the bulk of scoring in section 6 is concerned with the effect of this dysfunction on personal adjustment.

The development and testing of the Hearing Measurement Scale is described fully by Noble and Atherley (in press) and only a brief summary is given here. The scale is designed for use at an interview and the scoring of responses, generally on a five-point scale, varies from item to item. Judgements about the relative importance of the sections and questions were made by a panel of five people expert in assessment techniques and in audiology. The questions and scoring systems are given in more detail later. All interviews are tape recorded and scores are allocated by an independent observer from the tapes. In practice, one interviewer scores another's interview.

An estimate of the reliability of the scale was made from a re-application after 6 months in a group of 27 foundrymen all with at least 15 years of occupational experience but drawn from three trades of different noisiness. This was done to give as wide a range of hearing ability as possible. The correlation coefficient (Pearson) was 0·934 and indicated that the scale was highly reliable in a field test situation. There was no significant change in mean scale scores between the two applications.

The validity of the scale as a measure of hearing loss and handicap was established in a number of ways. First, as a test of its measurement of hearing loss, the results of the reliability sample were analysed according to the three subgroups of men. Of the 27, there were 13 moulders, 8 grinders and 6 chippers, matched for age and years of experience in the job. The scale scores of these subgroups were significantly different and corresponded to the noise immission levels associated with each type of job. The immission levels were derived, in accordance with the definition of Robinson (1968), from acoustic measurements and from estimates of exposure duration calculated from the men's case histories. The association between scale score and degree of noise exposure demonstrated that the scale was valid at least for the measurement of hearing loss.

The second validation study, to assess the scale as a measure of handicap, was carried out by comparing the scale scores from the reliability sample with an assessment of social interest among the men, made by an independent observer. It was found that the men could be divided into three groups corresponding to degrees of social withdrawal. It was seen that the centre group was indistinct from the two extremes and analysis was confined to the latter, therefore. Scale scores of the two extreme groups—the one, of 7 men, those who sought and enjoyed contact with others; the other, 9 men, those who preferred to be by themselves—were compared and found to be significantly different. Because we would expect, from studies of the deaf personality, that the greater the hearing loss the more the social withdrawal, we concluded that the scale was sensitive to such a handicapping effect.

A comparative study was then conducted on 46 foundrymen and results showed that most subsections related logically to different performance tests. Thus, the individual parts of the instrument were valid for the measurement of whichever quality they were stated to measure. Finally, a section total analysis was conducted using results from all the foundrymen ($N = 73$) and it was found that each subsection related closely to the total score. It was concluded that the scale was consistent and cohesive in its measurement and the more likely, therefore, to provide valid estimates of disability.

THE DROP-FORGERS

Thirty-eight drop-forgers took part in the study. They were selected from a complete list of employees, at random, on the grounds of age and occupational experience. They were not self-selected. The ages ranged from 36 to 53 years and the number of years of occupational experience ranged from 15 to 45. All 38 men were interviewed with the questionnaire and given an otological examination. Nineteen of the total were free from gross otological abnormality and on a second visit 18 of these 19 were given an audiometric test about 16 hours following the last exposure to occupational noise. The test was carried out using self-recording audiometers generating pulsed tones.

Results from two drop-forgers

The two men whose results are to be described in detail were aged 53 and 51. They were selected from the larger group because their results illustrate certain points which we wish to emphasize. Their years of experience in drop-forging were 19 and 24 respectively. Neither gave a history of exposure to the noise of military gunfire nor did they show any evidence of otological disorder other than occupational hearing loss. The two men are identified by the codes "mild" and "slight" respectively. These terms derive from a system of assessment using pure-tone performance which will be described below. Figure 59 shows the audiograms

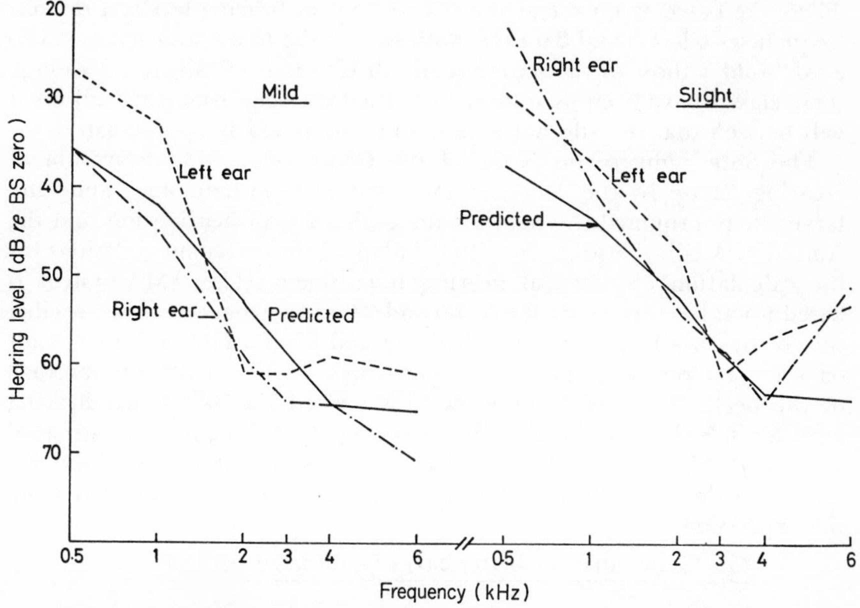

FIG. 59. Audiograms of two drop-forgers; left ears, right ears and predicted values.

from each ear of each man. Also shown in the figure are the "predicted audiograms" derived from a combination of noise measurements, conducted for us by A. M. Martin of the University of Salford and from Robinson's (1968) predictive equation. The predicted audiograms are based upon an equivalent daily exposure of 110 dB(A) and represent the median hearing levels corresponding to the men's years of exposure. The values at each test frequency which have been plotted include corrections for age worked out with the data given by Robinson. The agreement between observed and predicted values is good and supports the view that the men's hearing has been affected by the normal process of ageing and by noise but not by other factors.

Assessment of the hearing loss in the two men

There are in existence a number of schemes for the assessment of hearing loss which rely only upon knowledge of auditory thresholds. In our view, these share the disadvantages mentioned in connection with previously published questionnaires. They were derived from studies of conductive lesions and are inadequately validated for occupational hearing loss. However, it is of interest to test the two men against two such schemes.

In 1962, Davis described proposals for "classes of hearing handicap". These are based upon the arithmetic average of hearing levels at the test frequencies 0·5, 1·0 and 2·0 kHz. Both ears of the first man correspond to class "mild"; those of the second man fall into that of "slight". Although these classes have been used to identify the two men, from what follows it will be seen that they do not appear to be particularly appropriate.

The Subcommittee on Noise of the Committee on Conservation of Hearing set up by the American Academy of Ophthalmology and Otolaryngology proposed a system for the evaluation of hearing loss and the American Medical Association (1961) adapted these recommendations for the calculation of binaural hearing impairment. The AMA system is based upon hearing levels at 0·5, 1·0 and 2·0 kHz. From these the "decibel sum of hearing levels" (*sic*) is calculated and from a table the user reads off the corresponding "percentage impairment". The arithmetic average of the decibel sum of hearing levels is termed the "estimated hearing level for speech in decibels". The percentage impairments were adjusted so that 100% corresponds to 81·7 dB ASA estimated hearing level for speech in decibels. "Binaural Hearing Impairment" is calculated from the expression:

$$\frac{(5 \times \%\text{ impairment better ear}) + \%\text{ impairment worse ear}}{6}$$

When the results from the two drop-forgers are manipulated according to this system "mild" gives 24% and "slight", 19%. Thus, on the AMA system, there is little difference between the two men.

Results with the questionnaire from the two men

As part of the text the subsections of the Hearing Measurement Scale are set out in their order at interview. The questions are given more or less in the language in which they are put to the subject. Most questions require that the answer is fitted, by the scorer, into one of five categories:

"never" N, "hardly ever" HE, "sometimes" S, "nearly always" NA, "always" A. Some questions lead to only three categories (N, S or A) and others require "yes" or "no". Actual scores allocated to replies depend upon the weighting which, as previously mentioned, varies from question to question. Both responses and scores are given for the two men. At the end of the questionnaire results there is a summary of scores and following this there is an analysis of the results.

SECTION 1. Speech hearing

Question	MILD		SLIGHT	
	Reply	Score	Reply	Score
Participatory				
1.1 Do you ever have any difficulty hearing in a conversation with one other person?				
(i) at home	N	0	NA	7
(ii) outside	N	0	S	5
1.2 Do you ever have any difficulty hearing in a group conversation?				
(i) at home	N	0	A	8
(ii) outside	N	0	A	8
1.3 Do you have difficulty hearing conversation at work?	N	0	N	0
Is this due to your hearing, the noise or a bit of both?		—		—
Non-participatory				
1.4 Do you ever have difficulty listening to a public speaker?	NA	3	NA	3
1.5 Do you always hear what's being said on TV during				
(i) a play?	A	0	HE	5
(ii) the news?	A	0	HE	5
1.6 on Radio during				
(i) a play?	A	0		—
(ii) the news?	A	0		—
1.7 Do you have difficulty hearing what's said in a film at the cinema?	N	0	S	2

SECTION 2. Acuity for non-speech sound

Question	MILD		SLIGHT	
	Reply	Score	Reply	Score
Do you have any pets at home? Can you hear it when it...barks, mews, etc.?	A	0	A	0
Can you hear it when someone rings the doorbell/knocks on the door?	A	0	HE	5
Can you hear:				
a motor car horn?	A	0	A	0
the sound of footsteps outside?	A	0	A	0
the sound of a door opening?	A	0	A	0
the tick of a clock in the room?	no	1	no	1
the tap running?	A	0	A	0
water boiling in a pan?	A	0	A	0

SECTION 3. Localization

Question	MILD		SLIGHT	
	Reply	Score	Reply	Score
When you hear the sound of conversation, say in another room, can you always tell where it's coming from?	A	0	A	0
If you are in a group conversation and someone you can't see starts to speak, can you always tell where he is sitting or standing?	A	0	NA	1
If you hear a motor horn or a bell, can you always tell in which direction it is sounding?	N	6	A	0
Do you ever turn your head the wrong way when someone calls to you?	S	2	N	0
Can you usually tell how far away a person is when he calls out to you?	A	0	A	0
When you are walking outside have you ever noticed when a car that you thought, by its sound, was some distance away is in fact quite close?	HE	1	N	0
At work do you always move the right way to avoid something you can hear but cannot see coming?	NA	1	A	0

SECTION 4. Emotional response to hearing loss

Question	MILD Reply	MILD Score	SLIGHT Reply	SLIGHT Score
Do you think you are more irritable than other people, just the same or less so?	same	0	more	5
Do you ever give the wrong answer to someone because you have misheard them?	HE	1	S	3
If so, do you treat it lightly or do you get upset?	S	1	A	5
How do other people react? Do they tend to get irritated or do they make little of it?	N	0	HE	1
Do you think people are tolerant in this way or do they make fun of you?	N	0	N	0
Do you ever get bothered or upset if you are unable to follow a conversation?	N	0	A	8
Do you ever get the feeling of being cut off because of hearing difficulty?	N	0	N	0
If so, does this feeling upset you at all?	N	0	N	0

SECTION 5. Speech distortion

Question	MILD Reply	MILD Score	SLIGHT Reply	SLIGHT Score
Do you find that people fail to speak clearly?	N	0	NA	5
Do you find speakers fail to talk clearly on TV/radio?	N	0	N	0
Do you have difficulty understanding what someone's saying even though you can hear what's being said?	N	0	NA	5

SECTION 6. Tinnitus

Question	MILD Reply	MILD Score	SLIGHT Reply	SLIGHT Score
Do you ever get a noise in your ears?	N	0	N	0
Does this noise ever prevent you from sleeping?	N	0	N	0
Does it trouble you at all?	N	0	N	0

SECTION 7. Personal opinion of hearing

Question	MILD Reply	MILD Score	SLIGHT Reply	SLIGHT Score
Do you think your hearing is normal?	yes	0	no	3
Do you think your hearing difficulty is specially bad?	no	0	no	0
Does your hearing difficulty ever restrict your social or personal life?	N	0	NA	5

SUMMARY

	M	HAC (see text)	Mild	Slight
Speech hearing	76	23	3	43
Acuity	28	1	1	6
Localization	28	0	10	1
Emotional response	45	5	2	22
Speech distortion	20	0	0	10
Tinnitus	16	0	0	0
Personal opinion	13	1	0	8
Totals	226	30	16	90

The maximum possible score for each section is shown in column "M". The next column, "HAC", is the 10th centile score from a group of patients attending a hearing-aid clinic. This group, suffering from mixed and sensorineural lesions, is recognized to be disabled and the level of score shown in "HAC" is taken, for present purposes, as the criterion of impairment.

In terms of their replies to the questionnaire it is clear that one man is very much more affected by occupational hearing loss than the other. It is very interesting that "Slight", who on the audiometry-based systems has better hearing than "Mild" is, on the whole, the more seriously affected. "Slight's" overall score is very much in excess of the criterion HAC, whereas the other man fails to reach it by a considerable margin. There is no doubt that "Slight's" score on speech hearing, acuity, handicap, indirect speech and self-assessment puts him well into the range at which individuals feel the need of a hearing aid. Thus, there can be little doubt that he is disabled to some degree by his hearing loss. Indeed, the clinical picture as revealed by the questionnaire shows that this man is at a real disadvantage because of his hearing difficulty. However, he is not troubled by tinnitus, nor by much difficulty with the perception of direction in sound. The adequacy of function in these two areas, despite relatively severe effect in the others, illustrates the point that the areas of hearing are to some degree independent of each other.

The other man ("Mild") admits to little difficulty except in localization. Overall, he does not present a picture of a man disabled to any material degree.

From a clinical point of view it is clear that "Slight" can afford to lose no more hearing. "Mild", on the other hand, appears to have more reserve. Were judgements to be made on the audiometric results a different conclusion would be drawn. In this connection it is interesting that "Slight" had just started to use hearing protection at work whereas "Mild" felt no need of it.

General findings

A number of points emerge from the foregoing analysis and we have looked to the results from the entire group of drop-forgers for evidence of generalities. We have seen that two assessment schemes based upon average threshold level for pure tones at the frequencies 0·5, 1·0 and 2·0 kHz fail to predict which of the two men is worse affected. Two questions should be asked: the first, on the relationship between this average and the various subsections of the questionnaire, and the second, on the advantage to be gained from the use of threshold averages based on other frequencies.

These questions can be answered by reference to correlation analysis set out in Table XXVII. Inspection of the correlations between the various pairs of pure-tone averages shows that acuity at 0·5, 1·0 and 2·0 kHz relates significantly with acuity at all other frequency combina-

TABLE XXVII. Correlation coefficients between pure-tone hearing levels (averages at various frequencies) and scores in subsections of questionnaire

	0·5, 1, 2	0·5, 1, 2, 3	0·5, 1, 2, 3, 4	0·5, 1, 2 3, 4, 6	3, 4, 6
0.5, 1, 2	—	0·499*	0·89*	0·866*	0·692*
0.5, 1, 2, 3	—	—	0·953*	0·949*	0·812*
0·5, 1, 2, 3, 4	—	—	—	0·98*	0·888*
0·5, 1, 2, 3, 4, 6	—	—	—	—	0·928*
Speech hearing	0·506	0·489	0·401	0·402	0·282
Acuity	0·643*	0·583*	0·525	0·508	0·343
Localization	0·628*	0·531	0·691*	0·464	0·405
Handicap	0·519	0·559	0·528	0·55	0·502
Speech distortion	0·187	0·583*	0·594*	0·62*	0·547
Tinnitus	0·024	−0·125	−0·208	−0·148	−0·249
Personal opinion	0·187	0·491	0·48	0·539	0·381

* $P < 0{\cdot}01$.

tions presented in the table. Thus we should not expect any other pure-tone average to have a material advantage over the rest in respect of relationships with the subsections of the questionnaire. This is borne out by inspection of the correlations between pure tones and the questionnaire of which, as the table shows, only seven are significant. Overall, the values shown are consistent with quite large discrepancies between audiometric values and clinical picture, such as have been demonstrated with "Mild" and "Slight". Thus, as has been stated, we believe that an adequate clinical picture cannot be obtained from pure-tone thresholds alone.

CLINICAL PICTURE

The occupations with the greatest levels and durations of exposure that we have come across anywhere in industry are drop-forging and (with slightly lower levels) metal dressing with pneumatic chisels. Weavers are exposed to lower levels still, but similar durations. As a first step in the

TABLE XXVIII. Comparison of questionnaire scores for four subject groups

	Scores		
	75%	50%	25%
Hearing for speech and speech distortion			
Hearing-aid clinic	49	40	30
Drop-forgers	27·5	18	7
Dressers	27	14	7·5
Weavers	23·5	13	1
Emotional response, tinnitus and personal opinion			
Hearing-aid clinic	15·5	9	4·5
Drop-forgers	8·25	5	2
Dressers	5	3	3
Weavers	5·5	2·5	0
Acuity for non-speech sound			
Hearing-aid clinic	12	8	2
Drop-forgers	5	2	0
Dressers	2	1	0
Weavers	6·5	1	0
Localization			
Hearing-aid clinic	8	2	0
Drop-forgers	2	0	0
Dressers	4	2	0
Weavers	6	1	0

description of the clinical picture of occupational hearing loss in these groups their Hearing Measurement Scale scores have been compared with those of the hearing-aid clinic sample. Table XXVIII shows these comparisons. There were 23 subjects from the HAC, 19 drop-forgers, 13 chippers (metal dressers) and 12 weavers. The age structures of the occupational groups were similar. The seven sections of the questionnaire have been combined into four for this comparison and scores are shown at the median and upper and lower quartile. In general, the HAC scores are the highest and this trend is clearest for hearing for speech and speech distortion. However, it is clear that occupational hearing loss in moderate and severe degree is characterized by symptoms of disorder in the other areas of hearing. Further, although there are some differences between the occupational groups it is clear that the drop-forgers are not affected to a much greater extent than the other occupational groups.

From the drop-forgers' scores on the Hearing Measurement Scale the clinical picture of occupational deafness can be described. The median score provides an indication of the "average" picture and the upper quartile score provides a description of the more severely affected. The descriptions apply to men in their sixth decade of life who have spent more than half of their working lifetimes in a very noisy trade.

The average clinical picture

In conversation with groups of people both at home and outside some difficulty is experienced from time to time. Conversation with one person outside may also present occasional difficulty but there is none at home. On occasion wrong answers are given and sometimes, not often, speech in TV plays appears indistinct. Certain domestic sounds such as the clock ticking may be missed. The man is aware that his hearing is less than normal but at the same time he is not prepared to say that his hearing is abnormal for his age.

The severe clinical picture

Difficulty in conversation, individual and group, at home, work or outside is a common occurrence. There is difficulty in hearing what is said at public meetings. The man finds that people fail to speak clearly and very often the speech on TV is indistinct. The sounds of home and street are often missed and difficulty is sometimes experienced in the perception of direction and distance of sound.

He is aware that his hearing is not normal although he claims his difficulty imposes no restriction on his social or personal life. He knows that other people notice his difficulty in hearing. He quite often becomes irritated with himself because he is unable to follow conversations and there are occasions when he feels cut off. He does get tinnitus but it does not trouble him.

CONCLUSION

The purpose of this paper has been to give a description of the clinical picture of occupational hearing loss. We studied a group of drop-forgers in their sixth decade who had spent half their working lives in noise with exposures which are among the most severe we have encountered. There can be few industrial situations where these acoustical levels are exceeded. Two men, whose audiograms were similar, were shown to differ materially in the degree to which they were affected.

Examination of the relationships between pure-tone thresholds and sections of the questionnaire for the group as a whole showed that results from the performance tests and the clinical picture are incompletely related. For this reason, assessment of hearing loss cannot be based wholly upon audiometry.

The median clinical picture presented by the drop-forgers was of an essentially trivial disorder. For those at and beyond the 75th centile, that is, a minority, the effect was more serious. From comparisons with samples from other occupational groups there was no reason to suppose that the picture presented by the drop-forgers was in any way unusual.

Tinnitus and Noise-induced Tinnitus

By

T. I. Hempstock and G. R. C. Atherley

Department of Pure and Applied Physics, University of Salford, England

Summary

The disturbing consequences of tinnitus in the population at large and in noise-exposed populations in particular are discussed. Available evidence as to the disabling influence of tinnitus is conflicting and it is concluded that this confusion is due to the lack of an adequate criterion for assessing tinnitus.

As a preliminary to the establishment of a criterion, temporary threshold shifts were induced monaurally in normally-hearing subjects. The acoustical characteristics of the resulting tinnitus were investigated by matching it for pitch and loudness to a signal introduced into the non-stimulated ear. It was found that the pitch of the tinnitus bears a constant relation to the frequency of the stimulus for both $\frac{1}{3}$-octave-band noise and for pure tones. The pitch of the tinnitus is usually lower than the frequency of maximum threshold shift. In order to induce a measurable tinnitus the level of the pure-tone stimulus had to be higher than was necessary with the $\frac{1}{3}$-octave-band noise. However, the sensation level of the tinnitus does not depend upon the characteristics of the stimulating signal and is usually just above the threshold of hearing.

INTRODUCTION

The results of exposure to noise in so far as it affects the sensitivity of hearing have been thoroughly studied and are well documented. However, it may be that there are other consequences of noise exposure that are just as distressing to the sufferers as loss of hearing.

The purpose of this paper is to comment upon present knowledge of tinnitus which occurs as a result of exposure to noise.

Tinnitus is a common and unremarkable phenomenon which is experienced by many people with apparently normal hearing. In the majority of cases such tinnitus is neither long-lasting nor particularly troublesome but, without doubt, there are some who find it distressing. In the present state of knowledge it is difficult to assess the extent to which tinnitus can disturb those who experience it, either in the population at large or in populations exposed to excessive noise.

Data published by Hinchcliffe (1961) and shown in Table XXIX demonstrate that tinnitus is indeed a common experience. The table shows the percentage of individuals in different age groups from two random samples of the rural population of the United Kingdom who had at some time noticed noises in their ears or heads. Although the proportion is larger in the higher age groups, a significant percentage in the lower age groups report the experience.

TABLE XXIX. Prevalence of tinnitus as a function of age. Hinchcliffe (1961)

Age group (years)	History of tinnitus (per cent)
18–24	21
25–34	27
35–44	24
45–54	27
55–64	39
65–74	57

TABLE XXX. Sounds reported by normal and hard-of-hearing subjects in a quiet room. Heller and Bergman (1953)

	Hard-of-hearing patients		Normal subjects	
	Number	%	Number	%
Sound heard (tinnitus)	73	73	75	94
No sound heard (no tinnitus)	27	27	5	6
Total	100	100	80	100

It is interesting to compare these observations with those of Heller and Bergman (1953) shown in Table XXX. Two groups of people were placed in a quiet room and asked to describe any sounds they heard. One group of 80 adults had normal hearing and the other group of 100 were veterans of military service with diagnosed hearing losses. No suggestion was made to any of the subjects that the sound might originate within the subject himself. Of the group of normally-hearing subjects 75 (94 per cent) reported hearing a sound. Of the other group of 100, 75 reported hearing something. Heller and Bergman therefore suggested that tinnitus is in fact experienced by everybody but is usually masked by the ambient noise of the environment and is therefore inaudible. In a similar study Graham and Newby (1962) found only 10 out of 25 normal subjects reported tinnitus during a period of silence. The only difference between the two studies was that Heller and Bergman's criterion of normal was based solely on the subjects' own judgements of whether their hearing was normal or not, whereas Graham and Newby's criterion of normal was based on audiometric measurements. This helps to explain why a relatively large proportion of subjects with "normal" hearing reported tinnitus in Heller and Bergman's study. It also enables us to reconcile their findings with the view that tinnitus is an early symptom preceding impaired hearing. Indeed, this view can be extended by suggesting, as in fact Wegel (1931) has done, that the subsequent disappearance of the tinnitus is an indication that the degenerative processes have either been arrested or have reached completion. In none of the studies just discussed was an attempt made to assess the factor of distress in those who experienced tinnitus. It is interesting to note that there are few reports of tinnitus in children and none at all of children being disturbed by it.

The position is confused when the incidence of tinnitus in noise-exposed populations is investigated. In his studies, Hinchcliffe (1961) found no correlation between those who had experienced tinnitus and those who had worked for more than 1 year in an environment where the noise level was such that they had to raise their voice to be heard. There is support for this observation in the findings of Venters (1953) who, in a study of 254 clinical cases of tinnitus of differing ætiology, found only one, a boilermaker, whose tinnitus could be attributed with certainty to noise.

A wholly different view of the matter is expressed by Goldner (1953). He noted that among shipyard workers exposed to the noise of riveting hammers, tinnitus was the commonest complaint. It was often considered to be more disturbing than deafness and in some individuals it was disabling. Atherley (1967) in a study of foundrymen found that 33 out of 55 experienced tinnitus. Plomp (1967) found a clear relationship between the occurrence of tinnitus and the maximum threshold shift measured 2 hours after a group of 158 recruits had completed their first firing programme of small arms. Overall we can see that there is disparity in the evidence about the incidence of tinnitus. Furthermore, there is little information to establish whether the tinnitus caused by noise is disturbing or not. However, it does appear that the incidence of tinnitus is greatest where the exposure has been to noise of an impulsive nature. Apart from evidence from industrial studies of such noise it is also known that impulsive noise produced by explosions causes tinnitus. Henry (1945) reported tinnitus as being the most common complaint resulting from exposure to this type of noise during military service. In a large minority of cases tinnitus would last continuously for up to a year following exposure.

With regard to research into tinnitus generally, we think that much uncertainty stems from lack of adequate means of assessing the phenomenon. Research into both prevalence and severity would be very much more productive if there were an adequate descriptive criterion of tinnitus. Indeed, until there is available a reliable description of tinnitus associated with various states of hearing, it will not be possible to decide whether a history of tinnitus in a noise-exposed population is a matter of any importance.

Our own studies (Atherley *et al.*, 1968) have been intended as a preliminary to the establishment of such a criterion. A temporary loss in hearing was induced unilaterally in normally-hearing subjects by exposure to noise and the resulting tinnitus measured in order to find out whether any rules could be established which would enable the behaviour of tinnitus to be predicted.

PROCEDURE

Prior to stimulation the air-conduction thresholds of each subject were measured in both ears using a pulsed pure-tone self-recording audiometer. The stimulus was delivered monaurally for 5 minutes and consisted of $\frac{1}{3}$-octave bands of white noise centred at either 2, 3, 4 or 6 kHz set to a level of 110 dB SPL. Following the exposure a comparison tone was delivered to the non-stimulated ear and adjusted by the experimenter for both frequency and level until the subject reported that it matched his tinnitus. The frequency of this comparison tone was taken as the pitch of the tinnitus and its sensation level in the non-stimulated ear was taken as the sensation level of the tinnitus. A further determination of threshold was then made in the stimulated ear. The interval between the cessation of stimulus and this redetermination of threshold was about 2 minutes.

RESULTS

Occurrence of tinnitus and temporary threshold shift

None of the subjects complained of the tinnitus being severe and in most cases it disappeared within a few minutes of removal of the stimulus. We have therefore used the term "Noise-Induced Short-Duration Tinnitus" (NIST). For a small minority of subjects it lasted a few hours and on two occasions into the following day. Table XXXI shows the number of our subjects who experienced NIST for sufficient length of time for it

TABLE XXXI. Number of subjects with auditory fatigue (N_1) and with NIST (N_2) against stimulus centre frequency

Stimulus centre frequency (kHz)	N_1	N_2
2	8	7
3	28	25
4	7	7
6	14	12

to be measured in relation to the centre frequency of the stimulating signal.

Relationship between stimulus frequency and frequency of maximum threshold shift

As was to be expected, it was found that as the stimulus frequency increased, so did the frequency of maximum threshold shift (MTS). The change was highly significant ($P < 0{\cdot}001$). Figure 60 shows the values of

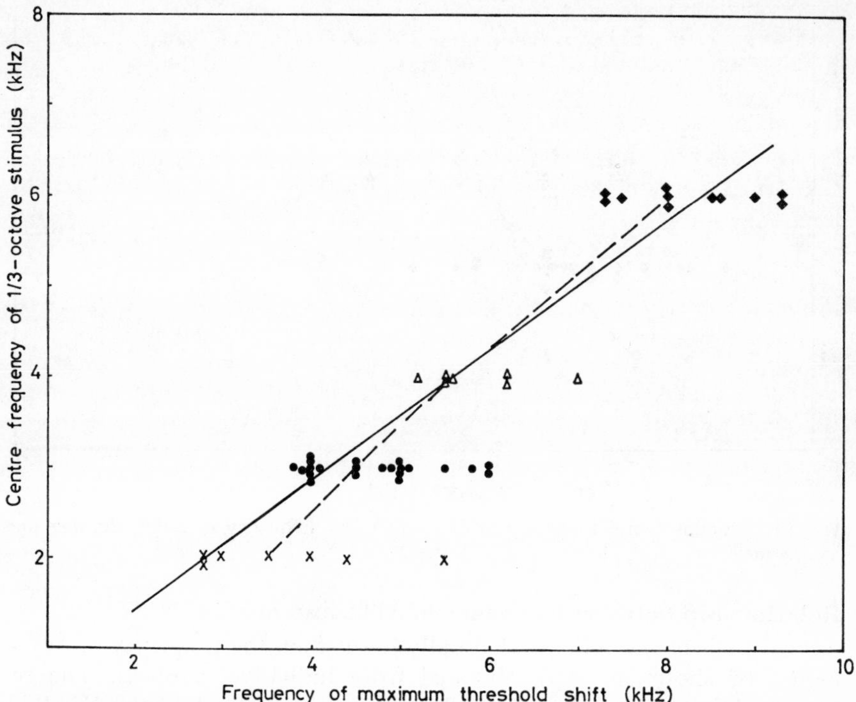

FIG. 60. Stimulus centre frequency against frequency of MTS showing line joining medians and line of ½-octave relationship.

MTS recorded by individual subjects at each stimulus frequency. The line joining median values for each stimulus is shown together with the line that would be obtained if the MTS were exactly half an octave above the stimulus frequency.

Relationship between stimulus frequency and pitch of NIST

Again, as the stimulus frequency rose so did the pitch of the NIST and the change was highly significant ($P < 0{\cdot}001$). Figure 61 shows the pitch of NIST recorded by individual subjects at each stimulus frequency. The line joining median values for each stimulus has again been shown.

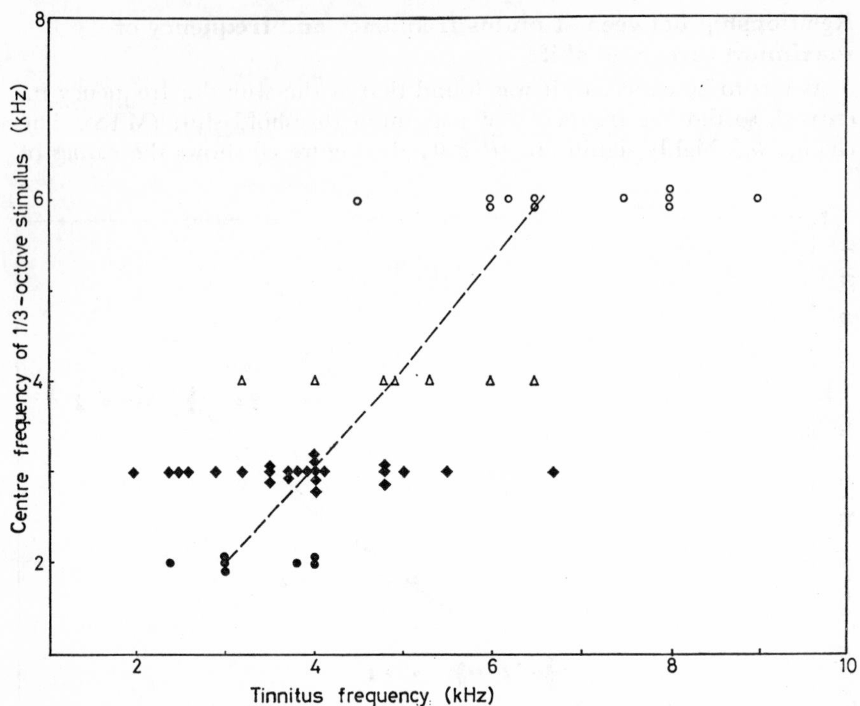

FIG. 61. Stimulus centre frequency against equivalent frequency of NIST showing line joining medians.

Relationship between frequency of MTS and pitch of NIST

The pitch of the NIST was usually lower than the frequency of MTS. Figure 62 shows the data obtained from individual subjects. The regression line represents $y = 0{\cdot}8x + 0{\cdot}3$ where y is the pitch of the NIST in kHz regressed on x, the frequency of MTS in kHz. The correlation coefficient between x and y is $+0{\cdot}82$.

Sensation level of NIST

The median values and interquartile ranges of the sensation level of NIST for each stimulus frequency are shown in Table XXXII. Despite the apparent differences in sensation level at different frequencies the distribution is not statistically significant ($0{\cdot}05 < P < 0{\cdot}1$). Over all frequencies the median sensation level was 9 dB. There did not appear to be any systematic variation of sensation level of NIST with the degree of MTS. In no instances was the sensation level of NIST greater than 25 dB.

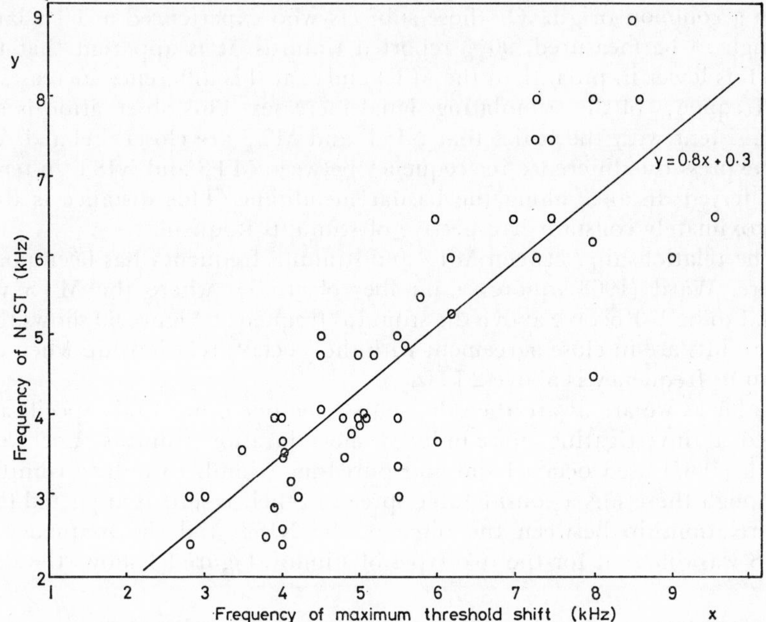

FIG. 62. Frequency of MTS (x) against equivalent frequency of NIST (y) showing regression line of y on x ($\frac{1}{3}$-octave-band stimuli).

TABLE XXXII. Sensation level of NIST (median and interquartile range) against stimulus centre frequency and at all frequencies

Stimulus centre frequency (kHz)	N	Sensation level (dB)	Interquartile range (dB)
2	7	11·0	8·0–18·5
3	25	5·0	2·0–11·0
4	7	8·0	4·0–12·0
6	10	12·0	10·0–16·0
All frequencies	49	9·0	5·0–15·0

DISCUSSION

The method of measurement of the tinnitus employed was similar to that used in audiometric studies by Reed (1960) and by Graham and Newby (1953). With unilateral tinnitus, introducing the matching signal into the contralateral ear simplifies the task for the subject. Most of our subjects had no difficulty in loudness-balancing and pitch-matching their tinnitus and they were agreed that the NIST was tonal rather than noisy.

The evidence of the data presented here suggests that NIST and TTS have a common origin. Of those subjects who experienced a TTS large enough to be measured, 90% reported tinnitus. It is apparent that the NIST is lower in pitch than the MTS and that this difference increases as the frequency of the stimulating signal increases. This observation is not inconsistent with the belief that NIST and MTS are closely related. We can express the difference in frequency between MTS and NIST in terms of inferred distance along the basilar membrane. This distance is then approximately constant irrespective of stimulus frequency.

The relationship between MTS and stimulus frequency has been noted before. Ward (1963) quotes a number of studies where the MTS was found to be $\frac{1}{2}$–1 octave above the stimulus frequency. Figure 60 shows that our results are in close agreement with the $\frac{1}{2}$-octave relationship when the stimulus frequency is above 2 kHz.

As far as we are aware there has only been one other study specifically aimed at investigating noise-induced short-duration tinnitus. Loeb and Smith (1967) used octave-band and pure-tone stimuli to induce tinnitus. Although there was a considerable spread in their results it appeared that the relationship between the pitch of the NIST and the frequency of MTS was different for the two types of stimuli. Figure 63 shows the data

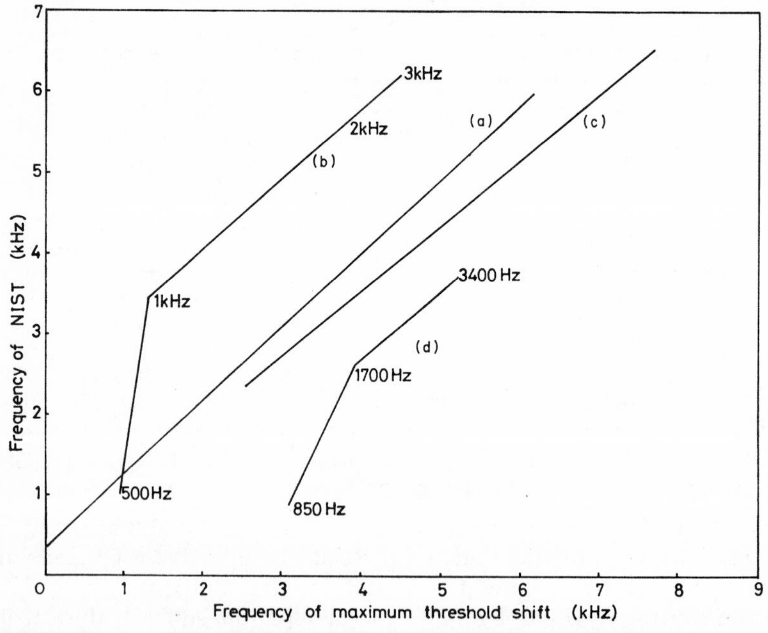

FIG. 63. Regression lines from Figs. 62 and 64 compared with data of Loeb and Smith (1960). (a) Pure tone, Hempstock and Atherley; (b) Pure tone, Loeb and Smith; (c) $\frac{1}{3}$-octave noise, Hempstock, Atherley and Noble; (d) octave noise, Loeb and Smith.

of Loeb and Smith which have been averaged for the purposes of plotting a graph, together with the regression line from Fig. 62 and a similar regression line obtained from a second set of experiments in which pure tones were used as stimuli. The figures relating to Loeb and Smith's data show the frequency of the pure-tone stimuli and the centre frequency of the octave-band stimuli used in their experiments. Figure 64 shows the

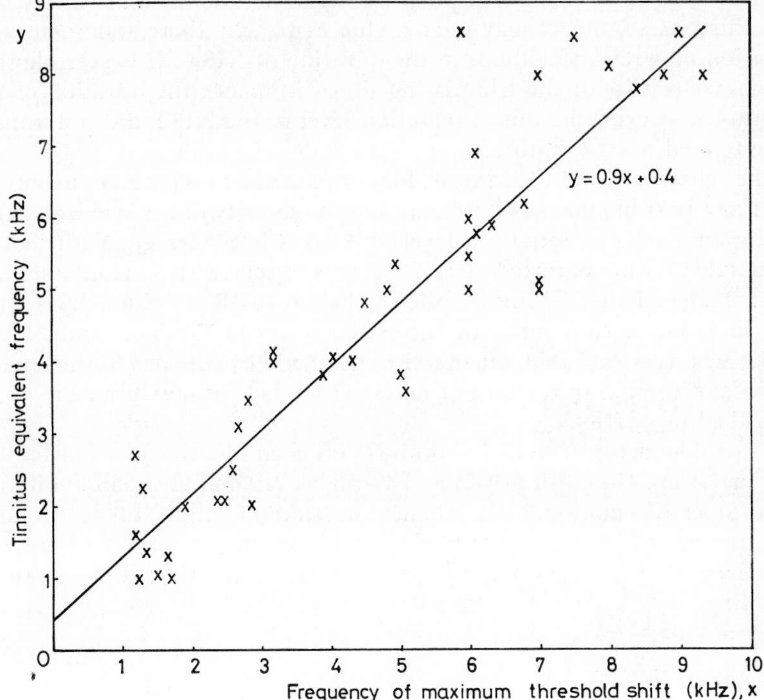

Fig. 64. Frequency of MTS (x) against equivalent frequency of NIST (y) showing regression line of y on x (pure-tone stimuli).

data obtained from individual subjects in our experiments when pure tones were used to induce the tinnitus. On this occasion the regression line represents $y = 0{\cdot}9x + 0{\cdot}4$, where y is the pitch of the NIST in kHz regressed on x, the frequency of MTS in kHz. The correlation coefficient between x and y is 0·93. Clearly the sets of data obtained from the $\frac{1}{3}$-octave band and pure-tone stimuli are not distinguishable and therefore our findings do not support those of Loeb and Smith.

One other relevant study was carried out by Davis *et al.* (1950). They were primarily concerned with an investigation of diplacusis produced by exposure to high-intensity sound, but they noted that tinnitus following exposure to high-level pure tones has a pitch above that of the pure tone. They also reported a diplacusis effect in the exposed ear, where the pitch was shifted upwards towards a pitch corresponding with that of the tinnitus.

In our experiment with pure tones the frequencies of the stimuli were 1, 2, 3, 4 and 6 kHz. It is interesting to note that the level had to be increased to 120 dB SPL in order to elicit tinnitus which lasted for a sufficient length of time for a pitch match to be obtained. It is not clear why this was so, but it may offer a clue as to why there was such wide variation between individuals in the duration of NIST. It is possible that the characteristics of the stimulating signal influence the duration of the tinnitus. However, the initial sensation level of the NIST did not appear to be related to its duration.

The sensation level of tinnitus does not appear to offer any encouragement as a possible means of ascertaining the severity of the symptom. Our finding of a median sensation level of 9 dB is in agreement with that of Reed (1960) who reported that 70% of subjects with various types of lesion matched their tinnitus to levels below 10-dB sensation level. It is also in broad agreement with the observations of Graham and Newby (1962) who reported that the descriptions made by subjects of the characteristics of their tinnitus do not necessarily relate to measurements of its acoustical properties.

A possible factor of some importance has been identified by Fowler and Fowler (1955), Goodhill (1950) and Kennedy (1953). They emphasize the importance of emotional disturbance or "state of mind" in determining the response of an individual to tinnitus, but none of them goes so far as to suggest that it offers a complete explanation of why tinnitus can be disabling.

CONCLUSIONS

We have found that there is a close relationship between the pitch of noise-induced short-duration tinnitus (NIST) and the frequency of maximum threshold shift (MTS). They are both related to the frequency of the stimulating tone, the relationship being independent of whether the stimulus is $\frac{1}{3}$-octave-band noise or pure tone. The median sensation level of the NIST is 9 dB; this is in agreement with findings of other studies of tinnitus accompanying a variety of otological lesions.

We are encouraged in the search for a criterion for tinnitus. Such a criterion would help to determine the degree to which tinnitus is an additional disabling factor in occupational hearing loss. It would help us to describe the wide variation in individual response to tinnitus and also to follow the progress of tinnitus in the same individual from time to time.

Occupational Hearing Loss and the Otologist

By

D. L. Chadwick

Department of Otolaryngology, University of Manchester, England

Foreword

It is with sadness that I preface my remarks by adding my own small tribute to that of other participants in memory of my colleague, the late Sir Terence Cawthorne.

He was to have chaired the present session of this Conference. His untimely decease leaves a gap in the ranks of otology which will not easily be filled. His loss is felt not only on account of his ever-present interest in noise and its effects upon hearing, but even more particularly for his wise counsel, kindliness and friendship. He was one of the few of whom it can truly be said, "He was a man, take him for all in all; we shall not look upon his like again."

It has been, however, a great personal pleasure to me to find the chair so ably filled at such short notice by my former chief and mentor, Air Vice-Marshal Dickson.

He it was who first aroused my interest in these problems at a time when realization was dawning that the jet engine had become a noise force to be reckoned with.

Over 20 years ago I remember examining with awe Sir Frank Whittle's original experimental turbo-jet engine. Small and insignificant by present-day standards, it had the appearance of a collection of tin cans welded together. Who could foresee that therein lay the potentialities which would lead to our current concern over supersonic flight and the sonic boom?

Having already listened to papers replete in their scientific exactitude, so fitting in this institute, dedicated as it is to measurements of a precise and detailed nature, it is with no little trepidation that I place on record some observations on occupational hearing loss as it presents in purely clinical guise to a mere ear, nose and throat surgeon.

INTRODUCTION

Occupational hearing loss has attracted increasing attention in recent years. The practising otologist obtains a somewhat biased view concerning this disease. He sees mainly the more advanced cases of noise-induced deafness, together with those unduly susceptible to noise. From a practical point of view, what is the incidence of this condition in present-day industrial civilization? To what extent does it prove a handicap in daily life? What relationship does it bear to other types of deafness in the community?

An attempt to answer these questions has been made by studying patients with occupational hearing loss seen over a 5-year period. The relationship between this kind of hearing loss is examined in the context of patients with deafness of other varieties attending the ear, nose and throat department of a teaching hospital serving a large and populous industrial area.

Industrial background

Within a radius of 25 miles of the Manchester Royal Infirmary dwells a population of 4¾ million. Contained inside the boundaries of its two largest cities, Manchester and Salford, are approximately 7800 factories and workshops. Placed more peripherally are numerous Lancashire cotton towns still retaining many traditional spinning and weaving mills.

Manchester is possibly one of the more noisy cities in the British Isles. I hope I am not betraying a confidence when I tell you that Dr. Glorig himself spent some of his very earliest days there.

It occurs to me that possibly memories of the sounds of our strident city impinging in unwelcome fashion on his infant ears might have been the driving force leading to his subsequent monumental studies in the field of noise and to the pre-eminent position which he now holds in his chosen subject.

The potential "at-risk" population

Of an estimated total of 412,825 employees in the principal industries, the number in the main occupations considered "at-risk" from industrial noise exposure are:

Engineering and electrical	39,930
Building construction	24,972
Textile industry	11,976
Metal manufacture	10,961
Timber, furniture	4,907
Mining	2,145

Adding to this figure of 94,891 those engaged in smaller noisy industrial processes, one-quarter of the working population labour in industrial noise environments potentially hazardous to hearing. The above were the official figures available when this study was commenced some 5 years ago.

An interesting side-light on current industrial population trends is evident when these figures are compared with the most recent statistics issued by the Department of Employment and Productivity. The number of textile employees has been reduced by over 2000, engineers and electricians by over 1000 and quarry workers and miners by 500.

On the other hand, despite the possession of the Manchester Docks, we are not particularly noted for either shipbuilding or marine engineering. Surprisingly, this labour force shows an almost 30% increase. The figures, however, must be viewed in their proper perspective; the numbers have in fact risen from 18 to 26!

From the geographical aspect, cotton mills and weaving sheds lie mainly to the north of the city. Centrally around the dock area are concentrated the heavy electrical and engineering industries, export of such products being facilitated by the Manchester Ship Canal with its links to Liverpool, the high seas and the New World.

More peripherally, light engineering factories are located in purpose-planned industrial estates and towards the south-west lie the quieter trades of the hatters, fur cutters and felt manufacturers.

Type of hearing loss

238 patients were examined: 215 showed industrial noise-induced hearing loss; 23, incidents of acute acoustic trauma.

RELATIONSHIP OF OCCUPATIONAL HEARING LOSS TO OTHER TYPES OF DEAFNESS

During the past year, 438 new patients with deafness were seen: 269 had a conductive hearing loss; 169 were perceptive. Of the latter, 48 were considered occupational in origin. The effects of noise therefore account for approximately 8% of all cases of deafness.

Diagnostic criteria

Diagnosis of "industrial noise-induced hearing loss" was arrived at in accordance with the recommendations of Burns and Robinson (1970). They state "The absence of any clear-cut diagnostic aid to the identification of permanent noise-induced threshold shift in individual cases forces one to fall back on a series of probabilities, based on such direct evidence as the audiogram, evidence which may be slightly less secure such as the supposed noise history, and fairly indirect evidence such as may be elicited by otoscopic and otological examination."

In the present investigation, other causes of sensorineural deafness were excluded as far as possible by radiological, serological, haematological and other examinations. There were 16% of occupational hearing-loss cases that had additional ear pathology.

OCCUPATIONS INVOLVED

The commonest occupations in which hearing losses occurred and the number in each group were:

Engineering	52	Sheet metal workers	8
Military service	38	Machinists	7
Diesel engineers	21	Printers	7
Weavers	21	Circular saw operators	6
Boiler-makers	17	Riveters	5
Spinners	15	Drillers	4

Note the preponderance of industries associated with intermittent and high-intensity impulsive noise, as opposed to continuous steady-state noise.

With regard to the operators of circular saws, some of the most severe hearing losses of all those encountered, extending down to involve the 500 Hz frequency, were seen in this group. In this context I would like to interpose a few comments relating to the paper read by Dr. Kylin since I had a particularly personal interest in his survey dealing with the hearing of forest workers.

Several summer vacations, before I qualified in medicine, were spent employed by the Forestry Commission. At that time, 30 years ago, working conditions in the woodlands of this country were primarily those of peace and quiet. In the pine woods of the English Lake District and the remnants of Shakespeare's Forest of Arden adjoining Stratford-on-Avon, tractors were little in evidence, most of the logs being hauled by horses. Power-saws were non-existent and trees were felled in traditional fashion with axe and two-handed band saws, the trunks cut into sections with a bushman's saw and trimmed with bill-hooks.

We are all well aware that the timber trade is one of Sweden's major sources of revenue. Dr. Kylin's report leaves no doubt in our minds that this is now a highly mechanized industry and Dr. Ward has commented on the high noise levels which have been recorded. These findings illustrate in no small measure just one area where to a formerly peaceful agricultural, or perhaps more correctly speaking, arboreal trade have in recent years been introduced mechanization, noise and resultant hazards to hearing.

In our own country, in a comparatively short space of time, this previously tranquil calling like so many other procedures has, in the name of speed, progress and efficiency, been automated, mechanized and supplied with power tools. In the process it has inevitably become far noisier.

Some of the early references to noise and deafness are concerned with the cannonading during naval engagements (Parry, 1825). Massive broadsides from Admiral Lord Rodney's flagship in 1782 and bombardments by Lord Nelson's fleet at the Battle of Copenhagen in 1801 have been instanced. These conjure up pictures of the "wooden walls", ships of those days being constructed entirely of timber.

In this sphere too, at least as far as noise levels are concerned, change has been for the worse. During my forestry days as far as this aspect is concerned I again encountered mute testimony to the change precipitated by the Industrial Revolution. Many fine trees had of necessity to be felled to meet the demands of the last war. Bishops Wood, a fine well-spaced plantation of sturdy oaks in Shropshire, had been laid out about the time of the Battle of Trafalgar. Their branches had been encouraged to twist and curve so that on reaching maturity they would supply timber for the complicated spars and beams required for constructing the wooden men-of-war of those days. Before they reached fruition, iron had taken the place of wood in the building of sea-going vessels and riveters' and boilermakers' deafness had by that time achieved a permanent place in medical nomenclature as the harsh noise of hammer and drill resounded throughout the shipyards of the world.

SEX-INCIDENCE

Males predominated, 202 subjects, the remaining 36 being female. The latter were all engaged in some aspect of the textile industry, weaving, spinning or as machinists.

AGE DISTRIBUTION

Other workers have postulated that:

(1) During the course of employment in a noise-hazardous environment, it takes 10 to 15 years for an initial temporary threshold shift (TTS) to become an established permanent threshold shift (PTS) (Glorig and Davis, 1961).
(2) Individuals may be unaware of a noise-induced threshold shift in early life. This may only constitute a disability when the effects of presbycusis are added later (Burns, 1968).
(3) This disability appears at an earlier age than would be expected as the result of presbycusis alone (Hinchcliffe, 1959b).
(4) Noise-free populations retain good hearing even late in life (Rosen *et al.*, 1962, 1964).

These findings receive confirmation from the following figures—the age at which treatment for symptoms associated with occupational hearing loss was sought.

Age in years	Number of cases
Under 20	1
20–30	14
30–40	35
40–50	65
50–60	72
60–70	42
70–80	9

Few cases present during the 15 years after leaving school—the one teenager suffered an acute acoustic accident. Most appear between 40 and 60, but an appreciable rise in numbers occurs from the age of 30 onwards.

SYMPTOMS

Deafness

A total of 90% attended because of deafness. Pure-tone audiometry demonstrated a high-tone loss involving the speech frequency range. In these, the V-shaped notch at 4 kHz, characteristic of acoustic trauma, had widened to encroach on the lower frequencies. A threshold shift of at least 30 dB was present at 2 kHz. In some cases the 1-kHz and 500-Hz frequencies were also involved.

Tinnitus

Subjective tinnitus occurred in some 30%. Sometimes this was the only symptom, the patient frequently being unaware of deafness. This hearing loss was frequently confined to a dip at 4 kHz.

Unsteadiness

Some disturbance of balance was reported by approximately 20%. Caloric testing often produced normal reactions.

Patients often noticed symptoms only on changing from one noisy occupation to another, or from a noisy job to a quiet one.

COMMENT

There are few more depressing or unrewarding patients than those with permanent occupational hearing loss. In the present state of medical knowledge, once the diagnosis is established, little can be done to alleviate matters. The answer lies in the realms of preventive medicine. The education of management and employees alike and the institution of Hearing Conservation Programmes, along lines too well known to be repeated here, should be vigorously pursued.

Finally, the suggestion is made that audiometry performed on school-leavers during their final year at school would prove an extremely valuable base-line, particularly for future entrants into industry or the armed forces. This would provide a useful reference level for any future hearing tests, especially if some method of recording the results in permanent form on a national basis could be devised.

SUMMARY

1. Eight per cent of all clinic cases of deafness in an industrial area were of occupational origin.

2. Diagnosis was by exclusion, based on assessment of history, noise-exposure, audiometry and clinical examination, etc.

3. Industries with steady-state noise environments appeared less damaging to hearing than those with high-intensity impulsive components.

4. Up to 15 years elapse before TTS becomes an established PTS.

5. Noise-induced threshold shifts may only amount to a disability when the effect of presbycusis is added.

6. This disability tends to occur earlier than that caused by presbycusis alone.

7. The value of final school year, pre-employment, audiometry is suggested.

On the Equal-energy Hypothesis relative to Damage-risk Criteria in the Chinchilla

By

W. Dixon Ward and D. A. Nelson
University of Minnesota, Minneapolis, Minnesota

Summary
Four groups of 4 chinchillas each were exposed to a 700–2800-Hz noise at 114 dB SPL for 4 hr, 117 dB for 2 hr, 120 dB for 1 hr, and 123 dB for 0·5 hr, respectively. These exposures all produced about 40 dB of permanent threshold shift (PTS) at all frequencies at and above the stimulus frequency. This equivalence supports, for single uninterrupted exposures, the so-called equal-energy hypothesis (EEH) which states that exposures of equal total energy (the product of power and time) are equally dangerous. However, the EEH is not applicable when exposures are intermittent in nature. Somewhat surprisingly, considerable PTS was also found at low frequencies (down to 125 Hz), and this PTS did increase with level. Presumably this reflects a grossly accelerated growth of distortion products as intensity is raised beyond 110 dB SPL.

With the steady accumulation of data relating hearing loss to years of 8-hour exposures to continuous industrial noises (e.g., Baughn, 1966; Robinson, 1968; Passchier-Vermeer, 1968), the specification of damage-risk criteria (DRC) for such exposures becomes based on increasingly firm ground. It seems clear from these surveys that common industrial noises below 80 dB(A) (80 dB on the *A*-weighted scale of the sound level meter) are quite innocuous, but that an increase in risk occurs, both in terms of the number of persons affected and the degree of hearing loss produced, as 80 dB(A) is exceeded. Whether one takes as the basic DRC for 8-hour exposures a level of 80, 85, 90 or 95 dB(A), therefore, depends only on an arbitrary decision as to just how much loss in how many people is considered tolerable. In the United States, for example, the most recent DRC is one of 90 dB(A) for continuous 8-hour exposure (the Walsh–Healey Act: Anon., 1969); this DRC will presumably result in some slight losses in the average worker after 20 years of exposure, but will produce compensable damage (an average hearing threshold level in excess of 25 dB ISO at 500, 1000 and 2000 Hz) in only a few ears.

The problem of how to treat shorter and intermittent exposures is still plaguing us, however. If the workers must be in the noise only half the workday, one can expect a slightly higher level to be tolerable. It also seems reasonable to expect that if this 4 hours of noise exposure were broken down into, say, eight 30-minute exposures with 30-minute rest periods between, an even higher level could be permitted. It is known that the *temporary* effects of noise conform to these expectations; the temporary threshold shift (TTS) produced by an intermittent exposure is less—under some conditions, much less—than that produced by the same total exposure in a single chunk (Ward, 1963). Furthermore, the shorter the exposure, the greater the level required to produce some fixed value of TTS. An entire set of DRC for continuous and interrupted noise exposures, the so-called CHABA DRC, was based on the relations governing the production of TTS—the underlying assumption was that all noise exposures that produce the same TTS_2 (the TTS measured 2 minutes after the end of the workday) are equally dangerous in regard to permanent threshold shift, or PTS (Kryter *et al.*, 1966).

Unfortunately, the CHABA DRC, essentially involving separate criteria for each octave band of noise, are very complicated. The trading relation between intensity and time for constant TTS simply is intrinsically curvilinear, and there is nothing we can do about it. The equivalent of an 8-hour continuous exposure to 1200–2400-Hz noise at 85 dB SPL, for example, is a 4-hour exposure at 87 dB, a 10-minute exposure at 105 dB, and a 5-minute exposure at 112 dB. In other words, the trading relation in TTS for this octave band of noise varies continuously from 2 to 7 dB per doubling time. And if the noise is on only in short (*ca.* 1 minute) bursts just half the time, an 8-hour exposure at 96 dB will produce the same TTS_2 as 8 hours of 85 dB steady noise (or 4 hours of 87 dB, and so on).

Because of this complexity, the CHABA curves are not widely accepted, and there is a movement afoot to return to the equal-energy hypothesis. This hypothesis, which served as the basis for assessing intermittent noises in one of the first DRC formally established in the U.S.A. (Air Force Regulation AFR 160-3, 1956), simply considers the total tolerable energy to be constant—regardless of level, duration or temporal pattern separately—so that the trading relation is always 3 dB per doubling time. As in the CHABA DRC, an 8-hour exposure to noise in the octave band 1200–2400 Hz at 85 dB SPL was considered in AFR 160-3 to be acceptable, but also 4 hours at 88 dB, 2 hours at 91, and so on, down to 5 minutes at 105 dB (compared to the CHABA DRC of 112 dB). Whether the 2 hours at 91 dB came in bursts or in one blast was ignored—only the total energy mattered.

The basis for adopting the equal-energy hypothesis (EEH) was a series of guinea-pig studies by Eldredge and Covell (1958). They found that, to a first approximation, the same amount of cochlear damage, as indicated by changes in the cochlear microphonic, was produced by a 500-Hz tone for 1 minute at 140 dB SPL and all exposures equivalent to it in energy, down to 118 dB for 160 minutes of exposure. The histological picture, it may be noted, was not nearly so clear; *all* the exposures they used, including some with somewhat less total energy, produced sizable areas of hair-cell destruction, so that the EEH could neither be confirmed nor denied.

There are no analogous data on hearing loss in man, because industrial exposures other than steady ones are generally so variable from person to person that it is difficult to get an adequate sample from which to draw conclusions. Indeed, hearing data associated with non-steady exposures are usually carefully eliminated from consideration. But even in animals. strangely enough, very little since Eldredge and Covell's early experiments has been reported that bears on the validity of the EEH, especially in terms of actual hearing losses as measured with behavioural techniques. One important exception is the study of Miller *et al.* (1963) on cats, in which the PTS produced by 2 hours of white noise at 115 dB SPL was three times as great when the exposure was continuous as when it was broken up into 16 7½-minute bursts with an hour of recovery between successive bursts.

In short, the truth or falsity of the proposition that equal amounts of acoustic energy (in a particular frequency region) will produce equal amounts of PTS is still undecided. I dare say that if one-tenth of the time and energy that has been squandered in standards committees arguing the point had instead been devoted to relevant experiments, we would have at least some idea of whether the EEH is reasonably accurate in some respects or only represents wishful thinking on the part of those who admire its one undeniably desirable aspect: its simplicity.

PROCEDURE

A series of exposures of monauralized chinchillas to a broad-band noise, specially tailored to give equal TTS at all frequencies from 1 to 8 kHz, had shown that a 2-hour exposure to 114 dB SPL just barely produced a significant PTS (after 1 week of recovery, the average remaining shift at 1, 2, 4 and 8 kHz had dropped to 10 dB) and that 123 dB for 2 hours produced an average PTS of 60 dB, which was somewhat more than we desired in our study of individual differences in susceptibility because some of the ears showed organs of Corti nearly devoid of hair cells everywhere except at the very apex (Ward and Nelson, unpublished data).

It was therefore decided to run a minor test of the EEH for PTS simultaneously with attempts to determine an optimum exposure for producing an average of 30 dB of PTS (which would, we estimated, give us a large range of individual PTS values without obliterating half of the organ of Corti). Accordingly, 4 groups of 4 chinchillas each were exposed to the following noises, respectively: 114 dB for 4 hours, 117 dB for 2 hours, 120 dB for 1 hour, and 123 dB for 30 minutes. In energy, these exposures were all twice as high as the 114-dB 2-hour exposure that just produced PTS. The noise was generated by passing white noise through a Peekel TF 823 filter set at "0" attenuation in the 1- and 2-kHz octave bands and "∞" at all others. For 123-dB total SPL, the octave-band levels at the animal's ear, measured by means of a standard Brüel and Kjær sound level meter at 250, 500, 1000, 2000, 4000 and 8000 Hz, were 76, 103, 120, 120, 107 and 79 dB respectively.

The animals were exposed in a special pillory-type restrainer that held the head in a relatively fixed position immediately in front of an Altec Voice of the Theatre speaker. Behavioural thresholds were obtained, using the method of conditioned avoidance (the animals jumped from one side of the cage to the other in order to avoid shock) before and for 3 months after the noise exposure. The pre-exposure thresholds were used in assigning animals to groups, so that each group had the same average pre-exposure threshold.

RESULTS

The final PTS's of the 15 chinchillas (1 died 3 weeks after exposure) at each test frequency are presented in Fig. 65. Each point represents the average of six threshold determinations made after the losses had stabilized. Group means are connected by the solid lines.

Considering first the higher frequencies, those at and above the cut-off frequency of the exposure noise (2 through 16 kHz), it can be seen that the EEH is reasonably well supported: the same PTS is produced by all four exposures. Although there is a 6-dB difference between the grand mean PTS's (averaging 2, 4, 8 and 16 kHz) of the 114 dB/4 hour and the 123 dB/30 minute groups, this difference is wholly due to the only animal in the entire experiment who failed to develop a PTS of at least 20 dB at some frequency, and of course is quite insignificant, statistically.

At the lower frequencies, however, the trend towards a greater PTS from the higher-intensity exposures is more pronounced. Although this trend reaches statistical significance only for 125 Hz (all four animals in the 114 dB/4 hour group showed less PTS than any animal in the 123 dB/30 minute group, an event that could occur by chance only once in 70 repetitions of the experiment if the exposures were really equivalent), its magnitude is relatively constant for all the frequencies; the former group has about 22 dB less PTS than the latter.

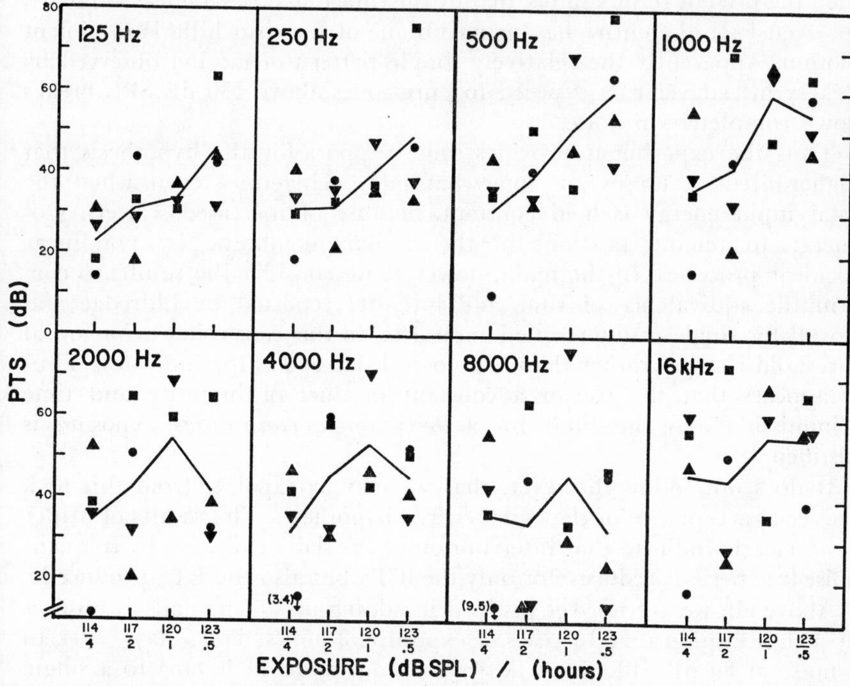

FIG. 65. Permanent threshold shifts of octaves of 125 Hz induced by single uninterrupted exposures to noise in the 700–2800 Hz band. Group means are connected by the solid line. Individual chinchillas within a group can be identified by means of the symbols employed.

DISCUSSION

What is curious here is not so much that there exists a gradation of effect (as a function of intensity) at frequencies below the range of the stimulus as the fact that so much PTS was produced at all. That is, it is known that as the energy in a high-frequency band of noise is gradually raised, the masking it produces at low frequencies also increases. Such "remote masking" (Bilger and Hirsh, 1956) may be interpreted as arising from the generation of non-linear distortion products due to interaction of frequencies within the pass band, and it is clear that at high intensities the "effective level" of these distortion products grows even more rapidly than the stimulus noise itself. Thus one would expect less effects in general at the remote frequencies with the less-intense but longer-duration exposures. But the fact that the PTS is nearly as great at 125 and 250 Hz as at 1, 2 and 4 kHz seems to imply that, at the levels involved here, these distortion products are just as intense as the noise from which they are derived. If PTS comes from mechanical overstimulation of the hair cells, then the present results imply that by the time one raises a noise to 120 dB (or even less), the entire basilar membrane of the chinchilla is in violent motion. Apparently the relatively simple pattern of motion observed by Békésy in cadaver ears exposed to pure tones above 130 dB SPL breaks down completely in noise.

Thus the experiment provides some support for the hypothesis that higher-intensity noises are somewhat more dangerous, even when the total input energy is held constant, because of increased scattering of energy to remote portions of the basilar membrane by non-linear cochlear processes. In the main, however, we consider the results to confirm the equivalence of time and intensity reported by Eldredge and Covell for single uninterrupted exposures, in this case using behavioural threshold changes rather than histological damage as the indicator. Thus it appears that the use of a constant product of intensity and time ("immission") as the limit for a *daily single continuous* exposure is justified.

It does not follow, however, that we may extrapolate from this to a universal acceptance of the equal-energy hypothesis. The results of Miller *et al.* clearly indicate that interruption of the daily exposure by frequent noise-free periods reduces not only the TTS but also the PTS produced.

Above all, we are not yet justified in adding up all the daily exposures in such a fashion that 10 years of exposure, 8 hours/day, 5 days/week to a noise at 80 dB SPL, is to be judged equivalent in hazard to a single 8-hour exposure to 114 dB, as the most extreme use of the EEH would indicate. In our original group of chinchillas, for example, daily 2-hour exposures to the 114-dB noise for a week produced neither a greater TTS_2 nor a slower recovery on Friday than on Monday, whereas the EEH would predict that *Tuesday's* exposure should be enough to produce the same PTS as in the 114 dB/4 hour group in Fig. 65. This shows unequivocally that recovery processes, especially those that are allowed to proceed for at least 16 hours, do have considerable effect on the ability of the auditory mechanism to withstand the next day's noisy onslaught.

It should be pointed out that by supporting the EEH, the results also tend to deny the existence of a "critical intensity". It has been theorized by Rüedi (1954) that the ear has, so to speak, a "breaking point"—an intensity above which categorically different processes are acting. This was suggested by experiments in which subjects were exposed to increasingly-intense noise bursts; the TTS produced showed a positively-accelerated growth curve that to Rüedi appeared to have an inflection, as if at a certain intensity the "elastic limit" of the ear were being exceeded. However, his experiments were run with a *constant* noise-burst duration; it seems certain that he would have found different "critical intensities" had he used different durations.

The outcome here does, however, imply the existence of a "critical single immission" (product of time and intensity) (Robinson and Cook, 1968) for the average chinchilla. An exposure to this particular noise is, from our earlier results, nearly safe when the SPL is 114 dB and the duration is 2 hours, but produces nearly 40 dB of PTS when the immission is doubled either by increasing the level to 117 dB or the time to 4 hours. It is interesting to note that a very similar discontinuity can be seen in the cat data of Miller *et al.*—the mean PTS produced by 115-dB noise jumped from 10 dB following 30-minute exposures to 35 dB after 2-hour exposures.

In summary, it seems clear that the equal-energy hypothesis is, to a first approximation, tenable for determining equivalent single uninterrupted daily exposures to noise. However, the need for further research on how damage cumulates from exposure to exposure is even clearer. Over a certain range of relative on- and off-times the 3-dB-per-doubling-time rule of the EEH may be nearly correct. In others the 5-dB-per-doubling-time relation adopted by the 1969 Walsh–Healey Act may be more appropriate; that particular relation was only a "guesstimate", a compromise more political than scientific in nature. For the shortest bursts and longest intervals, the trading relation may well even reach 10 dB or more.

ACKNOWLEDGEMENT

This research was supported in full by grants from the Public Health Service, U.S. Department of Health, Education, and Welfare. We extend our thanks to our patient chinchilla-testers: Barbara Evans, Jan Forfang, and Lonnie Sutherland.

Discussion on Papers in Section III

CHAIRMEN

E. D. D. Dickson W. D. Ward

PARTICIPANTS

G. R. C. Atherley	R. L. Kell
W. Burns	A. M. Martin
D. L. Chadwick	Mrs. W. Passchier-Vermeer
R. R. A. Coles	P. Ransome-Wallis
E. D. D. Dickson	D. W. Robinson
A. Glorig	S. D. G. Stephens
T. I. Hempstock	C. Wakstein
R. Hinchcliffe	W. D. Ward
J. D. Hood	

Dr. Hood: A point of importance which arises from Dr. Hinchcliffe's studies is the relationship of hearing level to the general state of health or otherwise of his subjects. Mention has earlier been made of the fact that persons with cochlear impairment are more susceptible to noise-induced hearing loss. Could one conclude, therefore, that in looking for susceptibility to noise-induced hearing loss, we need look no further than at the hearing level? In other words, would a person with remarkably good hearing be less susceptible to noise-induced hearing loss than one with a raised hearing threshold level?

Dr. Hinchcliffe: No, I do not think this is so; there are other factors than the hearing level of a subject.

Dr. Robinson: Evidence that bears indirectly on this point can be derived from our industrial studies (Burns and Robinson, 1970) by a kind of *reductio ad absurdum.* Suppose that variations in hearing acuity between individuals were due to differences in the transmission efficiencies of their acoustic pathways, their cochleae being alike. Then the insult due to a given amount of noise will be greater for a person with good hearing than for one with less good hearing, because more sound will reach his cochlea. Therefore he will appear to be more susceptible if we measure that by threshold shift from his own non-exposed base-line. Furthermore, the consequence of this will be that the dispersion of hearing levels in this hypothetical population will necessarily be smaller after exposure than it was before. This is contrary to the facts. Hence the supposed association of acute hearing with high susceptibility is false, and consequently the true situation is consistent with Dr. Hood's proposition.

Dr. Ransome-Wallis: Perception deafness from various causes is usually thought of as high-frequency deafness. There are, however, many instances of such deafness principally affecting the lower frequencies. Is there any information about this?

Dr. Hinchcliffe: Aside from the low-frequency sensorineural hearing losses due to endolymphatic hydrops, our population studies have shown that in many parts of the world flat sensorineural hearing losses may be associated with certain neurological disorders, which may also give rise to audiograms showing sharp peaks. The data presented by Mr. Kell are interesting in that, in contrast to ours for a rural population in Scotland, there is a tendency for the high-tone notch to disappear with increasing age. Did I understand Mr. Kell to say that some people had reported difficulty in hearing in spite of giving normal pure-tone audiograms? Also did these people have a discrimination loss on speech audiometry?

Mr. Kell: There appears to be a small proportion of people, with apparently normal hearing, who report that they are "slightly hard of hearing". These subjects are to be found in the group of controls aged less than 55 years, and they had normal speech audiograms for their age.

Professor Burns: One has come to associate with Dr. Davis the low fence at 25 or 26 dB ISO for the "3-average" criterion. Is Mr. Kell implying that he has in mind some equivalent low fence for the "4-average" figure, 0·5, 1, 2 and 3 kHz, and if so would he make a guess at the value?

Mr. Kell: We have presented our results here in terms of the low fence of 25 dB, but we doubt whether 25 would be the best fence for a "4-average" loss and our results, yet to be published, will include analyses at other fences.

Dr. Wakstein: In our study in Pittsburgh two years ago (Bugliarello *et al.*, 1968) we were interested in different assessment schemes that have been discussed, "3-average", "4-average", "5-average", and were very impressed by an assessment scheme described by the late N. Murray (1962) and which is evidently being used in Australia. What we did was to extrapolate the Wisconsin State Fair data; this may be inaccurate but we wanted to get a first-order estimate of the prevalence of hearing damage in the United States. Using the AAOO method we came to 4·9 million workers with hearing damage, defined as loss exceeding the AAOO "low fence". Using Murray's method we came to 14·2 million. Then, on the assumption that with the increased interest in pollution and degradation in the quality of the environment the compensation figures would be likely to rise, we took the third quartile compensation figure which was about $10,000 and the total claims came out at $6000 million and $13,500 million. We found it difficult to decide which of these methods was "right" and I formed the impression that many people here find it difficult to decide too.

Dr. Hinchcliffe: Dr. Atherley's very enjoyable paper prompts me to make three points as a basis for six questions. The points I wish to deal with are (1) the scales and the data analysis, (2) tinnitus, and (3) sound localization.

First, the scales probably correspond to a number of personality measures. It would be interesting to know what correlations Dr. Atherley obtained between the various scores. As regards the finding that the highest correlation between the scales and the hearing levels was with respect to the high frequencies, presumably this is what one would expect since this is where the hearing loss occurs?

Secondly, as regards the tinnitus. The last study that I did on this showed that in a particular hospital sample, whether tinnitus was present or not was correlated with the score on the hypochondriasis and hysteria scales of the MMPI (Hinchcliffe, 1965).

Thirdly, as regards sound localization. Since Nordlund (1964) has shown that localization difficulties arise in people with middle-ear or neuronal, but not with receptor-organ, lesions, one might enquire whether the presence of this symptom in one of his subjects indicates a non-receptor-organ component, that is a component in the hearing loss arising from factors other than noise. I would therefore ask (i) what are the results on the inter-correlation of the various scales? (ii) how do the various scales correlate with personality measures? (iii) was a factor, or principal component, analysis of the data performed? (iv) was there any significant correlation between tinnitus and personality measures? (v) was any tinnitus matching done? and (vi) in view of the fact that Dr. Atherley raised the question about localization, were there any sophisticated otological diagnostic measurements performed, apart from otoscopy, such as using acoustic impedance bridges, Békésy studies, and so on?

Dr. Atherley: Tinnitus will be dealt with by my colleague, Dr. Hempstock. He does, in fact, refer to some of the questions mentioned by Dr. Hinchcliffe. In my paper I omitted mention of another aspect of the questionnaire; what we called the non-scoring sections. These consist of questions of purely descriptive importance. We ask a man what his tinnitus is like, for example whether it is a rushing or a buzzing sound. From such questions we are building up a picture of tinnitus. This is of little value from the point of view of assessment but it may well have value in diagnosis in the future when we come to understand the relationship between description and diagnosis. In regard to localization I am aware of Nordlund's work (1962) but the answer to Dr. Hinchcliffe's question is no, we did not look at the diagnostic aspect of poor directional perception. Regarding personality and tinnitus, and indeed personality relationships within the questionnaire as a whole, Noble did a very thorough study of personality according to the precepts of the Manchester school. I say this carefully because I understand that there are differences of opinion between psychologists as to measures of personality and I am told that these have a regional orientation. From our study it came out clearly that the worse the overall score the more the men tended to be withdrawn. A battery of interrelations were done: among the sections of the questionnaire; and between the sections of the questionnaire and the various tests of hearing. From this meeting I have learned the importance of showing the poor relationship between the average of the audiometric frequencies 0·5, 1 and 2 kHz and certain sections of the questionnaire.

Dr. Coles: I would like to comment on the curious anomaly that Mr. Mild had a difficulty of localization which was not apparent in the other group. This is extremely worrying; it makes one begin to wonder possibly about the validity of the test at all, particularly if the person has bilateral high-tone lesions. These should not really affect localization very much, but I think there may be an explanation. If one has a borderline impairment, then perhaps the localization is the first thing to begin to go wrong. When the impairment gets more serious and begins to affect the hearing of everyday speech either in quiet or noise, then this becomes uppermost in the person's mind and seems so much more important that he tends to forget the localization loss. If this could be the explanation for Dr. Atherley's findings one should not weight too much the localization abnormality. As always when Dr. Atherley and I have discussed this subject we have differed a little on the value of case-taking, particularly when dealing with compensation cases. Dr. Atherley said there were some non-scoring questions but, in view of the fact that a person coming for compensation always wants to present the greatest possible disability and his best case, I wonder whether in that kind of case he feels that this would be sufficiently reliable.

Dr. Atherley: Looking back through the literature there is evidence that localization and other functions of hearing are, to a degree, separate. Jongkees and Groen (1946) showed that there was virtually no relationship between any measures of auditory threshold and localizing ability. However, in cases where the acuity is markedly different between the two ears one would expect some effect, although slight, on localizing ability. The relationships we have found (Atherley and Noble, 1970) are shown in Table XXXIII. They bear out the point that auditory thresholds and localizing ability are not closely related.

On the question of compensation, I avoided all mention of this subject in the paper because I recognized it as a controversial matter which is rather beyond the present scope. I think that in cases where compensation is being claimed the clinical history is of paramount importance. After all, it is very often the discrepancy between a man's story and the clinical findings that gives the clue that all is not as it should be. Of course, our questionnaire might be used in a non-scoring form; it would then lay down a standardized form of enquiry and this could be very useful in uncovering overstatement and exaggeration.

TABLE XXXIII. Correlation coefficients (Spearman) between pure-tone thresholds in either ear at six frequencies and score in a test of direction perception of a 1-kHz pure tone; 15 subjects. (Atherley and Noble, 1970)

Frequency (kHz)	Left ear	Right ear
0·5	0·054	0·433
1·0	0·044	0·180
2·0	0·303	0·459*
3·0	0·360	0·529*
4·0	0·409	0·451
6·0	0·343	0·538*

* $P < 0{\cdot}05$.

Dr. Ward: In his paper Dr. Atherley said that as far as he was concerned the test was valid in that it measures what he wants to measure. Could I then ask whether he is implying that he did some test to determine that a given person had trouble localizing sounds; in other words, correlating to determine that his answers were in fact a true mirror of the state of affairs?

Dr. Atherley: We made a comparability study. Foundrymen came to the laboratory and we performed a number of tests on them, including localization. Validity was assessed with a straightforward comparison between score on the test and the appropriate section of the questionnaire. Within the limits of our experiments we were satisfied that there was a relationship between answers to the questionnaire and performance at the localization test.

Dr. Ransome-Wallis: In his paper, Mr. Kell inferred that a large number of people did not use hearing aids as the aids were not very good. In my experience, the real problem is psychological. People will wear all manner of appliances, glasses, trusses, wooden legs, without demur but to wear a hearing aid signifies to them the ultimate decline. Another point is that the onset of presbycusis is usually a gradual process, the perception of background noise being the first to go, and the subject ultimately hears the voices he wants to hear against a "white" background. A hearing aid brings back to him normal background noise and so, usually at an advanced age, he has to re-educate himself to listen while ignoring the background. This often proves too difficult and the aid is put away in a drawer and forgotten. I should like to ask a question related to hearing against factory noise, namely what views are there about paracusis in this context?

Mr. Kell: I agree with Dr. Ransome-Wallis' stressing the importance of the social and other factors involved in wearing a hearing aid. At this stage, I wish only to draw attention to the very low use of hearing aids by our weavers.

Dr. Atherley: I have no views on paracusis. The literature is confusing on this subject and we were not sure how to approach paracusis through the questionnaire. We tried to ask about recruitment but we found that our questions were very often misunderstood and interpreted by our subjects in a way we did not intend. This was the value of the process of refinement in the early days of the questionnaire. It showed us that, whereas we thought we were asking questions about paracusis and recruitment, the subjects were describing unrelated phenomena.

Dr. Hood: I was much impressed by Dr. Atherley's statement that "the principal term 'hearing loss', with its connotation of reduced ability to receive sound, is inapplicable to those with acoustic trauma", because this is precisely the point I was trying to make in the discussion on the first session. It is an important one that is not given as much recognition as it ought to be, and I should like to illustrate it graphically. The first diagram (Fig. 66) shows the relationship between hearing loss and the degree of loudness recruitment, and is the result of a statistical study upon 200 cases of Ménière's disease (Hallpike and Hood, 1959). Note that as the hearing loss increases, the steepness of the recruitment curves progressively increases. The shaded areas are the 90% tolerance limits, and all the curves converge to a point in the region of about 100 dB. I do not know what Dr. Davis meant by two types of loudness recruitment but, just as one can predict these curves with some precision in Ménière's disease, so the same kind of prediction is applicable in the case of noise-induced hearing loss (Hood, 1960). There is exactly the same relationship between the steepness of the recruitment curve and the hearing loss in noise-induced hearing loss as in any other cochlear lesion, whatever its pathology. The other diagram, Fig. 67, shows the result of the effect of this distortion of the loudness function on speech discrimination. Above is shown a sample of curves taken from conductive-deaf subjects. The significant feature is that, whatever the degree of the hearing loss, their form is the same as the normal curve but displaced to the right by the amount of the deafness. There is a good correlation between this displacement and the average loss at 500, 1000 and 2000 Hz. Below are shown the average curves from a selection of subjects with end-organ deafness. Each is the average of about 10 patients and the number above each refers to the average hearing loss at 500, 1000 and 2000 Hz. With deafness below

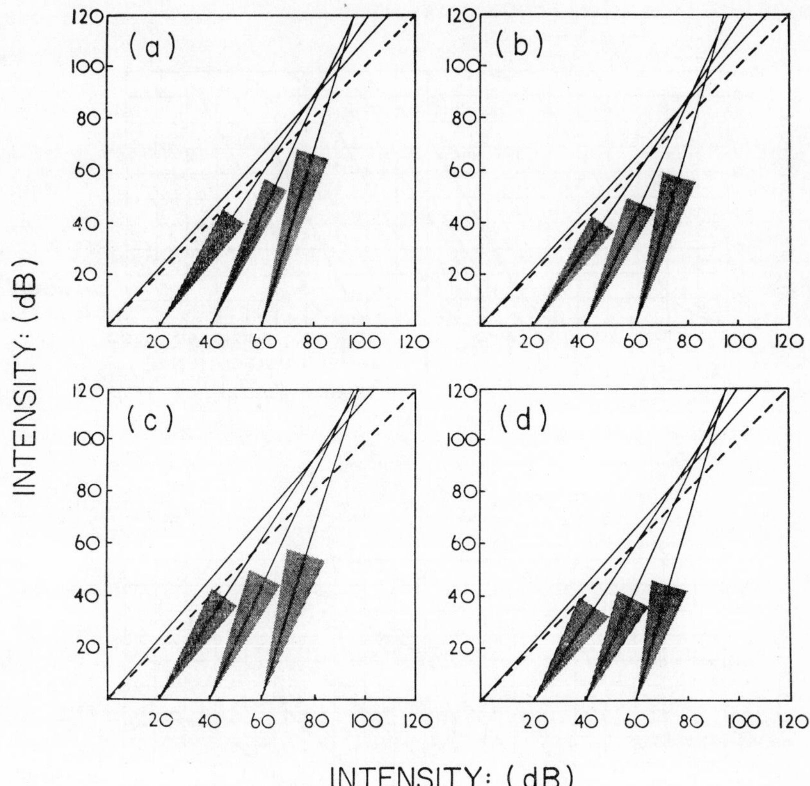

FIG. 66. Relationship between hearing loss and the degree of loudness recruitment, shown by the progressive steepening of the curves as the threshold intensity rises. (a) 500 Hz; (b) 1000 Hz; (c) 2000 Hz; (d) 4000 Hz.

20 dB, the shape of the curve is very much the same as the normal. It is interesting that this connects, in a kind of fortuitous way, with the AAOO "low fence", in that with hearing losses above about 25 dB redundant speech material has been completely eliminated as a result of the distortion of the loudness function. As the hearing loss increases the distorting effect becomes more marked, and when one reaches a deafness of 60 dB the speech discrimination is very poor indeed. It is true that these were taken for the most part from Ménière's disease but our experience with noise-induced hearing loss certainly leads us to believe that, as with loudness recruitment, so exactly the same kind of predictions apply in respect of speech discrimination. Dr. Davis made the point that in dealing with cases of noise-induced hearing loss one could, in a sense, consider them as conductive lesions and I would dispute this very strongly. It would imply that a subject with a given hearing loss would give the same

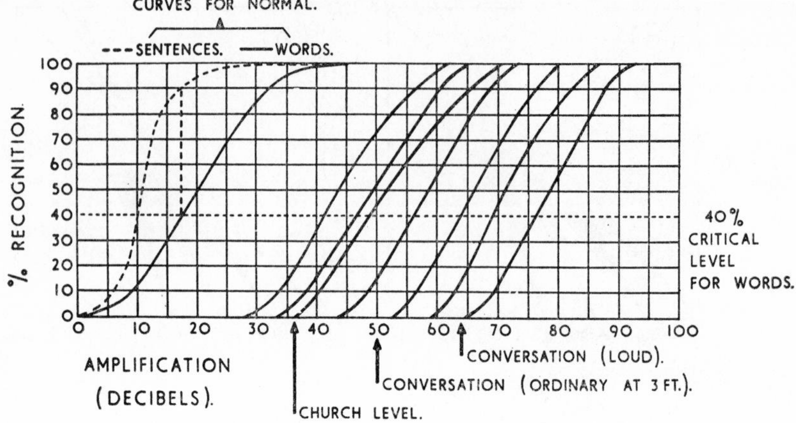

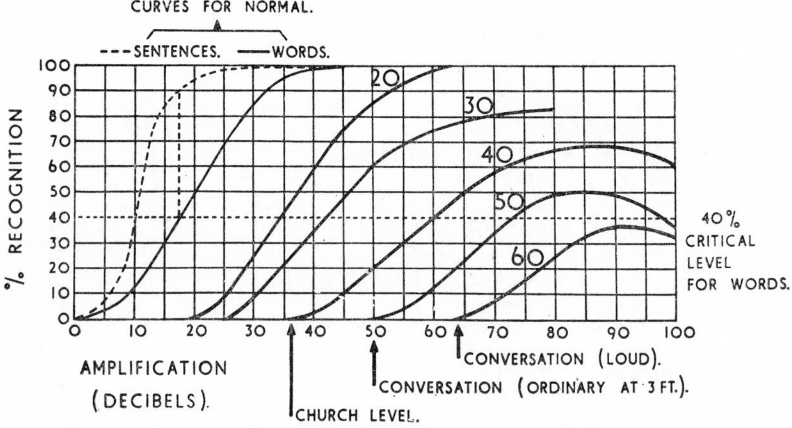

Fig. 67. Curves of intelligibility against speech level under various conditions. Normal hearing is depicted at the upper left. Seven typical cases of conductive-deaf subjects are shown at the upper right. The lower part of the figure shows results for normal hearing (left) contrasted with 5 cases with end-organ lesions (right) illustrating severe discrimination loss.

discrimination curve in the upper and lower parts of Fig. 67, whereas if he has a cochlear loss of say 60 dB he has a remarkably poor discrimination curve. It seems clear, therefore, that in devising scales of disability for noise-induced hearing loss this is another and most important factor that we have to take into account: it is not simply a question of hearing loss alone as has been suggested earlier in this symposium. Mr. Kell did not give us a great deal of information about his results on speech discrimination tests and I wonder if he could add to this. The question I would like to put directly to Mr. Kell and to Dr. Atherley is this: Do we treat these people as conductive hearing losses or as perceptive hearing losses, as suggested by Fig. 67?

Mr. Kell: I can confirm that the speech audiograms obtained among our noise-induced hearing loss subjects are similar in shape to those presented by Dr. Hood for his subjects with Ménière's disease, and they do not resemble the curves for those subjects with conductive hearing losses.

Dr. Atherley: In reply to Dr. Hood's point on speech discrimination tests, the information that we have is as given in Table XXXIV.

TABLE XXXIV. Correlation coefficients (Spearman) between speech tests and questionnaire items on speech

	Left ear	Right ear
Speech reception threshold for:		
disyllables	0·563*	0·430*
continuous discourse	0·324	0·412*
Speech discrimination loss for:		
monosyllables	0·509*	0·496*

Values marked * are highly significant, $P < 0{\cdot}01$.

I think that these figures support Dr. Hood's observations.

Dr. Hinchcliffe: May I add that, from studies in a hospital population, we found (Hinchcliffe, 1967a) a high correlation ($r{\sim}0{\cdot}6$) between the speech discrimination loss and the hearing levels for the frequencies 2, 4 and 8 kHz. This might be interpreted as due to the fact that speech intelligibility depends primarily on consonants, which have their important formant frequencies in this particular region. As regards the interrelationship of speech discrimination and loudness recruitment, Pestalozza and Shore (1955) showed that a marked discrimination loss can exist in the absence of any loudness recruitment. Conversely, a high discrimination score does not always predict the absence of recruitment (Hirsh *et al.*, 1954).

Dr. Glorig: I would like to ask Dr. Hood how he explains the loss of discrimination in acoustic neurinoma in the absence of recruitment, if he is assuming that the discrimination problem is directly related to recruitment.

Dr. Hood: Dr. Glorig's question is getting a little away from the main subject under discussion but, very briefly, I would have thought that the poor discrimination in acoustic tumours is due to the derangement of the nerve fibre itself. I do not see that this presents any great difficulty, but there is one item I would add on the correlation between speech discrimination and loudness recruitment. In attempting this correlation elsewhere (Hood, 1968), we found that there is in fact a better correlation between the recruitment angle and the speech discrimination than there is between hearing loss and speech discrimination, so that one can really consider the relationship between the loudness recruitment angle and speech discrimination completely independently of the hearing loss.

Dr. Wakstein: I would like to pursue the question of assessment scales. Mr. Kell said that the percentage impaired, based on the "3-average", was around 25% and the percentage impaired, based on the "4-average", was around 10%. It seems to me that this comparison reduces to the relation between how bad the impairment is, which is in effect a value judgement, and what the percentage of people having that impairment is. Could Dr. Atherley say how his assessment of social adequacy compares with Davis' social adequacy index?

Dr. Atherley: I would like to reiterate a general point. Virtually all schemes for predicting the effects of hearing loss on people, including the social adequacy index, are based upon studies of conductive lesions. We think that a new start is required. If we were to produce numerous correlations between the many schemes and our results we would only be providing ammunition against ourselves. This may appear a cynical view but it must be remembered that we were not trying to assess our work in the light of what has gone before. From the evidence of our research we believe that sensorineural lesions behave in many respects differently from conductive ones. We are not enthusiastic about theories or systems derived from studies of conductive lesions being applied to sensorineural ones. For example, we believe that the so-called social effects of hearing cannot be assessed completely and adequately from knowledge of pure-tone thresholds no matter what range or averages are used.

Dr. Stephens: I would like to return to Dr. Atherley's Mr. Slight and Mr. Mild. Could I suggest that the difference between Mr. Slight with his score of about 90, and both Mr. Mild and the hearing-aid group may be explained by the results of the "indirect" scale? This scale seems to be essentially a measure of neuroticism, Mr. Slight thus being seen as a rather neurotic individual who gives high response scores to most general questionnaires and uses ear defenders; whereas his more stable colleague does not.

Dr. Atherley: I am sorry that Dr. Noble has emigrated to Australia and is not here to deal with this question. My answer is that the Manchester school is not keen on the classification of mankind into four categories. The withdrawal shown by our subjects might be what Dr. Stephens would call neuroticism. However, Noble studied these men in detail and one of his colleagues gave the following summary of the findings:

"The men don't give very much away, although on the other hand, there may not be all that much to give away. They seem to be a fairly balanced lot, within a rather narrow range of interests. Aware of the monotony of their job they do, however, get some satisfaction out of earning their livelihood and doing a day's work. They live quiet lives.... Perhaps hearing loss doesn't matter all that much since they don't seem to make any great demands on life ... on the whole the men seem to view themselves as not too irritable (or wouldn't like to be thought so) and as being reasonably content while at the same time not liking to be disturbed by unusual or unacceptable experience. A quiet life is the aim ... not Living Theatre.... One question is whether this 'quietness' would be a natural feature of people like these or whether they have become so because of hearing loss."

I would go so far as to say that the working pattern is not conducive to what might be called extraverted behaviour. The group as a whole showed the pattern described above, not just the high scorers in a particular section. In other words there were no great personality differences among the individuals and the group as a whole showed the tendency to withdraw.

Dr. Glorig: When Dr. Atherley said that he had done all speech tests and other kinds of tests to evaluate hearing in the usual way, he did not report any correlations between those tests and what his questionnaire showed. It looks as though Mr. Slight is better motivated than Mr. Mild, and I wonder whether or not he did, in fact, have more problems as assessed by the usual testing methods. In Dr. Atherley's studies was the person's environment checked, and if so did the people he lives with agree with what he said?

Dr. Atherley: We did, in fact, make a laboratory study of inter-relationships between the sections of questionnaire and all the performance tests and the details of these are given by Noble (1969). In regard to the differences between the two men there is a point that I would like to emphasize: these men did not come forward of their own accord. Our method for obtaining subjects is first to seek general approval from both sides of industry. Following this, we ask for lists of employees showing names, ages and years of employment in particular jobs. From this list we select names; we then approach these men and ask them to take part in our research. In this way we avoid some of the more serious effects of selection bias. Thus the two men I was describing were not volunteers in so far as they were not self-selected. Certainly they were not motivated by any question of compensation. The results of the threshold tests on the two men are, as Dr. Glorig said, contradicted by the questionnaire results. Which are correct can only be shown by further research. Checking of the environment was done in an earlier study. We related the men's scores with what the wives said about their husbands' hearing and the agreement was good, so good in fact that we stopped using this technique. We were pleased to discontinue it because it often required visits to the wives while the men were at work.

Dr. Ward: An occupational hazard!

Mr. Chadwick: I would like to congratulate Mr. Kell and his colleagues on their careful study, particularly the way they have so clearly demonstrated the importance which attaches to inclusion of the hearing level at 3 kHz when assessing social disability. One question I would like to ask relates to a previous study on Dundee jute workers (Taylor *et al.*, 1967). In the homes of retired weavers, teenagers were frequently found listening to pop music with the radio turned on full blast, experiencing no obvious signs of discomfort. On the other hand, the weavers with their considerable degrees of hearing loss were unable to tolerate such levels—this obviously being an indication of recruitment. The question of possible auditory damage from pop music is currently very topical. I wonder whether Mr. Kell has any comments to make on what one might term the *recreational* element, as opposed to the *occupational* element, in noise-induced hearing loss and whether any allowance for, or assessment of, this factor was made in his present studies?

Mr. Kell: Yes, we did ask our subjects whether they listened to radio and TV and, if so, whether they liked to have the sound volume set high and higher than other members of the family. Those weavers with hearing impairment usually preferred the volume to be loud, but many stressed that they could not tolerate the volume at very loud, which provides evidence for the recruitment phenomenon. A number of weavers mentioned, in passing, that they could not tolerate the level at which young people in their family operated record players, etc.

Dr. Hinchcliffe: Since we now all seem to be aware of the importance of auditory measures other than those related to tonal hearing levels, might I suggest that projected studies in the area that we have been discussing should also include some or all of the following measures: speech discrimination loss, comfortable and uncomfortable loudness levels, and aural harmonic thresholds.

Dr. Coles: I would like to ask Mr. Kell whether it is too late to have the computer examine a few more frequency combinations. The ones given will be extremely useful and revealing, but if one is going to take three upper frequencies I would have thought it worthwhile to look at 1, 2 and 4 kHz as well as 1, 2 and 3 kHz. The former are evenly spaced at octave intervals. Also of interest would be the combination 0·5, 1, 2 and 4 kHz which has been mentioned by Dr. Davis and is also in the Australian method. The whole study has tremendous implications and importance for possible future legislation in this country; it would seem, therefore, a great pity not to analyse the results of these additional frequency combinations if it entails only a bit more computer programming and a few more minutes' running time.

Dr. Robinson: I should like to underline the comment made by Dr. Coles and encourage Mr. Kell and his collaborators to extract the maximum from their sociological data. I would go further and not restrict the analysis to frequency averages from the pure-tone audiogram. After all, one routinely performs more sophisticated operations in other branches of acoustics. For example, to calculate the loudness of a complex sound we are not content simply to average certain octave-band sound pressure levels; in that case we are not afraid of non-linear transformations and a strange algebra of addition in order to obtain the correct answer. There appears to me to exist already the appropriate algebra for doing what is necessary in the present context, namely to calculate the articulation index from the pure-tone audiogram. Could Mr. Kell and his colleagues at Dundee be persuaded to program their computer to include something like this in their correlation analysis?

Mr. Kell: Here I have only presented the results on two frequency averages, but other combinations of the audiogram are being assessed. Further analysis of the results by discrimination analysis and order ranking are in progress and will be reported in *International Audiology*.

Professor Burns: I should like to support what has already been said about the handling of the data, namely that all reasonable explorations should be done. The pioneering work of Dr. Taylor on this particular population started us thinking about the implications some years ago. I think it would be unfortunate if otological and other opinion crystallized prematurely in this country on any particular formula. However much Dr. Robinson and I have been influenced by the desire for reasonable simplicity in some of the conclusions that we have drawn, I do not think that one should be afraid of using rather more elaborate formulations in deciding on a form of numerical index for disability. This is without prejudice to any other ways of achieving the result, such as Dr. Atherley has outlined.

Dr. Ward: I would like to return to the question of recruitment on which I have done a little work, as Dr. Glorig mentioned earlier. At one time we did a study on some men who had high-frequency hearing loss (Ward, Fleer and Glorig, 1961). Half the losses had been caused by gunfire as best we could determine, and half by steady noise. One of the things measured was recruitment, and the curves that we got were in every way, including slope, identical to those that Dr. Hood has presented here. So there is no question but what recruitment, measured in the normal way, will come out to be the same in Ménière's disease and in noise-induced hearing loss. The only possible difference between the two conditions is suggested when we consider alternative theories as to what is going on in recruitment; perhaps there *are* two kinds of recruitment. If, in fact, these high-frequency hearing losses are characterized by only relatively refractory nerve fibres, which at high intensities of stimulation fire in a normal manner, one would expect speech eventually to reach normal intelligibility as the intensity is increased. On the other hand, suppose the areas concerned are completely dead. In this case one generally accounts for recruitment on the basis that as the intensity of the test tone is raised, more and more of the normal portion of the basilar membrane is involved. At high intensities the contribution that would have been provided by these dead fibres would no longer be appreciable in terms of the total so that loudness would be "normal". In this latter case one would not expect full intelligibility to be reached no matter how high the intensity were raised. I think that in noise-induced hearing loss normal firing does not occur. There are several lines of evidence and one of these is diplacusis, the shift in pitch of a pure tone in the vicinity of a tonal gap. In a case of noise-induced hearing loss one will usually find that a barely supraliminal tone presented in this region is shifted quite a way upward in pitch. This can be taken to mean that the fibres which are firing are those on the basal side of the affected area. If it were a matter of relatively refractory fibres one would expect that the firing pattern, and hence the pitch, would gradually return to normal as one raised the intensity, but that is not what seems to happen. The test must be done with a person who has a tonal gap in one ear and normal hearing in the other, and then one finds that a tone of say 6000 Hz appears to have the pitch of a normal 9000 Hz tone not only at threshold but all the way up to the point at which transcranial conduction enters in, after which the tone delivered to the bad ear is heard in the good one. It is then very difficult to make pitch judgements. The point is that one does not get a gradual return to normality of pitch; the shift seems to be relatively independent of intensity. Thus, if a person has a hearing loss at 3 and 4 kHz so severe that he cannot tell the differences among *t*, *p* and *k* acoustically then he will not be able to distinguish them no matter how high the intensity is raised, and 100% intelligibility for isolated words will never be reached. I think this is one of the considerations involved when discussing the meaning of recruitment in diagnosis.

Dr. Hood: As to the question of loudness recruitment and its basis, I am very much in the dark. Like others, I have my theories, and my suggestion is that it is due to a specificity for loudness amongst the hair cells, that is to say a grading such that the external hair cells are specific to low-intensity sounds and the inner hair cells to high-intensity sounds. This was put forward a great many years ago by Tumarkin and if one considers recruitment in these terms then it is easy to see, assuming that in cochlear deafness it is the external hair cells which are more susceptible to damage whether the cause be disease or injury, that this leaves the inner hair cells preserved with their own specificity for a particular loudness level. This would account for a certain deficiency of loudness even at high intensities, but I am not sure about the significance of it for intelligibility.

Dr. Ward: My point was that no matter how high the intensity is raised, the missing areas cannot contribute in the same way as a normal cochlea to the intelligibility. As a specific example, if one gives the word "tick" a person with high-frequency loss will call it "pick", irrespective of the level. His discrimination reaches an asymptote and he can never do any better.

Dr. Hood: I quite agree that loudness recruitment is not the be-all and end-all of speech intelligibility debasement in these patients; there must be other factors too. Diplacusis is probably a case in point, as is the frequency characteristic of the hearing loss. I do not doubt that these all make their own particular contribution.

Air Vice-Marshal Dickson: Tinnitus, as every otologist knows, is a distressing complaint. Many letters to the Royal National Institute for the Deaf are from patients who ask, "What can you do to relieve me of my tinnitus?" I had therefore hoped when I saw the title of the paper by Dr. Hempstock and Dr. Atherley that they would produce some kind of answer. Tinnitus is so difficult to localize—whether it is central or whether it is peripheral in origin—and so I hope that the discussion may bring out some contribution towards alleviation, that is, of tinnitus which has not been induced deliberately.

Dr. Ransome-Wallis: I find the subject of tinnitus fascinating, especially in the manner in which it is described by individual patients. The assortment of noises described appears to be more varied in female patients than in men. I have, on occasion, been able to alter completely the character of tinnitus by giving the patient a course of nicotinic acid. Any comment on these phenomena would be most helpful.

Dr. Hempstock: The intention in our paper was to deal with the assessment rather than the treatment of tinnitus, and I agree with Dr. Ransome-Wallis about the wide variety of descriptions that sufferers give for the symptom. The only tangible piece of evidence to come from a study of the literature is the observation that tinnitus associated with a perceptive hearing loss is predominantly high-pitched and that tinnitus associated with conductive losses is predominantly low-pitched. Otherwise the patient's description of his tinnitus is not of very much diagnostic value.

Dr. Coles: When commenting on the duration of the tinnitus, Dr. Hempstock said that in most cases it disappeared within 5 minutes; presumably in some cases it did not? My question is whether this correlated to any extent with the degree of TTS, that is, did the tinnitus have a more prolonged recovery time when there was greater auditory effect or TTS? I ask this question because for a long time I have used a criterion of 5 minutes of TTS as an indication of severity of gunfire noise exposure. This has proved, in quite a number of studies, to be a fairly reliable indication of past exposure to noise hazards; individuals who got more than 5 minutes' tinnitus tended to have average hearing losses rather greater than those who had not experienced such tinnitus. To illustrate this I may refer to one study on Royal Marine recruits carried out before proper ear protection was introduced. We knew that the noise was hazardous and gave the men ear protectors, but at that time it was not a disciplinary offence if they did not use them, and the amount of their actual use was very variable. It was interesting that those who got tinnitus lasting more than 5 minutes after the first occasion of shooting were the men who used their ear protection subsequently. This partly answers the question of what can be done about the alleviation of tinnitus: to some extent it alleviates itself in this kind of situation if one provides ear protection. Perhaps a psychologist might argue that this showed something else, about anxiety for example. But the group who had the more tinnitus, and used their ear protectors more, in the end also showed more permanent threshold shift. So I return to my question: did Dr. Hempstock's subjects with the prolonged recovery from tinnitus also have larger temporary threshold shifts?

Dr. Hempstock: In reply to Dr. Coles, the amount of temporary threshold shift did not seem to affect the period of recovery from tinnitus; in fact, there were some subjects whose tinnitus lasted several hours on one occasion but who would only experience it for a few minutes following the next exposure, although their TTS was the same on both occasions. The duration of tinnitus is clearly an important parameter in assessing its disturbing potential. It is interesting to note that occupational hearing loss following exposure to impulsive noise appears to be associated with longer-lasting tinnitus than that following exposure to continuous noise. As similar observations are made in the laboratory when temporary threshold shifts are produced by impulse noise, it may be that the high peak sound pressures present in impulse noise are particularly effective in producing tinnitus.

Dr. Hinchcliffe: I would like to congratulate Dr. Ward on his paper on the chinchilla studies and at the same time present some data obtained from a comparable noise-exposure experiment on cats. The three points on the graph (Fig. 68) each represent the median noise-induced persistent threshold shift (NIPTS) for a group of three cats; the NIPTS for each cat being in turn the average for nine frequencies (125, 250, 500 Hz; 1, 2, 4, 8, 12 and 16 kHz). One group had been exposed to white noise of 105 dB SPL for 8 hours, another to 105 dB SPL for 4 hours and the third

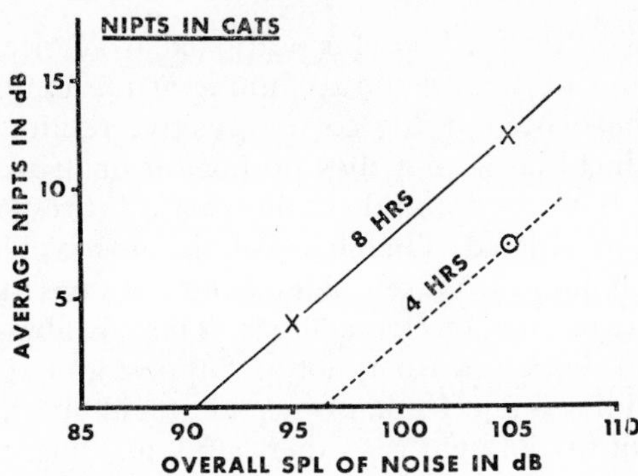

FIG. 68. Noise-induced PTS in 3 groups of 3 cats, determined by Hinchcliffe and Sokolovski). The horizontal intercept between the curves is 6 dB, suggesting a trading relation of 6 dB per twofold change in the duration of exposure.

group to 95 dB SPL for 8 hours. For the purpose of this tentative analysis it was assumed that, over the range studied, the NIPTS averaged in decibels would be a linear function of the overall sound pressure level of the noise to which the animals were exposed. Moreover, it was also assumed that the family of curves with exposure time as parameter would lie parallel to one another. The actual experimental work was executed by Dr. Alexander Sokolovski* on a research grant that I had from the Science Research Council. Although the data are presented somewhat differently from those for Dr. Ward's chinchillas, and they are for small numbers only, they would indicate a 6-dB trading relationship. Moreover, I detect a tendency among the medians of the chinchilla data points suggesting that Dr. Ward's results could be held comparable to our own.

Dr. Ward: That would be an equal-pressure trading relationship and long ago Spieth and Trittipoe (1958) also suggested that it should be 6 dB. The Walsh–Healey Act has adopted 5 dB and a group in Germany has championed 4 dB. Here, with the chinchilla and Robinson's (1968) work, we have 3 dB, so perhaps we can now compromise at $4\frac{1}{2}$ by averaging them all together! The one animal in our experiment who did not get more than 15 dB of PTS happened to be in the lowest intensity group.

* Now at the University of Giessen, German Federal Republic.

This means that perhaps if one ran enough animals one could confirm the reality of the apparent slope that Dr. Hinchcliffe mentioned, which would be in the direction of confirming Rüedi's original notion of a critical intensity. But I think this evidence bears much more on the notion of a critical immission.

Mr. Martin: I would like to ask Dr. Ward, how does one obtain an audiogram from a chinchilla and how accurate is it?

Dr. Ward: We used the method of conditioned avoidance, mainly because Miller used it and developed the technique at the Central Institute for the Deaf. We have been trying to use positive reinforcement, but the trouble with chinchillas is that they do not eat or drink much, so when one tries to give them food and drink in reward for responding correctly, they are very soon satiated. Therefore conditioned avoidance is what we used: the animals jump from one side of the test cage to the other when they hear a tone, or they receive a shock. There is always a problem in deciding when to shock and when not to. Suppose an animal really heard the tone and did not jump. In that case, one would give him a little shock to remind him of his job. On the other hand, one does not want to give the animal a shock if he really did not hear because then the animal begins "ping-ponging" back and forth as he can always circumvent the shock by doing so. As a result, this type of testing is still as much an art as a science. If, however, one employs a single tester, who is not allowed to see the previous results beyond a base-line audiogram to give him some idea where to begin, there may be anything from 5 to 15 dB difference between successive thresholds. One must therefore take an average of four or five runs, after assuming that the threshold has reached equilibrium, to get a threshold that one can be sure of to ± 5 dB. However, by averaging the shifts at a number of frequencies, the variance goes down accordingly.

Mrs. Passchier: We have examined Dr. Ward's data in terms of the most probable regression line. Although Fig. 65 of his paper shows the results for the 15 chinchillas at each octave frequency from 125 to 16,000 Hz inclusive, the data available to us at the time were the average values of PTS over only part of the range, namely 500 to 8000 Hz inclusive as given in Dr. Ward's preprint. However, this partial analysis is correct so far as it goes. The most probable regression line, fitted by least-squares, turned out to have a slope of 4·5 dB per halving of the time. On this evidence it seems that the shorter exposure to a higher noise level, keeping noise immission constant, results in a larger PTS. The difference over an eightfold duration ratio seems to be as much as 13·5 dB averaged over the five frequencies. Admittedly, the 95% confidence limits on the slope of 4·5 dB/half-time are $-2{\cdot}2$ and 11·2, and since the equal-energy hypothesis requires a zero slope, this hypothesis cannot be rejected. However, it is clear that a lot of alternative hypotheses could not be rejected either, and the results of Dr. Ward's experiment do not seem to contribute very much to resolving this question. The inclusion of the frequencies that we omitted, namely 125, 250 and 16,000 Hz would not change this argument very much.

Dr. Ward: This is a perfectly legitimate criticism, although the force of the argument can be made stronger or weaker depending on which frequencies one examines, and on whether one believes that the exceptionally "tough-eared" animal in the 114-dB group has distorted the result simply because he happened to fall in that group. However, I still think sixteen animals are better than none, but if Mrs. Passchier does not choose to accept the equal-energy hypothesis over this range on the basis of our data I cannot really quarrel. My only rejoinder is that the 7 dB difference between the medians of the first and last groups is not statistically significant. The scatter and overlap are so large as hardly to justify regression analysis; about all that one can do is to apply a non-parametric test and then one cannot get anywhere near a probability level of $P=0{\cdot}05$ for the difference between the first and fourth groups. So I have to agree that further research is necessary, but I hope that somebody besides us is willing to undertake it!

Dr. Hinchcliffe: That was the point that I also tried to bring out in relation to our cat experiments, at the Institute of Laryngology and Otology: whilst the results do not contradict the equal-energy hypothesis, they do not contradict the equal-pressure hypothesis either.

Dr. Robinson: Without entering into the arguments as to the statistical significance of Dr. Ward's and Dr. Hinchcliffe's results, I would like to make the comment that the equal-energy principle occupies a unique position. There can be very good reasons why energy might be the essential agent, as it is in molecular physics and chemistry. I do not think the same applies to any other trading relationship and if it turns out that the relation is anything else this would be evidence of more complicated things happening. As regards Mrs. Passchier's analysis of Dr. Ward's data, I think it is worth remarking that her inference as to the relative damaging effects of the four exposures of equal noise immission is contrary to the widely-accepted viewpoint that if one packs a just-permissible 8-hour steady-noise exposure into a shorter period then the permitted noise level may rise higher than that indicated by the equal-energy trade-off. In terms of Dr. Ward's diagram (Fig. 65), one would expect the regression line to be horizontal or downward sloping. The evidence of a contrary trend is the first I have yet seen that the allegedly over-conservative equal-energy principle may not be conservative enough. In this regard, the data obtained by Dr. Ward and by Drs. Hinchcliffe and

Sokolovski are in conflict and if Dr. Ward's chinchillas truly reflect what is going on in man current ideas of damage risk for intermittent noise will need revising.

A Summing-up

By

A. Glorig

Director, Callier Hearing and Speech Center, Dallas, Texas

First of all I would like to compliment the organizers of the Conference. I think Dr. and Mrs. Robinson have put together one of the finest Conferences I have ever attended in this field. I should make one or two suggestions, however. Some members of the audience might have been helped with some primer courses on noise and noise-measurement. These Conferences, even though some are really bad, remind me of a story I heard not long ago. Many of them are like sex—when it's good it's very good and when it's bad it's usually still pretty good. I think these Conferences should be looked on as milestones, particularly this one, and I would like to thank Dr. Robinson personally.

Dr. Davis talked about a very important subject. When we set damage-risk criteria, what are we trying to prevent from damage? This is a question that has been discussed over a good many years. Despite the fact that some people feel that some of the conclusions we have reached may be wanting, I would like to say that the basis of the criteria used in our country has proved quite useful. Very little complaint has come from its use. We should certainly look at it as at least an excellent beginning towards a method of evaluating hearing loss, for compensation purposes. When you are deciding about a method for your country remember we were conserving hearing for ordinary speech as heard in quiet and the most practical way to compare, in terms of going from pure tones to speech, was through averaging the hearing level at 500, 1000 and 2000 Hz. We discussed that it would probably be better if we could weight the frequencies differently. At the time we made this decision we did not know how to weight them. We did not have sufficient information about going from pure tones to speech. I am not so sure that our method can be improved a great deal. The original concept was to compensate for wage loss. A man really suffers no wage loss, nor a potential wage loss, if he can carry on ordinary everyday communication.

Mrs. Passchier's paper about the relations of hearing loss to steady and fluctuating noise seemed to show that there is a direct relation between steady noise, and probably fluctuating noise, which is reasonably close to the equal-energy concept. There are some differences that were mentioned that we must look into further, but until those differences are defined better we probably should stay with equal-energy. Whether it is correct or not remains for time to show. Some of the studies that Dr. Ward has been referring to may produce data which will help us to refine this concept, as he suggested himself a while ago. In my own opinion and as Dr. Chadwick said, that of a mere otologist—I like to look at it in a simplified way. After all the ear is being exposed to a form of energy, and the effect of this energy should be dependent on time and effective intensity. We may evolve what I have formerly called a Noise Exposure Index but which Dr. Robinson has called "noise immission". I didn't even know there was a word like "immission" until he brought it up.

I was very much interested in Dr. Kylin's paper on forest workers. I did a brief study of this in the United States, but I was mostly interested in the operation of the saw. The hearing data are being gathered now and I hope to be able to study the audiograms in the near future. I am interested in discovering just how much time the saw is actually running. We made a time study of several saws and found that out of the 8-hour day the saw was actually on at maximum level not more than an hour to an hour and a half. This means that the bursts of speed don't last very long. Usually the cutting time is a function of how large the log is. When one starts converting this kind of exposure into total energy one begins to see why these subjects don't show as much hearing loss as would be expected from the noise levels present. The on-time is a very small part of the 8-hour day so we need to examine these intermittent noises much better.

As always, I was very much impressed with Dr. Robinson's paper and I would like to compliment him on his report this time which, for this type of audience, was the best he's done—at least in my opinion. I'm not going into detail on his paper because I think it speaks for itself. The thing that I would like to say is that it appears from his "mathematical shenanigans" —as I call them—that he is heading toward a fundamental concept I spoke about earlier. It should eventually result in a sort of an energy/time or level/time (whichever it turns out to be) index, which can be used as a unit to predict what will happen, at least to the group ear. I'm not convinced yet that we can use it for the individual ear.

Professor Burns too has, as always, given us something to think about. Dr. Ward and I can be blamed for all the talk about TTS and PTS relationships. Some time ago therefore I was delighted to see that Professor Burns agreed that in groups there seemed to be a direct relation between TTS and PTS, although he was not sure that it was related to individuals. On the other hand Dr. Nixon and I studied the same men working in five different noises for 5 years. These men had been previously exposed to the noise for less than 3 years, and we did PTS and TTS studies over a 4-year period. Actually the study was designed to last 5 years but in the fifth year California started instituting an ear-protection programme and we had to be content with data over 4 years. In this particular study there emerged some mathematical functions that made it possible to predict individual PTS from TTS.

Dr. Coles has been talking about impulsive noise for some time and I think rightly so since he has probably done most of the recent work on this. I would like to make it clear that gunfire is not the same noise that is produced by a drop-hammer even though they are both impulsive. This is summed up in his final words: when one looks at impulsive noise there are three things which are most important: the peak value, the duration of the impulse and the rate at which the peaks occur. All must be accounted for when damage-risk criteria are involved.

I was fascinated by Mr. Surböck's paper. The work going on in Austria is indeed interesting. When I see such studies I become jealous because in our country it is impossible to do them. I think the kind of service one can give industry in a small country like Austria should produce a lot of very fine data over the years. I only wish that we could do the same thing in the United States. I was quite fascinated with the number, 91,000 subjects, that he had tested. This is a large number of audiograms and the Austrians should not fail to examine them in every way possible, particularly with respect to the amount of risk involved as a function of level and years of exposure. "Percentage risk" is a most important concept: the development of tables to predict, at least in groups, what will happen to a specific number of people over a known number of years as a function of "equivalent exposure". I think the studies by Mr. Surböck and Dr. Raber should give us much more confidence in our "percentage risk" tables. The compensation that Mr. Surböck mentioned is a little different than we have in the United States. I noted the 66% for total disability relative to wages, and the 50% for total deafness relative to the whole man. We feel that if the man is what we call a "basket-case", that is, a case who requires service for all his needs, he is 100% disabled. Total hearing loss is only about 35% when referred to the total man.

Next was Dr. Delany's paper. As always he has presented some highly technical and very precise data. His are very nice studies that I wish I were able to do myself. But I wonder if, in the clinical context, the variations that Dr. Delany mentioned would be significant. The kind of clinical audiometry usually done in an industrial situation would not allow for such precision. In studies of normal hearing, where one is using good psychoacoustic techniques such variations are quite significant but I am not so sure what they mean in terms of variations in serial audiograms. We reported as much as 25 to 30 dB differences in either direction depending on which audiogram one examined. This was on 400 subjects who had from 6 to 15 audiograms each over a period of 10 years. One could prove that noise actually improved hearing if one used the right audiograms! We studied these data at some length and came to the conclusion that in about 85 to 90% of the subjects involved in serial audiograms the results could be reasonably stable and dependable. In the remainder sizeable variations in any direction could be found. I am not sure what the problem is but I suppose it is somewhat related to what Dr. Stephens mentioned. We have called it the "set" of the subject at the time the audiogram was made. Just what we mean by "set" I have never been able to define to my own satisfaction, but I do know that when you test an individual who is a naïve listener the result depends on his attitude—his motivation—his particular set at the time the audiogram is done. These variations have no relation to the effects of noise and poor testing technique. I am talking about an individual who is tested by an expert over a period of years in good quiet conditions. I wish somebody would explain this to me; I don't know why it happens.

These kinds of technical problems remind me of a story. It seems quite appropriate when one is talking about highly technical subjects to an audience that is not highly technically oriented. A couple went to a judge to be married and the judge said, "You must first have a licence before I can marry you." They obtained a licence and came back. The judge looked at the licence and said, "Well, I'm sorry but there's no date on the licence." So they went back to the licence bureau for a date and returned to the judge. This time the judge said, "Well, I'm more distressed now, today's the 16th, not the 17th, you must return and have this corrected." They did so and returned to the judge for the third time and he said, "Well, the date's all right but now you've got the groom's name where the bride's name should be. You must have that corrected." After doing this and returning to the judge for the fourth time the judge said, "Now the licence is correct, but I would like to know who this little boy is that you have with you." So the man said, "Why, that's our little boy, judge." At this time the judge looked quite distressed and told the man that even though he was being married today the boy would be a technical bastard. The man looked at the judge with a large smile on his face and said, "I don't think we'll mind that at all, judge, that's what the man down the street said you were." I wonder sometimes if some of our high-level technical scientists find themselves, at the end of a meeting of this kind, in the same unhappy position as the judge.

My friend Floyd Van Atta did his usual good job. He gave a fairly good digest of what's going on in our country with respect to regulations through the Federal Government. The thing I like about Van Atta's attitude is that he feels it is not his business to tell industry what to do, it is his business to tell them that they have a problem. If government regulation can stay with this role and leave industry to call in consultants to help make the essential changes, the results would be good; goodness knows, in our country we get interference enough from the Federal Government. One of the things that came out of Van Atta's paper which impressed me very much was something that our Committee on Hearing Conservation has been advising for some time—and that is "education". Most of us feel that there should be a period of education before we insist that people wear ear protection. Just making a programme mandatory isn't going to succeed. I have had a great deal of experience with this matter and find that if one initiates an educational programme for 6 to 9 months and then makes the wearing of ear protection mandatory one will obtain a great deal more co-operation from the men involved.

I was interested in the protection methods that Mr. Forrest mentioned. I have heard about this in our own country where someone sent me a set of plugs claiming that they would allow speech to pass but would keep out high-level sounds. I was not sure what to think about this being rather naïve in this respect, but according to Mr. Forrest these plugs depend on the acoustical properties of a small hole and some sort of a resonant chamber and they do seem to work in high levels, particularly with impulsive kinds of noise. However, I would like to be sure that Mr. Forrest looks at these protectors over a long period to see whether the protection really is adequate. It's a little bit hard for me as an otologist to feel that if one can hear speech one will not sustain any damage from high-level noise so I would like to see a little more evidence that they work. I hope they do, but on the other hand, in most cases where one needs to hear speech, the ordinary ear protector is really not good enough to prevent hearing speech, unless one speaks quite softly. I wonder if there ever is a time when speech cannot be heard, thereby causing an accident? I can see why Mr. Forrest would feel this way. I have been asked about the need to hear speech while wearing ear protection many times and I usually reply that I wished ear protection were that good. If one raises his voice moderately, speech can be heard through the best protectors.

That brings me to Dr. Bruton's paper. He describes the hearing conservation programme as it exists at the BOAC and BEA. I am very familiar with this programme since I have been visiting the BOAC for more than 10 years, assisting in organizing the programme. The things he mentioned should be remembered. Even though one may be forced to conduct the kind of hearing conservation programme that BOAC is recommending there are problems that one should be aware of before starting such a programme. Don't be too discouraged, because such programmes are working in a large number of industries in our country. I have known Mr. Fowler, who is in the audience here and who has since become an Englishman, for many years and I know that Chrysler Corporation had a good programme while he was there. He can confirm that a programme if properly executed will work. We are beginning to get evidence of how well it works in terms of the differences in the hearing of people who wear ear plugs and those who do not. I recently tested

100 men that work in a bottle factory and this is the fourth test on the same men over a 17-year period. When a man has a good hearing threshold and you ask him, "Do you wear anything in your ears?" the answer is always, "Yes, I wear ear plugs." Every one of these men who wears ear plugs shows good thresholds. It is very convincing evidence that ear plugs will work, despite what people think of them.

Dr. Bryan's talk about liability was very interesting to me. I had never heard that liability could be related to ignorance: I have always heard that ignorance was no excuse although I had heard about the Devon case prior to hearing Dr. Bryan's talk. Since these people were not aware of the general recommendations that were made regarding noise they were not held liable. If they had read the literature or even the newspapers and the magazines I think they would have discovered a lot more about noise than they appear to have known at the time.

As usual, Dr. Hinchcliffe has given one of his exhilarating papers. One of the things that always amazes me about him is how versatile he is. I am not so sure he goes to these exotic places because he wants the data or because they are very nice places. I notice he has never gone to the North Pole or Greenland and Iceland; it is always to some nice South Sea area where the climate is good and the tans are very evident. I am not going to say much about presbycusis, but I do feel that a correction is unwarranted in terms of what we know with respect to the amount of change that is a function of ageing. It is well known that some people have more presbycusis than others but I don't know how one can decide which individual it is. If one must correct for presbycusis one should start from audiometric zero because starting from the low fence would mean that 25 dB had already been deducted.

The paper by Dr. Taylor and his colleagues, as given by Mr. Kell, presents some interesting findings. I would like to make only one or two remarks with respect to caution when extrapolating from 3-, 4-, or 5-frequency averages, to hearing "difficulty". I think one must be careful about how one defines difficulty. Ask the right questions and almost anyone will admit having difficulty, depending on what one means by difficulty. These researchers should think carefully about their questionnaires before they begin to say that one average is better than another. The right questionnaire can correlate with almost anything.

I was very much impressed with Dr. Atherley's delivery. He gave a very nice paper and gave it in a scholarly manner. I'm always impressed with these young Englishmen and the way they can talk. His questionnaire was an ingenious one, although I think the same warning applies here. When the questionnaire appears to come out with different results than one would expect from looking at the man's hearing levels, there is probably something wrong with the questionnaire. When Mr. Mild, who by audiogram had more hearing loss than Mr. Slight—and Mr. Slight was the one who was complaining the most—it seems to me that one should look a little more carefully at how the questions were asked. I know Dr. Atherley did this on purpose because it was a reversal of what one would expect. I also know, and I agree with him, that he should not form a questionnaire on the basis of presently-used routine tests or other questionnaires. I think, however, that he should first decide upon definite criteria for what he wants and then try to make comparisons. The usual way, as we did some years ago, is to compare answers to pure-tone audiograms, to discrimination scores and with questions concerning environment. However, I agree that the kind of studies Dr. Atherley did are very important. Somehow we must be able to test a single individual and find out just what difficulty he is having. It doesn't work just from pure-tone averages, although it does look fairly good in a large majority of cases. If a man has a certain loss at 1000 Hz he will have a certain amount of "difficulty", depending, of course, on how one defines difficulty.

Dr. Ward is one of the most reasonable people I've had the privilege of knowing. We worked together for some years and then he left me, for which I have been eternally sorry, and wish he'd come back. I think his data on chinchilla are a good way to arrive at some probable answers that we can't get from humans. I agree with him 100% that trying to get the kind of data on equal-energy and intermittency on humans is almost impossible. I have tried for years now to find a group of people where we could do this. We can find some people exposed to steady noise, where the noise is on 8 hours and where they are in it for approximately 8 hours; but it is very difficult to find people where there is noise exposure with regular intermittency. Probably the coal mines come the closest to this. Even there the intermittency is not the same from day to day over a period of months. I certainly agree with Dr. Ward that more research is needed to determine the factors that are involved when trying to assess intermittency.

The paper that Mr. Chadwick gave about the otologist was very interesting and amusing as well as being very informative. I was interested in some of the numbers that he gave. He said about 25% of the population of Manchester was exposed to noise. I would like to make two other comparisons where he said that 8% of his office practice was due to noise-induced hearing loss, but that the large majority of the cases he saw, according to the numbers he gave, were conductive losses. Well, obviously, conductive losses would be more apparent in a surgeon's office because that's where they go to get something done about it. It's very difficult sometimes for otologists to conceive the idea that there are more neurosensory losses by far than there are conductive losses. Most of the losses they see in their offices are conductive losses. I would also like to compare two other numbers. If one looks at the latest National Health Survey made by the U.S. Public Health Service there are about 3% of the population in the United States that have losses greater than 30 dB in the three frequencies. In another population similar to Manchester, that is Milwaukee, where we did the Wisconsin State Fair, this 3% becomes 16% with greater than 30 dB average. I think one would find that this holds in Manchester also. I should like to remark about the use of the term "acoustic trauma" for the single-incident kind of exposure and noise-tried to separate acoustic trauma and noise-induced hearing loss because of the differences involved in the kinds of hearing loss that occur from a sudden exposure versus a long-term exposure. I believe it is better to use "acoustic trauma" for the single-incident kind of exposure and noise-induced hearing loss for the long-term exposure.

Finally, Dr. Hempstock's paper on tinnitus was very interesting to me since I am presently writing a chapter on tinnitus for a book. These data are extremely good; the study is well done and nicely presented. I don't know of any other data about tinnitus that is as good. Tinnitus is a very baffling phenomenon. After reviewing the literature I found that we knew as much about tinnitus in 1800 as we know now, which was and is very little.

In closing, I would like to tell a story about someone that illustrates who is responsible and how responsibility is designated for some of these industrial-type hazards. It's a story about a soldier who was in Viet Nam for a couple of years and came home and, as soldiers do when they come home, he started going out with one of the local girls. He was home about two months and was notified that he had been named the father of her unborn child. He thought, "Well, I don't see how I can be because I've been away two years and she's already about four months pregnant and I've only been home two months." Anyway, when the case was tried the judge held him responsible and named him the father of the child. The young man said, "I don't understand this, judge, I'd like an explanation." The judge answered, "Son, in this court if we can't find the first signer of the note we hold the last endorser responsible."

Closing Remarks

By

Air Vice-Marshal E. D. D. Dickson

Chairman, Royal National Institute for the Deaf, London, England

Dr. Glorig has given a masterly summary of what has taken place over the three days of this very interesting and profitable symposium. There should be no difficulty, after all we have heard, to convince our legislators that noise does cause deafness. At this time they are in the process of considering the question of noise-induced hearing loss from the point of view of compensation, so I hope that some of what we have discussed here will reach their ears. At the same time, another conclusion from this meeting is that we can, with some measure of certainty, predict what is going to take place—at least under certain circumstances—and thereby provide the necessary protection and safeguards. In the rarefied atmosphere which one would expect in such surroundings as the NPL, I make a plea that, in the final assessment of disability or damage sustained by a patient or claimant, the ultimate assessment must be a clinical one and that differential diagnosis must play a very important part. And I think that role is bound to fall sooner or later on the shoulders of the otologist. He, unfortunately, is the final arbitrator of causes, and must apportion what moiety is due to noise and how much is due to the other contributory factors which have been so objectively enumerated here.

Audiometry, I must say, is a useful adjunct but we must be certain that diagnosis is not made purely and simply on audiometry alone. The personality of the patient must be considered, to say nothing about the judgement and experience of the examiner: we must remember that the patient is an individual and not a laboratory specimen. I was very interested to hear the remarks being made about speech audiometry and I had hoped that this subject would have been elaborated a little more, because I cannot help feeling that, when it comes to assessing handicap, the disability which an individual has sustained as a result of hearing loss will be assessed on speech audiometry. Pure-tone audiometry and other evidence that we can collect will, of course, be taken into account, but it is speech that the person wants to hear. The test should, I think, be carried out binaurally, in a free field if possible, and with a certain amount of conditioned background noise. I have never been convinced that the pure-tone test—the ability to hear a tone of a certain pitch and intensity—will tell us whether a person can understand or discriminate speech according to what *he* thinks should be understood and discriminated. One knows from clinical experience that two audiograms showing the same kind of curve do not necessarily represent the same kind of disability, and this particularly applies to the sensorineural type of hearing loss, or inner-ear deafness. In the final consideration of the procedure to be adopted, I think one must be careful not to lay down definite criteria at present but to give them serious consideration, because once these things are written in the Statute Book they are extremely difficult to eradicate at a later date.

I was intrigued with Dr. Hallowell Davis's remark about benign and malignant recruitment. I was under the impression that recruitment is one of the manifestations of a lesion of Corti's organ and that this is in fact the basis of one of our main differential diagnostic procedures to determine whether a lesion is in Corti's organ or whether it is a neurinoma of the VIII nerve. I think recruitment plays a very important part in the discrimination of speech, particularly under noisy conditions. This is illustrated by the fact that a lot of patients who have sensorineural hearing loss and are given a hearing aid are all right kept under quiet conditions when they can follow what is said. The moment one puts them into a background of noise, a cocktail party for example, they take off their hearing aids saying, "I just cannot stick this noise, because I cannot understand what's being said, and the noise worries me more than anything else."

Finally, I hope that the problem of tinnitus is given more consideration because, as I said earlier, it is one of the most distressing conditions with which we as otologists have to deal. A little more thought should be exercised when exposing experimental subjects to noise; this, at any rate, is an avoidable cause of tinnitus.

With these few remarks I would like to add my congratulations and sincere thanks to the organizers of this important meeting for such an excellent programme, and I now declare the Conference closed.

Bibliography

Acton, W. I., Coles, R. R. A. and Forrest, M. R. (1966). Hearing hazard from small-bore rifles. *Rifleman*, **74**, 9.

Acton, W. I. and Forrest, M. R. (1968). Noise and hearing: further experiments and conclusions. *Rifleman*, **76**, 5. (See also *J. Acoust. Soc. Amer.*, 1968, **44**, 817.)

Air Force Regulations (1956). Hazardous noise exposure. AFR No. 160-3, October 29th. Department of the Air Force, Washington, D.C.

American Medical Association (1942). Tentative standard procedure for evaluating the percentage of useful hearing loss in medicolegal cases. *J. Amer. med. Ass.*, **119**, 1108.

American Medical Association (1947). Tentative standard procedure for evaluating the percentage loss of hearing in medicolegal cases. *J. Amer. med. Ass.*, **133**, 396.

American Medical Association (1961). Committee on Medical Rating of Physical Impairment: ear, nose, throat and related structures. *J. Amer. med. Ass.*, **177**, 489.

American Standards Association (1954). "The Relations of Hearing Loss to Noise Exposure." Report by Exploratory Sub-committee Z24-X-2. New York.

Anon. (1953). Noise in industry. *Scope*, 42, October. Creative Journals Ltd., London.

Anon. (1955a). The curse of noise. *The Times*, Part I, October 24th; Part II, October 25th.

Anon. (1955b). Noise dangers in industry. *The Times*, April 29th.

Anon. (1955c). Move for protection against noise. *The Times*, November 26th.

Anon. (1955d). Effect of noise on health. *The Times*, December 3rd.

Anon. (1969). Revision of Part 50-204 of Title 41 (Walsh-Healey Public Contracts Act); Sub-section 50-204.10. Occupational Noise Exposure. Federal Register Vol. 34 No. 96 Part II, 20th May. Washington D.C.

Argyle, M. and Robinson, P. (1962). Two origins of achievement motivation. *Brit. J. soc. clin. Psychol.*, **1**, 107.

Atherley, G. R. C. (1967). "Chronic Acoustic Trauma." M.D. Thesis, University of Manchester.

Atherley, G. R. C. and Noble, W. G. (1969). Present hearing and past military gunfire experience. *Appl. Acoust.*, **2**, 199.

Atherley, G. R. C. and Noble, W. G. (1970). Effect of ear-defenders (ear-muffs) on the localization of sound. *Brit. J. indust. Med.*, **27**, 243.

Atherley, G. R. C., Hempstock, T. I. and Noble, W. G. (1968). A study of tinnitus induced temporarily by noise. *J. acoust. Soc. Amer.*, **44**, 1503.

Babbitt, J. A. (1947). In "Nelson's Loose-Leaf Surgery of the Ear". Kopetzky, S. J. (ed.).

Barr, T. (1886). Enquiry into the effects of loud sounds upon the hearing of boiler-makers and others who work amid noisy surroundings. *Proc. Glasgow phil. Soc.*, **17**, 223.

Baughn, W. (1966). Noise control: percent of population protected. *Int. Audiol.*, **5**, 331.

Baughn, W. (1968). Unpublished report dated 29th February. Medical Arts Research Corporation Inc., Anderson, Ind.

Beagley, H. A. and Knight, J. J. (1968). The evaluation of suspected non-organic hearing loss. *L. Laryng. Otol.*, **82**, 693.

Berry, G. (1962). Noise in machinery. *New Scientist*, No. 283, 19th April, p. 89.

Bilger, R. C. and Hirsh, I. J. (1956). Masking of tones by bands of noise. *J. acoust. Soc. Amer.*, **28**, 623.

Bitterman, M. and Holtzman, W. (1952). Conditioning and extinction of the galvanic skin response. *J. abnorm. soc. Psychol.*, **47**, 615.

Blaha, V. and Slepicka, J. (1967). Klinický a hygienický rosbor risika hluku v kamenouhelných dolech. *Cs. Hyg.*, **12**, 521 (in Czech.). Abstracted in *Excerpta Medica*, 1968, No. 2780.

Blumenfeld, V. G., Bergman, M. and Millner, E. (1969). Speech discrimination in an aging population. *J. Speech Hear. Res.*, **12**, 210.

Bocca, E. (1958). Clinical aspects of cortical deafness. *Laryngoscope*, **68**, 301.

Bochenek, Z. and Jachowska, A. (1969). Atherosclerosis, accelerated presbyacusis and acoustic trauma. *Int. Audiol.*, **7**, 509.

Boenninghaus, H.-G. and Röser, D. (1958). Prozentuale Hörverlustbestimmung des Sprachghehörs und Festsetzung der Minderung der Erwerbsfähigkeit. *Zeit. f. Laryng. Rhinol. Otol.*, **37**, 719.

British Standards Institution (1954). "Threshold of Hearing for Pure-Tones by Earphone Listening." BS 2497. (Superseded by BS 2497:1968, Pt. 1 and BS 2497:1969, Pt. 2.)

British Standards Institution (1958). "Pure Tone Audiometers." BS 2980.

British Standards Institution (1966). "Specification for Cartridge Operating Fixing Tools." BS 4078.

British Standards Institution (1968). "A Reference Zero for the Calibration of Pure-tone Audiometers. Part 1, Data for Earphone Coupler Combinations maintained at certain Standardizing Laboratories." BS 2497, Pt. 1.

British Standards Institution (1969). "A Reference Zero for the Calibration of Pure-tone Audiometers. Part 2, Data for certain Earphones used in Commercial Practice." BS 2497 Pt. 2.

Browd, V. L. (1953). "A New Way to Better Hearing." Faber and Faber, London.

Brown, R. E. C. (1948). Experimental studies on the reliability of audiometry. *J. Laryng. Otol.*, **62**, 487.

Bugliarello, G., Wakstein, C. *et al.* (1968). "Noise Pollution." Report prepared for Resources for the Future, Inc., Washington D.C.

Bunch, C. C. (1937). Nervous deafness of known etiology. *Laryngoscope*, **47**, 615.

Burns, W. (1968). "Noise and Man." John Murray, London.

Burns, W. and Hinchcliffe, R. (1957). Comparison of auditory threshold as measured by individual pure-tone and by Békésy audiometry. *J. acoust. Soc. Amer.*, **29**, 1274.

Burns, W., Hinchcliffe, R. and Littler, T. S. (1964). An exploratory study of hearing loss and noise exposure in textile workers. *Ann. occup. Hyg.*, **7**, 323.

Burns, W. and Littler, T. S. (1960). Noise. In "Modern Trends in Occupational Health" (ed. Schilling, R. S. F.). Butterworth, London.

Burns, W. and Robinson, D. W. (1970). "Hearing and Noise in Industry." H.M.S.O., London.

Burns, W., Stead, J. C. and Penney, H. W. (1970). The relations between temporary threshold shift and occupational hearing loss. In Burns and Robinson (1970), Appendix 13.

Carhart, R. (1957). Clinical determination of abnormal auditory adaptation. *Arch. Otolaryng.*, **65**, 32.

Cattell, R. B. (1962). "Handbook for the IPAT 8-Parallel-Form Anxiety Battery." Inst. for Pers. and Abil. Testing, Univ. of Illinois.

Chaiklin, J. B. and Ventry, I. M. (1963). Functional hearing loss. In "Modern Developments in Audiology" (ed. Jerger, J.). Academic Press, New York.

Cohen, A., Kylin, B. and LaBenz, P. (1966). Temporary threshold shifts in hearing from exposure to combined impact/steady-state noise conditions. *J. acoust. Soc. Amer.*, **40**, 1371.

Coles, R. R. A. (1969). A legal action for noise deafness. *Sound*, **3**, 69.

Coles, R. R. A., Garinther, G. R., Hodge, D. C. and Rice, C. G. (1968). Hazardous exposure to impulse noise. *J. acoust. Soc. Amer.*, **43**, 336.

Coles, R. R. A. and Rice, C. G. (1966). Auditory hazard from sports guns. *Laryngoscope*, **76**, 1728.

Coles, R. R. A. and Rice C. G. (1967). Hazards from impulsive noise. *Ann. occup. Hyg.*, **10**, 381.

Coles, R. R. A. and Rice, C. G. (1970). Towards a criterion for impulse noise in industry. *Ann. occup. Hyg.*, **13**, 43.

Committee on Conservation of Hearing (1959). Guide for the evaluation of hearing impairment. *Trans. Amer. Acad. Ophthal. Otolaryng.*, **63**, 236.

Committee on Conservation of Hearing (1964). Guide for conservation of hearing in noise. *Trans. Amer. Acad. Ophthal. Otolaryng.*, Suppl.

Committee on Conservation of Hearing (1965). Guide for the classification and evaluation of hearing handicap in relation to the International audiometric zero. *Trans. Amer. Acad. Ophthal. Otolaryng.*, **69**, 740.

Committee on Hearing, Bioacoustics and Biomechanics (CHABA) (1968). Proposed damage-risk criterion for impulse noise (gunfire). Report of Working Group 57 (ed. Ward, W. D.). U.S. National Academy of Sciences—National Research Council, Washington D.C.

Committee on the Problem of Noise (1963). "Noise; Final Report." Cmnd. 2056. H.M.S.O., London.

Cooper, D., Hill, L. T. Jr. and Edwards, E. A. (1967). Detection of early arteriosclerosis by external pulse recording. *J. Amer. med. Ass.*, **199**, 449.

Copeland, W. C. and Robinson, D. W. (1967). An investigation of the noise exposure due to air and ground operations at London Airport (Heathrow). NPL. Aero Special Report 004. National Physical Laboratory, Teddington.

Corcoran, D. W. J. (1965). Personality and the inverted-U relation. *Brit. J. Psychol.*, **56**, 267.

Counter, S. A. and Tobin, H. (1969). Is there a critical duration? Paper presented at the American Speech and Hearing Association meeting, Chicago, 15th November.

Crowe, S. J., Guild, S. R. and Polvogt, L. M. (1934). Observations on the pathology of high-tone deafness. *Bull. Johns Hopkins Hosp.*, **54**, 315.

Dahlstrom, W. G. and Welsh, G. S. (1960). "An MMPI Handbook." Univ. of Minnesota Press, Minneapolis.

Davies, T. A. Lloyd (1957). "The Practice of Industrial Medicine." Churchill, London.

Davis, H. (1948). The articulation area and the social adequacy index for hearing. *Laryngoscope*, **58**, 761.

Davis, H. (1962). Opening address. Report of the 1962 Conference. Royal National Institute for the Deaf, London.

Davis, H., Morgan, C., Hawkins, J., Galambos, R. and Smith, F. (1950). Temporary deafness following exposure to loud tones and noise. *Acta Oto-laryng.*, Suppl. 88.

Davis, H. and Silverman, S. R. (eds.) (1970). "Hearing and Deafness." Holt, Rinehart and Winston, New York.

Delany, M. E. (1970). On the stability of auditory threshold. NPL Aero Report Ac 44. National Physical Laboratory, Teddington.

Delany, M. E. and Whittle, L. S. (1966). A new artificial ear and mastoid. *J. sci. Instrum.*, **43**, 519.

Delany, M. E. and Whittle, L. S. (1967). Reference equivalent threshold sound pressure levels for audiometry. *Acustica*, **18**, 227.

Delany, M. E., Whittle, L. S. and Knox, E. C. (1966). A note on the use of self-recording audiometry with children. *J. Laryng. Otol.*, **80**, 1135.

Departmental Committee on Compensation for Industrial Disease (1907). Report. H.M.S.O., London.

Department of Health and Social Security (1969). "Industrial Noise and its Effects on Hearing." Cmnd. 4145. H.M.S.O., London.

Dickson, E. D. D. (1953). Some effects of intense sound and ultrasound on the ear. *Proc. Roy. Soc. Med.*, **46**, 139.

Dickson, E. D. D., Ewing, A. W. G. and Littler, T. S. (1939). The effects of aeroplane noise on the auditory acuity of aviators. *J. Laryng. Otol.*, **54**, 531.

Dieroff, H. G. (1966). The problem of impulse-rich working noise, its measuring, and the hearing losses resulting from it. *Int. Audiol.*, **5**, 339.

Eldredge, D. H. and Covell, W. P. (1958). A laboratory method for the study of acoustic trauma. *Laryngoscope*, **68**, 465.

Evans, E. J. (1947). Noise in the factory. *The Times Review of Industry*, February 6th.

Eysenck, H. J. (1967). "The Biological Basis of Personality." Charles C. Thomas, Springfield, Ill.

Fabinyi, G. (1931). Morphological and functional changes of internal ear in arteriosclerosis. *Laryngoscope*, **41**, 633.

Fieandt, H. von and Saxén, A. (1937). Pathologie und Klinik der Altersschwerhörigkeit. *Acta Oto-laryng.*, Suppl. 23.

Fleischer, K. (1952). Uber Vorgänge des Alterns am Gehörorgan. *Z. Altersforsch.*, **6**, 147.

Fletcher, H. (1929). "Speech and Hearing." Van Nostrand, New York.

Fosbroke, J. (1831). Pathology and treatment of deafness. *Lancet*, **19**, 645.

Fowler, E. P. and Fowler, E. P. (1955). Somatopsychic and psychosomatic factors in tinnitus, deafness and vertigo. *Ann. Otol. Rhinol. Laryng.*, **64**, 29.

Fry, D. B. (1961). Word and sentence tests in use in speech audiometry. *Lancet* ii, 197.

Gaeth, J. H. (1948). "Study of Phonemic Regression in Relation to Hearing Loss." Ph.D. Thesis, North Western University, Chicago.

Gallo, R. and Glorig, A. (1964). Permanent threshold shift changes produced by noise exposure and aging. *Amer. ind. Hyg. Ass. J.*, **25**, 237.

Gannon, R. P. and Tso, S. S. (1969). The occult effect of kanamycin on the cochlea. *Proc. IX Int. Cong. Oto-Rhino-Laryng.*, Mexico City.

Glorig, A. (1958). "Noise and Your Ear." Grune and Stratton, New York.

Glorig, A. and Davis, H. (1961). Age, noise and hearing loss. *Ann. Otol.*, **70**, 556.

Glorig, A. and Nixon, J. (1960). Distribution of hearing loss in various populations. *Trans. Amer. otol. Soc.*, **48**, 94.

Glorig, A., Ward, W. D. and Nixon, J. (1962). Damage-risk criteria and noise-induced hearing loss. In "The Control of Noise." NPL Symposium No. 12. H.M.S.O., London.

Glorig, A., Wheeler, D., Quiggle, R., Grings, W. and Summerfield, A. (1957). "1954 Wisconsin State Fair Hearing Survey." Amer. Acad. Ophthal. Otolaryng.

Goldner, A. I. (1953). Deafness in shipyard workers. *Arch. Otolaryng.*, **57**, 287.

Goodhill, V. (1950). The management of tinnitus. *Laryngoscope*, **60**, 442.

Graham, J. T. and Newby, H. A. (1962). Acoustical characteristics of tinnitus. *Arch. Otolaryng.*, **75**, 82.

Gray, J. A. (1964). "Pavlov's Typology." Pergamon Press, Oxford.

Greenwood, W. (1933). "Love on the Dole." Jonathan Cape, London.

Hahlbrock, K. H. (1957). "Sprachaudiometrie." Georg Thieme Verlag, Stuttgart.

Hallpike, C. S. (1962). Vertigo of central origin. *Proc. Roy. Soc. Med.*, **58**, 364.

Hallpike, C. S. and Hood, J. D. (1959). Observations upon the neurological mechanism of the loudness recruitment phenomenon. *Acta Oto-laryng.*, **50**, 472.

Hansen, C. C. and Reske-Nielsen, E. (1965). Pathological studies in presbyacusis. *Arch. Otolaryng.*, **82**, 115.

Hansson, J.-E., Kylin, B. and Gustavsson, B. (1967). Skogstraktorn som arbetsplats år 1967. Research Notes No. 32, Royal College of Forestry, Sweden. (In Swedish.)

Harris, C. M. (ed.) (1957). "Handbook of Noise Control." McGraw-Hill, New York.

Harvey, B. and Murray, R. (1958). "Industrial Health Technology." Butterworth, London.

Heller, M. F. and Bergman, M. (1953). Tinnitus Aurium in normally-hearing people. *Ann. Otol. Rhinol. Laryng.*, **62**, 73.

Henry, G. A. (1945). Blast injuries of the ear. *Laryngoscope*, **55**, 663.

Heron, A. (1956). A two-part personality measure for use as a research criterion. *Brit. J. Psychol.*, **47**, 243.

High, S. W., Fairbanks, G. and Glorig, A. (1964). Scale for self-assessment of hearing handicap. *J. Speech Hear. Dis.*, **29**, 215.

Hinchcliffe, R. (1959a). The threshold of hearing as a function of age. *Acustica*, **9**, 303.

Hinchcliffe, R. (1959b). The threshold of hearing of a random sample rural population. *Acta Oto-laryng.*, **50**, 411.

Hinchcliffe, R. (1961). Prevalence of the commoner ear, nose and throat conditions in the adult rural population of Great Britain. *Brit. J. prev. soc. Med.*, **15**, 128.

Hinchcliffe, R. (1962a). Aging and sensory thresholds. *J. Geront.*, **17**, 45.

Hinchcliffe, R. (1962b). The anatomical locus of presbycusis. *J. Speech Hear. Dis.*, **27**, 301.

Hinchcliffe, R. (1965). A psychophysiological investigation into vertigo. Unpublished Ph.D. Thesis, University of London.

Hinchcliffe, R. (1967a). Intercorrelation of some auditory measurements on a vertiginous population. *Int. Audiol.*, **6**, 63.

Hinchcliffe, R. (1967b). Occupational deafness. *Proc. Roy. Soc. Med.*, **60**, 1111.

Hinchcliffe, R. (1967c). Personality profile in Ménière's disease. *J. Laryng. Otol.*, **81**, 477.

Hinchcliffe, R. (1968). Population studies concerned with presbyacusis. *Ind. J. Otolaryng.*, **20**, 52.

Hinchcliffe, R. and Littler, T. S. (1958). Methodology of air conduction audiometry for hearing surveys. *Ann. occup. Hyg.*, **1**, 114.

Hirsh, I. J., Palva, T. and Goodman, A. (1954). Difference limen and recruitment. *Arch. Otolaryng.*, **60**, 525.

Hood, J. D. (1960). A comparative study of loudness recruitment in cases of deafness due to Ménière's disease, head injury and acoustic trauma. *Acta Oto-rhino-laryng. Belgica*, **14**, 224.

Hood, J. D. (1968). Speech discrimination and its relationship to disorders of the loudness function. *Int. Audiol.*, **7**, 232.

Hood, J. D. (1969). The role of deranged metabolism in susceptibility to noise-induced hearing loss. *Sound*, **3**, 58.

Hsi-Kuei, T., Fong-Shyong, C. and Tsa-Jung, C. (1958). On changes of ear size with age, as found among Taiwanese Formosans of Fukienese extraction. *J. Formosan Med. Ass.*, **57**, 105.

Hughson, W. and Westlake, H. (1944). Manual for program outline for rehabilitation of aural casualties both military and civilian. Amer. Acad. Ophthal. Otolaryng.

Igarashi, M., Schuknecht, H. F. and Myers, E. N. (1964). Cochlear pathology in humans with stimulation deafness. *J. Laryng. Otol.*, **78**, 115.

Industrial Welfare Society (1961). "Industrial Noise." I.W.S. Summary No. 83, London.

Ingard, U. and Ising, H. (1967). Acoustic nonlinearity of an orifice. *J. acoust. Soc. Amer.*, **42**, 6.

Ingham, J. G. (1966). Changes in MPI score in neurotic patients: a three-year follow-up. *Brit. J. Psychiat.*, **112**, 931.

International Electrotechnical Commission (1961). "Recommendations for Sound Level Meters." Publication 123, Geneva.

International Electrotechnical Commission (1965). "Precision Sound Level Meters." Publication 179, Geneva.

International Electrotechnical Commission (1970a). "IEC Provisional Reference Coupler for the Calibration of Earphones used in Audiometry." Publication 303, Geneva.

International Electrotechnical Commission (1970b). "An IEC Artificial Ear of the Wide-band Type for the Calibration of Earphones used in Audiometry." Publication 318, Geneva.

International Organization for Standardization (1964). "Standard Reference Zero for the Calibration of Pure-tone Audiometers." ISO Recommendation R389, Geneva.

International Organization for Standardization (1970). "Assessment of Noise Exposure during Work for Hearing Conservation Purposes." ISO Draft Recommendation DR1999. Geneva.

Jackson, J. E., Fassett, D. W., Riley, E. C. and Sutton, W. L. (1962). Evaluation of the variability in audiometric procedures. *J. acoust. Soc. Amer.*, **34**, 218.

Jerger, J. F. and Carhart, R. (1956). Temporary threshold shift as an index of noise susceptibility. *J. acoust. Soc. Amer.*, **28**, 611.

Jerger, J. and Herer, G. (1961). Unexpected dividend in Békésy audiometry. *J. Speech Hear. Dis.*, **26**, 390.

Jongkees, L. B. W. and Groen, J. J. (1946). On directional hearing. *J. Laryng. Otol.*, **61**, 494.

Jones, H. H. and Oser, J. L. (1968). "Farm Equipment Noise Exposure Levels." Office of Public Information, Environmental Control Administration, Cincinnatti, Ohio. (See also *Amer. ind. Hyg. Ass. J.*, **29**, 146.)

Jönsson, M. (1967). Siebaudiometrische Untersuchungen von Lärmarbeitern. *Deut. Gesundh.-Wes.*, **22**, 2286. (Abstracted in *Excerpta Medica* 1968, No. 2347.)

Kell, R. L., Pearson, J. C. G. and Taylor, W. (1970). Hearing thresholds of an Island population in North Scotland. *Int. Audiol.*, **9**, 334.

Kennedy, A. (1953). Discussion on tinnitus. *Proc. Roy. Soc. Med.*, **46**, 832.

Kirikae, I., Sato, T. and Shitara, T. (1964). Study of hearing in advanced age. *Laryngoscope*, **74**, 205.

König, E. (1966). Das Problem der Sprechaudiometrie im deutschschweizerischen Sprachgebiet. *Pract. oto-rhino-laryng.*, **28**, 39.

Konigsmark B. W. (1968). "Hereditary Deafness in Man." Johns Hopkins Univ. Sch. of Med.

Korenchevsky, V. (1961). "Physiological and Pathological Ageing." Karger, Basel.

Kosten, C. W. and van Os, G. J. (1962). Community reaction criteria for external noises. In "The Control of Noise', NPL Symposium No. 12, H.M.S.O., London.

Kryter, K. D. (1963). Exposure to steady-state noise and impairment of hearing. *J. acoust. Soc. Amer.*, **35**, 1515.

Kryter, K. D. and Garinther, G. R. (1965). Auditory effects from acoustic impulses from firearms. *Acta Oto-laryng.*, Suppl. 211.

Kryter, K. D., Ward, W. D., Miller, J. D. and Eldredge, D. H. (1966). Hazardous exposure to intermittent and steady-state noise. *J. acoust. Soc. Amer.*, **39**, 451.

Kuiper, J. P. and Visser, F. (1969). Gehoorbeschadiging bij machinale houtbewerkers (Hearing damage of machine wood workers). Report of the Labour-Inspectorate, Voorburg, Netherlands.

Kylin, B. (1960). Temporary threshold shift and auditory trauma following exposure to steady-state noise. *Acta Oto-laryng.* Suppl. 152.

Kylin, B. *et al.* (1968). Hälso- och Miljöundersökning bland Skogsarberare. Research Notes No. 5. National Institute of Occupational Health, Stockholm. (In Swedish.)

Kylin, B. and Johansson, B. (1964). Vilket buller bör föranleda hörselskyddande åtgärder. *Sv. Läkartidningen*, **61**, 1962. (In Swedish.)

van Laar, F. (1966). Results of audiometric research at some hundreds of persons, working in different Dutch factories. Publication AG/SA C23, N.I.P.G.-TNO.

LaBenz, P., Cohen, A. and Pearsson, B. (1967). A noise and hearing survey of earth-moving equipment operators. *Amer. ind. Hyg. Ass. J.*, **28**, 117.

Legge, T. (1934). "Industrial Maladies." Oxford University Press, London.

Lehnhardt, E. (1967). The C^5-dip: its interpretation in the light of generally known physiological concepts. *Int. Audiol.*, **6**, 86.

Lisland, T. (1967). Støgmålinger på skogstraktorer. Driftsteknisk Rapport No. 6. Det Norske Skogsforsøksvesen. *Tids. för Skogbruk*, No. 1, 123.

Littler, T. S. (1962). Techniques of industrial audiometry. In "The Control of Noise", NPL Symposium No. 12. H.M.S.O., London.

Littler, T. S. (1965). "The Physics of the Ear." Pergamon Press, Oxford.

Littler, T. S. (1966). Contribution to discussion on Chadwick, D. L., Acoustic trauma—clinical presentation. *Proc. Roy. Soc. Med.*, **59**, 963.

Loeb, M. and Smith, R. P. (1967). Relation of induced tinnitus to the physical characteristics of the inducing stimulus. *J. acoust. Soc. Amer.*, **42**, 453.

Loeper, J., Orcel, L., Lion, J. and Beurlet, J. (1961). Etude histologique des stades initiaux de l'athérosclérose. *C.R. Soc. Biol.*, **155**, 466.

McKelvie, W. B. (1927). Annual report of the Chief Inspector of Factories. H.M.S.O.

McKenzie, D. (1925). Discussion on labyrinth deafness. *Brit. med. J.*, **ii**, 867.

Mayer, O. (1920). Das anatomische Substrat der Altersschwerhörigkeit. *Arch. f. Ohren.*, **105**, 1.

Miall, W. E. and Lovell, H. G. (1967). Relation between change of blood pressure and age. *Brit. med. J.*, **ii**, 660.

Miller, J. D., Watson, C. S. and Covell, W. P. (1963). Deafening effects of noise on the cat. *Acta Oto-laryng.*, Suppl., 176.

Ministry of Labour (1963). "Noise and the Worker." Safety, Health and Welfare Series, No. 25. H.M.S.O., London.

Monro, D. B. (1926). Homer. *Encyclopaedia Britannica*, 13th Edition, **13**, 626.

Mrass, H. and Diestel, H. G. (1959). Bestimmung der Normalhörschwelle für reine Töne bei einohrigem Hören mit hilfe eines Kopfhörers. *Acustica*, **9**, 61.

Murray, N. E. (1962). Hearing impairment and compensation. *J. otolaryng. Soc. Aust.*, **1**, 135.

National Physical Laboratory (1962). "The Control of Noise." Symposium No. 12, H.M.S.O., London.

Nixon, J. and Glorig, A. (1961). Noise-induced permanent threshold shift at 2000 cps and 4000 cps. *J. acoust. Soc. Amer.*, **33**, 904.

Noble, W. G. (1969). "A Scale for the Measurement of Hearing Loss and Disability." Ph.D. Thesis, University of Manchester.

Nordlund, B. (1962). Angular localisation. *Acta Oto-laryng.*, **55**, 405.

Nordlund, B. (1964). Directional audiometry. *Int. Audiol.*, **3**, 186.

Parry, C. H. (1825). Collection from unpublished medical writings, **1**, 544. Underwood, London.

Passchier-Vermeer, W. (1968). Hearing loss due to exposure to steady-state broadband noise. Report 35, Institute for Public Health Engineering TNO, Netherlands.

Pestalozza, G. and Shore, I. (1955). Clinical evaluation of presbyacusis on the basis of different tests of auditory function. *Laryngoscope*, **65**, 1136.

Plomp, R. (1967). Hearing losses induced by small arms. *Int. Audiol.*, **6**, 31.

Ramazini, B. (1713). "De Morbis Artificium." Padua (1964 edition entitled "Disease of Workers", publ. Hafner, New York).

Ramazini, B. (1740). "A Treatise on the Diseases of Tradesmen" (trans. Dr. James). Osborne, London.

Rapin, I. and Costa, L. D. (1969). Test-retest reliability of serial pure-tone audiograms in children at a school for the deaf. *J. Speech Hear. Res.*, **12**, 402.

Reason, J. T. (1968). Individual differences in auditory reaction time and loudness estimation. *Percept. Mot. Skills*, **26**, 1089.

Reed, G. F. (1960). An audiometric study of two hundred cases of subjective tinnitus. *Arch. Otolaryng.*, **71**, 84.

Rice, C. G. and Coles, R. R. A. (1966). Design factors and the use of ear protection. *Brit. J. indust. Med.*, **93**, 194.

Robinson, D. W. (1968). The relationships between hearing loss and noise exposure. NPL Aero Report Ac 32. National Physical Laboratory, Teddington. (Available as Appendix 10 in Burns and Robinson, 1970.)

Robinson, D. W. and Cook, J. P. (1968). The quantification of noise exposure. NPL Aero Report Ac 31. National Physical Laboratory, Teddington. (Available as Appendix 11 in Burns and Robinson, 1970.)

Rosen, S. (1969a). Epidemiology of hearing loss. *Int. Audiol.* **8**, 260.

Rosen, S. (1969b). Dietary prevention of hearing loss; long-term experiment. *Proc. IX Int. Cong. Oto-Rhino-Laryng.*, Mexico City.

Rosen, S., Bergman, M., Plester, D., El-Mofty, A. and Satti, M. H. (1962). Presbycusis study of a relatively noise-free population in the Sudan. *Ann. Otol. Rhinol. Laryng.*, **71**, 727.

Rosen, S. and Olin, P. (1965). Hearing loss and coronary heart disease. *Arch. Otolaryng.*, **82**, 236.

Rosen, S., Plester, D., El-Mofty, A. and Rosen, H. V. (1964). High frequency audiometry in presbycusis. *Arch. Otolaryng.*, **79**, 18.

Rosenblith, W. A. and Stevens, K. N. (1953). "Handbook of Acoustic Noise Control." Office of Technical Services, Washington D.C.

Rosenthal, R. (1969). Task variations in studies of experimenter expectancy effects. *Percept. Mot. Skills*, **29**, 9.

Rosenwinkel, N. E. and Stewart, U. C. (1957). The relationship of hearing loss to steady-state noise exposure. *Amer. ind. Hyg. Ass. Q.*, **18**, 227.

Röser, D. (1963). Sprachgehör und Tonaudiogramm. *Zeit f. Laryng. Rhinol. Otol.*, **42**, 851.

Rüedi, L. (1954). Different types and degrees of acoustic trauma by experimental exposure of the human and animal ear to pure tones and noise. *Trans. Amer. otol. Soc.*, **42**, 186.

Sappington, C. O. (1943). "Essentials of Industrial Health." Lippincott, Philadelphia.

Sataloff, J., Vassallo, L. and Menduke, H. (1969). Hearing loss from exposure to interrupted noise. *Arch. env. Health*, **18**, 972.

Schilling, R. S. F. (ed.) (1960). "Modern Trends in Occupational Health." Butterworth, London.

Schmidt, P. H. (1967). Presbycusis. *Int. Audiol.*, Suppl. 1.

Schuknecht, H. F. (1964). Further observations on the pathology of presbycusis. *Arch. Otolaryng.*, **80**, 369.

Schuknecht, H. and Tonndorf, J. (1960). Acoustic trauma of the cochlea from ear surgery. *Laryngoscope*, **70**, 479.

Sercer, A. and Krmpotić, J. (1958). Über die Ursache der progressiven Altersschwerhörigkeit. *Acta Oto-laryng.*, Suppl. 143.

Shambaugh, G. E., Jr. (1960). Chairman's remarks. *Arch. Otolaryng.*, **71**, 511.

Shepherd, D. C. and Goldstein, R. (1966). Relation of Békésy tracings to personality and electrophysiologic measures. *J. Speech Hear. Res.*, **9**, 385.

Shepherd, D. C. and Goldstein, R. (1968). Intrasubject variability in amplitude of Békésy tracings and its relation to measures of personality. *J. Speech Hear. Res.*, **11**, 523.

Silverman, S. R., Thurlow, W. R., Walsh, T. E. and Davis, H. (1948). Improvement in the social adequacy of hearing following the fenestration operation. *Laryngoscope*, **58**, 607.

Smith, S. L. (1968). Extraversion and sensory threshold. *Psychophysiology*, **5**, 293.

Spieth, W. and Trittipoe, W. J. (1958). Intensity and duration of noise exposure and temporary threshold shifts. *J. acoust. Soc. Amer.*, **30**, 710.

Spoor, A. (1967). Presbycusis values in relation to noise induced hearing loss. *Int. Audiol.*, **6**, 48.

Spoor, A. and Passchier-Vermeer, W. (1969). Spread in hearing levels of non-noise exposed people at various ages. *Int. Audiol.*, **8**, 328.

Stamler, J. (1960). Current status of the dietary prevention and treatment of atherosclerotic coronary heart disease. *Cardiovasc. Dis.*, **3**, 56.

Stein, J. (1928). Die Arteriosklerose des Gehörorganes. In "Handbuch der Neurologie des Ohres".

Stephens, S. D. G. (1969). Auditory threshold variance, signal detection theory and personality. *Int. Audiol.*, **8**, 131.

Stephens, S. D. G. (1970a). Personality and the slope of loudness function. *Q. J. exp. Psychol.*, **22**, 9.

Stephens, S. D. G. (1970b). Studies on the uncomfortable loudness level. *Sound*, **4**, 20.

Svenska Elektriska Kommissionen (1969). "Estimation of Risk of Hearing Damage from Noise: Measuring Methods and Acceptable Values." Proposal SEN 590111, Stockholm. (In Swedish.)

Swets, J. A. (1961). Is there a sensory threshold? *Science*, **134**, 168.

Taylor, W., Pearson, J. C. G. and Mair, A. (1967). Hearing thresholds of a non-noise-exposed population in Dundee. *Brit. J. indust. Med.*, **24**, 114.

Taylor, W., Pearson, J. C. G., Kell, R. and Mair, A. (1967). A pilot study of hearing loss and social handicap in female jute workers. *Proc. Roy. Soc. Med.*, **60**, 59.

Taylor, W., Pearson, J. C. G., Mair, A. and Burns, W. (1965). Study on noise and hearing in jute weaving. *J. acoust. Soc. Amer.*, **38**, 113.

Taylor, G. D. and Williams, E. (1966). Acoustic trauma in the sports hunter. *Laryngoscope*, **76**, 863.

Venters, R. S. (1953). Discussion on tinnitus. *Proc. Roy. Soc. Med.*, **46**, 825.

Walker, J. G. (1970). Temporary threshold shift from impulse noise. *Ann. occup. Hyg.*, **13**, 51.

Ward, W. D. (1962). Effect of temporal spacing on temporary threshold shift from impulses. *J. acoust. Soc. Amer.*, **34**, 1230.

Ward, W. D. (1963). Auditory fatigue and masking. In "Modern Developments in Audiology" (ed. Jerger, J.). Academic Press, New York.

Ward, W. D. (1965). The concept of susceptibility to hearing loss. *J. occup. Med.*, **7**, 595.

Ward, W. D., Fleer, R. E. and Glorig, A. (1961). Characteristics of hearing losses produced by gunfire and by steady noise. *J. aud. Res.*, **1**, 325.

Wegel, R. L. (1931). A study of tinnitus. *Arch. Otolaryng.*, **14**, 158.

Weissler, P. G. (1968). International standard reference zero for audiometers. *J. acoust. Soc. Amer.*, **44**, 264.

Weston, T. E. T. (1964). Presbycusis. *J. Laryng. Otol.*, **78**, 273.

Whittle, L. S. and Robinson, D. W. (1961). British normal threshold of hearing. *Nature*, **189**, 617.

Wilkinson, R. T., Morlock, H. C. and Williams, H. L. (1966). Evoked cortical response during vigilance. *Psychon. Sci.*, **4**, 221.

Zwaardemaker, H. (1893). Über das Presbyacustische Gesetz an der untere Grenze unseres Gehörs. *Arch. f. Ohren.*, **35**, 299.

Zwislocki, J. (1952). New types of ear protectors. *J. acoust. Soc. Amer.*, **24**, 762.

Zwislocki, J., Maire, F., Feldman, A. S. and Rubin, H. (1958). On the effect of practice and motivation on the thresholds of audibility. *J. acoust. Soc. Amer.*, **30**, 254.

Name Index

Numbers in italic indicate page where reference is listed

Subject Index